For Patients of Moderate Means
A Social History of the Voluntary Public General Hospital
in Canada, 1890–1950

Between 1890 and 1910 scientific and technological innovation transformed the custodial Victorian charity hospital for the sick poor into the primary source of effective acute medical care for all members of society. For the next half century hospitals coped with relentlessly escalating demands for accessibility by both medical indigents and a new clientele of patients able and willing to pay for hospitalization. With limited statutory revenues and unpredictable voluntary support, hospitals taxed paying patients through ever-increasing user fees, offering in return privacy, comfort, service, and medical attendance in private and semi-private wards that were more appealing to middle-class patients than the stark and grudging service of the public wards.

The Great Depression, however, finally exhausted the average patient's ability to pay and engendered a national health-care crisis. A public hospital insurance scheme was first achieved in Saskatchewan in 1947 and nationally in 1957. Universal accessibility without fear of the financial consequences of hospitalization reflected concern for both the medical health of Canadians unable to pay for hospital care, and the economic health of the paying "patient of moderate means" threatened with medical pauperization. It also provided the resources necessary to address the modern epidemic of lifestyle diseases and to accommodate the demands of the post-war therapeutic revolution.

Employing the historical records of selected hospitals, reports and data from all levels of government, a wide range of professional medical, nursing, hospital, and public health journals, and the international historiography of hospital history, David and Rosemary Gagan describe and account for the invention, rise, decline, and rebirth of the modern Canadian hospital between 1890 and 1950. They pay particular attention to the evolving interdependence of doctors and hospitals in the struggle to legitimate the social and cultural authority of scientific medicine, the evolution of hospital-based nursing, and the experiences of patients.

DAVID GAGAN, a professor of history at Simon Fraser University, is the author of *A Necessity Among Us: The Owen Sound General and Marine Hospital, 1891–1985*.

ROSEMARY GAGAN, an instructor in Women's Studies at Simon Fraser University, is the author of *A Sensitive Independence: Canadian Methodist Women Missionaries in Canada and the Orient, 1881–1925*.

MCGILL-QUEEN'S ASSOCIATED MEDICAL SERVICES (HANNAH INSTITUTE)
Studies in the History of Medicine, Health, and Society
Series Editors: S.O. Freedman and J.T.H. Connor

Volumes in this series have financial support from Associated Medical Services, Inc., through the Hannah Institute for the History of Medicine program.

For Patients of Moderate Means

A Social History of the Voluntary Public General Hospital in Canada, 1890–1950

DAVID GAGAN and
ROSEMARY GAGAN

McGill-Queen's University Press
Montreal & Kingston · London · Ithaca

© McGill-Queen's University Press 2002
ISBN 0-7735-2436-3

Legal deposit third quarter 2002
Bibliothèque nationale du Québec

Printed in Canada on acid-free paper that is 100% ancient
forest free (100% post-consumer recycled), processed chlorine
free.

This book has been published with the help of a grant from
the Humanities and Social Sciences Federation of Canada,
using funds provided by the Social Sciences and Humanities
Research Council of Canada.

McGill-Queen's University Press acknowledges the financial
support of the Government of Canada through the Book
Publishing Industry Development Program (BPIDP) for its
publishing activities. We also acknowledge the support of
the Canada Council for the Arts for our publishing program.

**National Library of Canada Cataloguing in Publication
Data**

Gagan, David, 1940–
      For patients of moderate means : a social history of the
  voluntary public general hospital in Canada, 1890–1950 /
  David Gagan and Rosemary Gagan

      (McGill-Queen's/Associated Medical Services
  (Hannah Institute) studies in the history of medicine, health,
  and society; 13)
  Includes bibliographical references and index.
  ISBN 0-7735-2436-3

  1. Public hospitals—Canada—History.
  I. Gagan, Rosemary Ruth   II. Title.   III. Series.

  RA983.A1G34 2002   362.1'1'09710904   C2002-901875-7

Typeset in 10/12 Palatino by True to Type

For Mary and Madeleine

Contents

Preface

In the nineteenth century during times of illness, hospitalization was the last resort of the destitute and the homeless. For everyone else, hospitals represented an unsavoury, potentially lethal, conjunction of poverty, pain, infection, medical ineffectiveness, and social regimentation. Between 1890 and 1914, hospitals, and popular perceptions of them, underwent a startling transformation. Propelled by the new standards of institutional *asepsis,* by diagnostic and surgical innovation, by the growth of medical specialization, and by the emerging science of professional nursing, hospitals became the preferred source of medical treatment and care for people of all classes. Hospital-based community health care emerged as a new industry that even adopted the model and the language of scientific industrial management to define its objectives and organize its complex activities. Popular enthusiasm for hospitalization was accompanied by a frenzy of hospital construction amid predictions that the twentieth century would witness the successful exploitation of the full potential of hospital-centred medical science. The costs would be high, but the rewards – measured by the production of health – would be even greater; and in any event, it was argued, institutional efficiency and scientific innovation would keep the costs of health easily within the grasp of the patient of average means.

Within one generation, however, the promise of affordable hospital medical treatment and care – hospitalization that did not create severe financial distress – had already eluded more than half of Canada's households. Driven by inflation, by the cost of repetitive

expansion to meet demand, by the costs of treating inadequately subsidized indigents, by the legal and social necessity of accommodating
too many patients for whom hospitalization was deemed inappropriate, and by the tariff on medical innovation, relentlessly rising
expenditures had become a fixture of hospital economics by 1930.
Inevitably, expenditures outstripped the principal source of hospital
income, the fees of patients willing and able to pay premium prices
for care qualitatively differentiated from the spartan service available
to indigents in the public wards. Patients in revolt against this regime
blamed hospital boards. Boards blamed doctors. General practitioners blamed specialists. Middle-class patients blamed medical indigents. They all blamed provincial governments, which wrestled
ineffectually with the problem of hospital funding throughout the
1920s and then could not afford a solution when one became essential during the Great Depression. Only the redefinition of the social
objectives of Canadian federalism, and the legislative intervention of
the federal government to maintain a minimum standard of hospital
and medical services for all Canadians regardless of income, forestalled the collapse of Canada's first community-based health care
"system" and replaced it with another, many of whose current problems are, in retrospect, all too familiar.

That, however, is another story. This study is concerned with the
invention of the modern Canadian public general hospital and with
the interaction among its major protagonists – trustees, administrators, physicians, nurses, and patients. It was their objectives, activities, and experiences that shaped the hospital's characteristics as a
developing community medical and social institution, between 1890
and the advent of a national system of universal health care.

In the course of completing this book we have accumulated many
debts which we gratefully acknowledge. Our research has been fund-
ed by the Social Sciences and Humanities Research Council of
Canada, by the Hannah Institute for the History of Medicine, by the
University of Winnipeg, and by Simon Fraser University. Cornwall
General Hospital, Owen Sound General and Marine Hospital, St
Catharines General and Marine Hospital, Toronto General Hospital,
Vancouver General Hospital, the Simon Fraser Health Region (Royal
Columbian Hospital), the British Columbia Medical Association, and
the College of Physicians and Surgeons of Ontario generously grant-
ed access to their historical records. We experienced unfailingly help-
ful archival access and assistance at the City of Vancouver Archives,
the Public Archives of British Columbia, Manitoba, and Ontario, the
Legislative Library of Manitoba, and the University of Manitoba
Archives, where Anne Thornton-Trump's advice was especially

welcome. The Interlibrary Loan unit at Simon Fraser University deserves special thanks as well. Peter Twohig generously shared his unpublished research with us. Our research assistants, Matthew Neufeld and Tanya Miller, facilitated our project through their ability to work independently following up good ideas. Sarah Gagan, Rebecca Gagan, Abigail Gagan, and Halcyon Meiers retrieved, deciphered, and interpreted for us on short notice obscure documents from distant sources. The insights and advice of our manuscript's anonymous assessors profoundly improved the final version. The staff of McGill-Queen's University Press, especially Roger Martin, and our copy editor, Jane McWhinney, made the entire process of submission, revision, and publication as non-threatening as it is ever likely to be. None of the foregoing people share our responsibility for errors of fact or interpretation that may have eluded us or are attributable to our scholarship.

D. P. G.
R. R. G.

For Patients of Moderate Means

History and the Hospital

In the last twenty-five years, historians have substantially remapped the landscape of Canadian social history. Their inquiries have identified in particular the high ground of change and continuity in the social history of late nineteenth- and early twentieth-century Canada: the role of industrialization, immigration, and urbanization in redefining the essential context of social experience; the emergence of the working class; the changing role of the family in society; the reinterpretation of childhood and adolescence and their association with formal education; the successes and failures of movements of social and moral reform; the impact of first-wave feminism; the interplay of religion, spirituality, and social criticism; ethnicity, gender, occupation, and class as determinants of individual social and economic experience; and the relationship between social policy and social control. The formidable scope of this historiography notwithstanding, some major social developments have remained largely unexplored. One of these is the wholesale transfer of the care and treatment of the sick from the home to the hospital, which took place between 1890 and 1920, and the subsequent rise and fall of the modern public hospital as a doctors' workshop of medical science for all members of the community, between 1920 and 1950.

In 1880 there were eleven general hospitals in the province of Ontario. They admitted just 5,116 patients from a population rapidly approaching two million. In 1900 the number of general hospitals in Ontario had increased to fifty in thirty-one cities and towns, and one of every hundred Ontarians was hospitalized for treatment. Thirty years later, every Ontario town large enough (and some that were not) to support a community general hospital boasted such a facility, and these hospitals provided health care to one in fifteen Ontarians in 1930.

This pattern of hospital development was repeated elsewhere in Canada. In 1897 Manitoba had just four hospitals, two of which were in Winnipeg. In the next thirty years two dozen new hospitals were added in twenty communities. By 1930 yearly in-patient usage represented nearly 8 per cent of Manitoba's population. In British Columbia, hospitals and hospitalization experienced similar growth. At the end of the nineteenth century there were twelve general hospitals in ten communities but two decades later, the province boasted sixty-four general hospitals, to which one of every ten British Columbians was admitted annually.

The simplest explanation for this phenomenon was the urban population growth that resulted from immigration and industrialization. This growth necessitated a concomitant expansion of community health-care facilities to accommodate the industrial population that was incapable of providing domestic care for its sick. But demographic and economic changes were neither the only – nor the most important – reasons for the emergence of the general hospital as an essential Canadian institution between 1890 and 1920. Even before 1890, hospitals had been established in every Canadian city. No self-respecting citizen, however, could be induced to voluntarily enter an institution associated with high mortality rates from hospital-induced infections, and with the custodial care of sick paupers, transients, and carriers of highly contagious diseases – patients for whom medical charity or isolation from the general population provided a non-therapeutic alternative to personal indignity or a concession to public safety. Respectable urban Canadians by choice, the rural population out of necessity, received medical attention from their family physician at home or in the doctor's surgery, or from a practitioner of alternative "medicine," and convalesced among their relatives, or, for the well-to-do, in the care of private nurses and domestic servants. The middle and upper classes patronized hospitals only as charitable subscribers to the improbable medical relief of the dependent but deserving poor. Their individual benevolence augmented the medical charity of doctors and the meagre subsidies provided for indigent care by provincial and municipal governments.

By 1920, however, Canadians from all walks of life were clamouring to be admitted to public hospitals; in just two decades, they had become centres of diagnostic efficacy, technological innovation, and surgical accomplishment. Moreover, many patients were by now willing to pay premium fees not only for medical treatment but for personalized hospital care. They sought treatment for a rapidly expanding catalogue of major and minor illnesses and they had a well-developed set of expectations and criticisms of hospital-based health care that already identified them as knowledgeable consumers of institutional medicine. Simultaneously, hospital privileges became the *sine qua non* of medical practice in Canada; physicians, who had once eschewed hospital service as assiduously as their middle-class patients had avoided hospitalization, sought to enhance their professional authority, limit competition, better their standard of living, and promote the science of medicine as an essential determinant of national efficiency. Out of this interplay of newly discovered mutual dependencies – paying patients, aggressive doctors, and development-driven hospitals – arose a new model of hospital-based community health care. But after a brief period, perhaps twenty years, of relative success, the redefined hospital's ultimate failure – exacerbated, though not created, by the Great Depression – to sustain quality and accessibility with its historical sources of income eventually provided the impetus for the introduction of the Canadian variant of state medicine.[1]

Why did the local general hospital become, in just one generation, a medical and social necessity with a mission to heal the sick irrespective of social condition rather than an institution dedicated merely to doing the sick poor no harm? How did this transformation in health services and public attitudes occur? What explains its timing? Who were the principal stakeholders in this transition? What roles did patients, doctors, nurses, administrators, trustees, and governments play, and how were they, in turn, affected by events? How, in the longer term, did this essential transformation set the stage for the subsequent evolution, especially the apparent failure by 1940, of the Canadian system of hospital-based medical care, and with what result? These are the broad questions pursued in this study of the Canadian general hospital from 1890 to 1950.

Whether it is possible to formulate a generic social history of the Canadian voluntary general hospital remains to be seen. Founded to address community needs and conditions, sustained in part by private benevolence and municipal taxes, governed by citizen volunteers, and patronized principally by the local populace, each hospital was a unique institution. Nevertheless, these institutions also exemplified an international phenomenon that occurred throughout western Europe and North America at the end of the nineteenth century. Whatever their exceptional individual characteristics might have been, their medical priorities, as well as their operating standards, therapeutic capabilities, business practices, internal cultures, and relations with their external communities, were informed by common scientific, professional, social, and economic contexts that defined the appeal, the scope, the efficacy, and the limitations of hospital-centred community health care. These shared contextual elements and the effects they produced are the raw materials of a collective hospital history with national and local variations.[2]

The expanding international historiography of that history has made a significant contribution to the social history of medicine. For the historian of medicine, the hospital is a medical institution whose significance lies in its organization, operation, and ideals as they relate to medical practice, medical education, and scientific innovation.[3] To the social historian, the hospital is "an organ of society, sharing its characteristics, changing as the society of which it is a part is transformed, and carrying into the future evidence of its past."[4] It is for this reason that much of the recent historiography relating to the history of hospitals has focused on that critical period between 1880 and 1930, when hospitals experienced a transition as fundamental as the wholesale transformation of society itself. Historians have interpreted the emergence and the acquired characteristics of the modern hospital as a conservative response to the needs and demands of a rapidly growing and changing society, by doctors and hospital authorities determined to preserve medical authority over and institutional control of a highly desirable new commodity – health. The nineteenth-century hospital's function as a medically marginal, supposedly "interest free" benevolent institution for the relief of the sick poor gave way, in just one generation, to a new identity derived from its participation in, even dominance of, the marketplace for medical treatment and care for all classes in society. The hospital's appeal to a new class of users who could, and would, pay for its services was based on its recent claim to diagnostic and therapeutic superiority, which was rooted in advances in applied medical science and technology that made the hospital a safe, effective, and preferred environment for the treatment of, and recovery from, acute illness. Aided, abetted – and often impelled – by an emerging medical profession that was determined to control entry to medical practice, and its standards and rewards, hospitals' organizational structures, medical priorities, business practices, and internal cultures changed to reflect their new medical mission, their new clientele, and the newly recognized interdependence, for individuals and hospitals alike, of health and wealth. When, for the first time in history, scientific and technological progress enabled individuals to purchase health,[5] hospitals, it may be argued, progressed from "treating the poor for the sake of charity to treating the rich for the sake of revenue."[6]

One immediate result of the medicalization of the hospital was that it became at least a two-class institution, discriminating between patients who could pay for differentiated care and treatment and its traditional population of medical indigents, supported by inadequate public and private charity, whom neither the hospital nor the medical profession could abandon. Indigent victims of infectious and chronic diseases became the objects of a grudgingly economical service not because they sought and deserved charity, but because they occupied space and resources that otherwise could generate hospital revenues and medical fees from middle-class patients who tended to be briefly hospitalized with treatable acute illnesses that usually required surgery, the focus of the new medicine. Thus, the quality of a patient's life on the wards, indeed the whole experience of hospitalization, became associated with degrees of relative independence, defined in terms of ability to pay, from medical and institutional benevolence and control. In short, the social realities of the modern hospital became a microcosm of the social structures, processes, and conditions of everyday life.[7]

The extent to which users were either beneficiaries or victims of this new culture of institutional medicine depended principally on the evolving relationship between doctors and hospitals. Hospitals relied on the historical altruism of the medical profession to meet their obligations to indigent patients, and on doctors' diagnostic and surgical skills to attract paying patients and produce health for all patients – the new hospital's vigorously promoted *raison d'être*. The medical profession quickly identified the modern hospital as the doctors' workshop. There, all the tools essential to the new orthodoxy of "scientific" medicine's limited, but increasingly valued and sought after, ability to intervene successfully in the course of acute diseases were brought together. The medical workshop was designed to enhance the surgeon's skill and the physician's art, advance the leading edge of medical education, improve the efficiency of medical practice, and, above all, promote the patient's confidence in and respect for the authority of the practitioner and of traditional (as opposed to alternative) medical science. These elements should have led to a productive symbiotic relationship among hospitals, doctors, and users.

But the seeds of disharmony were sown early in the transitional process. Hospitals' successful pursuit of their new mandate to produce health for all social classes increasingly depended on their ability to finance the care of indigents, the modernization and expansion of buildings, and a rapidly evolving scientific infrastructure from patient fees – which they relentlessly inflated. As public and private benevolence waned, paying patients became the principal source of hospital income. The hospitals' priorities inevitably became defined by their preference for short-stay patients paying premium fees for differentiated care in expensive private and semi-private wards relative to what were seen as malingering indigents consuming unrecoverable resources in the free wards. The result, however, was the gradual estrangement of patients, especially middle-class patients, from hospitals, as their willingness and ability to pay for hospitalization were outdistanced by hospitals' revenue requirements. Paying users first began to resist the perpetual inflation of hospital charges in the 1920s, and then either abandoned hospitals altogether when the Great Depression assailed their incomes, or reluctantly reappeared in hospitals among the medical paupers of the public wards. The departure of paying patients, the resurgence of medical indigence, and hospitals' growing financial instability inevitably initiated a struggle between hospital trustees and medical staffs to determine hospital priorities. Boards and administrators, who were converts to the popular ideology of industrial efficiency, insisted on the primacy of managerial authority in all matters affecting the institution. This meant reining in the aspirations, expectations, and hard-won privileges of the medical profession, especially general practitioners, after their successful twenty-year campaign for open hospitals and collegial governance. For their part, private practitioners, who were neither employed nor appointed by hospitals, increasingly insisted on their role as intermediaries between their patients and the hospital, on the hegemony of medical authority in, and physician control of, the hospital, and on their right to determine both the intent and the extent of the hospital's medical altruism.[8]

In North America, the medical profession's most notable successes were twofold: first, wresting hospital practice from the control of board-appointed attending physicians and surgeons and opening it to all of the private general practitioners in the community; and, second, the implementation of the hospital standardization movement of the 1920s, which established internationally recognized benchmarks for medically accredited hospitals and signalled the ultimate triumph of medicalization. The profession's obvious failures were its ultimate inability to curb the historical hospital preference for the medicine practised by elite specialists at the expense of general practitioners, and doctors' equivocal political response, as independent business men in a highly competitive environment, to alternative strategies – especially contributory hospital and medical insurance schemes – for the equitable provision of health care to all as the anti-dote to the threatened medical disenfranchisement of their principal client, the so-called "patient of moderate means," after 1930. In Canada, the growing estrangement of doctors from hospitals, and of patients from both, was at once the cause and the effect of a health-care crisis that contributed to a re-examination of public policy on the costs and distribution of a minimum standard of health care for all on the eve of the modern therapeutic revolution. [9]

These, in broad outline, are the themes that define recent explanations of the social history of the hospital in Western society since the late nineteenth century, and more particularly the history of hospitals in the United States. In spite of the growing proliferation of celebratory histories of Canadian hospitals, these larger themes remain relatively unexplored by Canadian historians, with some notable exceptions. Normand Perron's *Un siècle de vie hospitalière au Québec* (1984), and J.T.H. Connor's *Doing Good: The Life of the Toronto General Hospital* (2000) are exemplary models of institutional social history, while Geoffrey Reaume's *Remembrance of Patients Past: Patient Life at the Toronto Hospital for the Insane, 1870–1940* (2000) is a path-breaking study of the daily experience of hospitalized patients.[10] More generally, the potential for research into the emergence of the modern Canadian hospital has been significantly enhanced by the rapidly accumulating historiography of the history of Canadian medicine, nursing, medical technology, and paramedical services, and by the growing imperative to preserve institutional records.[11] Drawing upon the inventory of this recent scholarship, as well as on selected institutional, professional, and government sources, our task is to determine whether the historical evolution of Canadian hospitals replicates these larger international processes or represents a uniquely Canadian phenomenon. Given the historical environment in which the modern hospital emerged in Canada as a social as well as a medical necessity imbued, for better or worse, with the aura of an essential and benevolent community public utility, it seems highly unlikely that the Canadian hospital would have become anything less than a microcosm of the shifting social and economic realities that alternately sustained and threatened its – and the nation's – quest for social efficiency, order, and purpose.

This study focuses on the history of voluntary public general hospitals. They were not the only form of hospital organization in Canada, where hospitals and hospices founded and managed by religious orders, specialized hospitals for lying-in, women, children, and incurables, hospitals funded and managed by municipal corporations, public sanatoria, asylums, and private hospitals were also commonplace and provided the same services as voluntary community hospitals. Indeed, the history of the confessional hospital in Canada demonstrably deserves a critical evaluation in its own right, given its unique mission, funding, and administrative arrangements, and the evolving tensions between its spiritual imperatives and its developing medical environment between 1880 and 1960.[12] The secular voluntary general hospital, however, was the most widespread form of hospital organization in Canada and, arguably, given its dependence on popular support for its financial viability, for the diversity of its medical activities, and for the quality of its services, the most sensitive to the interplay of forces and interests, internal as well as external, that shaped the evolution of hospitals everywhere in North America. Voluntary general hospitals were originally founded, governed, and financed by local patrons to create a visible community social asset sustained by public and medical altruism. They were re-invented, socially and medically, after 1890 by patients and doctors in response to health- and health-care crises and opportunities; and their effectiveness, until at least 1950, continued to be measured largely by the local availability of adequate resources with which to achieve their purposes.

To illustrate, give substance to, and test the relevance of the themes and patterns that emerge from the historiography of Canadian hospitals and of medicine between 1890 and 1950, we have generalized from the experience of a limited, but diverse, range of Canadian institutions. Their surviving records have afforded the broadest possible resource base for an analysis whose goal is to contextualize provincially, nationally, and even internationally, events and processes that transpired, historically, at the level of the local hospital. In his comprehensive study *Mending Bodies, Saving Souls: A History of Hospitals*, Guenter Risse describes the essential outline of the history of the hospital in terms of its mission, sources of support, and internal organization, the institutional experience of staff and patients, and the hospital's "ritualized caring activities."[13] The historian's relative success in addressing these themes depends, lamentably, on the availability and scope of archival sources that until very recently have been indifferently preserved.[14] Patient records, especially records that reveal patients' responses to the experience of hospitalization, are notoriously slim. On the other hand, admissions registers, surgery inventories, and detailed hospital morbidity reports combined with quantitative methodology have allowed us to reconstruct patient populations and hospital usage at least from an epidemiological perspective. Similarly, with the exception of nursing school records, hospital employment records tend to render hospital workers invisible while,

for reasons that will become obvious from our analysis, extant hospital financial records are both meticulous and detailed. These archival
biases are necessarily reflected in the substance of our analysis, which
relies heavily on sources external to the hospital – government documents and professional journals in particular – to achieve a themati-
cally balanced discussion without committing the sin of the first
history of an English-Canadian hospital, a history with the hospital
left out.[15]

Within this documentary and methodological context, our analysis
is organized both chronologically and topically. The first three chapters provide a history of the Canadian voluntary general hospital
from the late-Victorian era until the advent of national hospital insurance. In three subsequent chapters we examine evolving relationships among hospitals, the medical profession, nurses, and patients.
We have restricted our inquiry to the period 1890–1950, that is, from
the beginning of the movement to reshape the public general hospital as the primary health-care centre for the whole community until
the advent of national hospital insurance, which fundamentally
altered the political, economic, and social determinants of the hospital's mission. Still, some things have not changed. The current Canadian health-care crisis has ample precedent. Its roots are firmly
entrenched in society's ambiguous and reactive responses to the
problems of equitable health-care delivery since the modern hospital
first institutionalized the promise of freedom from the fear of sickness and premature death.

Our analysis of the historical foundations of the modern hospital
describes an institution ready, willing, and able at the end of the nineteenth century to cast off its Victorian identity as a charnel house for
the sick poor and to become, in the new era of industrial and scientific progress, an efficient factory for the production of scientifically
mitigated health for public consumption at a fair price commensu-
rate with its value. It was a vision ultimately thwarted, however, by
hospitals' inability to cast off their historical responsibilities for the
medically indigent, by the ineluctable social and economic realities of
Canadian society between the wars, by territorial disputes between
hospital managers and the medical profession – and within the medical profession – for control of the hospital's mission, and by the failure of hospital authorities, the medical profession, and governments
to agree about the limits to the capacity of middle-class patients to
underwrite, for the whole population, the relentlessly inflated costs
of medical determinism. Among the possible solutions to the ensuing
crisis of hospital funding and accessibility, access on demand, sustained by a national scheme of compulsory public hospital insurance,

eventually, though not inevitably, emerged as the Canadian solution to this dilemma just when the modern therapeutic revolution was poised to alter indelibly the promise and the expectation of hospital-centred medical science, and, consequently, to redefine the now firmly entrenched dependence of health on wealth.

1 Hospital Fever

The nineteenth-century general hospital was a medically marginal but socially essential agency of voluntary charity. Sustained by private benevolence and government grants, the hospital provided indoor, largely custodial, care for sick indigents. Their dependent and submissive relationship with hospitals characterized them as inmates, not patients, the subjects equally of medical and public curiosity and of social stigmatization, because they both required and accepted confinement in an institution, and the care of strangers, that no "respectable" citizen would endure. Hospitals were associated with the most repugnant circumstances of disease and death. Respectable Canadians received medical treatment, and convalesced, at home in the care of trusted family physicians, attentive female relatives, and domestic servants. By the end of the Victorian era, however, the fundamental social change manifested through industrialization, immigration, urbanization, the increasingly critical state of public health, and a growing economic inequality not only had vastly accelerated the demand for medical charity but had also limited the ability of all but the most affluent families to provide home care for the sick.

This social transformation coincided with several important developments in the evolution of medical science and health care. Medical acceptance of germ theory and its clinical application, *asepsis*, made hospitalization in general, and invasive surgery in particular, relatively safe. At the same time, the emergence of professional nursing as the science of patient care promoted effective convalescence following the doctor's skilled diagnosis and successful surgical intervention in acute diseases. Scientific advances in biology and chemistry, and technological innovation, x-rays and electrocardiograms for example, enhanced diagnostic accuracy and added to medicine's reputation as a rigorous scientific discipline. All of these developments in turn strengthened the appeal of medicine as a profession, in particular with its opportunities for medical specialization, and led to a growing supply of, and competition among, doctors eager to seize every professional and economic advantage.

These social and medical factors coalesced in the 1890s around the hospital, which became both the source of, and the marketplace for, the new scientific medicine for all classes in society, and especially for a new clientele of patients. Their ability to pay for medical treatment and care, and their growing confidence in, and demand for, the highest standard of hospital care rather than home care, created opportunities and problems for the emerging alliance of medical and hospital professionals. The result, in any event, was the modern public general hospital.

There is no obvious watershed that conveniently separates the era of the charity hospital from the age of the community hospital in Canada. The varied pace of local and regional developments dictated the timing of change as much as national or international events. The charity hospital of the nineteenth century never entirely disappeared. Intimations of the modern hospital could be found in the best of the late-Victorian metropolitan hospitals like the Toronto General or the Montreal General. But an observation from Ontario's Inspector of Hospitals and Charities in his report for 1894 offers a convenient benchmark. "Our hospitals," he noted, "are now ... being patronized by the wealthier classes ... as paying patients" whose satisfaction with their treatment and care was being translated into great enthusiasm for hospital philanthropy.[1] To the inspector, this was a new phenomenon with the potential to change dramatically the financial status and the medical performance of the province's hospitals as providers of health care to the poor. A decade later his successor commented on the progress of this development. Community hospitals were springing up everywhere. "It is not too much to hope," he said, "that before long every physician in Ontario will be able to command hospital facilities for his patients within easy reach of their homes ... It is surely not visionary to predict that the time will come when a hospital in every town of 3,000 inhabitants will be regarded as a necessity and demanded by every thriving, progressive community." He offered three reasons for his opinion: "civic pride" made hospital progressivism a "social" imperative in every community; "increase[d] public confidence" in the medical efficacy of hospitals had induced "the well to do class" to embrace hospital treatment; and providing for the "needy sick" would continue to be a matter of "supreme [public] importance."[2] But there was already disturbing evidence that the indigent and the working poor were not equal beneficiaries of this transformation in community health care, and that humanitarianism was no longer the leading source of the "hospital spirit" among Ontarians that it had been just two decades earlier.[3]

For a few nineteenth-century communities as disparate as Halifax, Toronto, Hamilton, Owen Sound, St Catharines, Winnipeg, and New Westminster, hospitals had become essential institutions long before they became medically indispensable; but their purpose was limited. It was defined equally by the state of medical science, the enlightened self-interest of the prospering classes, and the ever-present realities of a growing urban working-class population among whom a marginal material existence, transience, the diminishing prospect of social mobility, and repetitive dependence on charity were common milestones of their life cycle.[4] Victorian hospitals were built for the provident poor through the generosity of the better classes and their elected representatives, whose motives as public men, voluntary subscribers, and hospital governors or visitors were both altruistic and practical. Explaining the purpose of Ontario's *Charity Aid Act* (1874) which formalized provincial government support for hospitals, J.W. Langmuir, Ontario's first inspector of prisons and asylums, noted that "[the] class of persons that Government aid is designed to relieve, are the sick and diseased ... but more especially those who have neither the means to pay for medical treatment, nor suitable lodgement and surroundings during sickness. These sick poor have a special claim upon the sympathy and assistance of Government that those of the well-to-do portion of the community do not."[5]

If medical charity was a public responsibility, it was also a personal, Christian moral obligation. The comfortable classes could readily agree with Mayor John Frost of Owen Sound, Ontario, that to "be good, it [is] necessary to do good. To be happy, it is necessary to make others happy. Hospitals [afford] a great opportunity of doing good."[6] Medical charity reflected, in the respective roles of giver and receiver, the appropriate order of a society structured along the fault line between prosperity and dependence, success and failure, status and invisibility. But it was also a society fearful that the fault line might crack, violently, if thrift, industry, temperance, respectability, and deference – the Victorian mantra of success – failed the deserving poor.

Hospitals were just one aspect of a widespread voluntary movement meant to contain, and relieve, human distress and ensure social stability at a time when, for example, 60 per cent of Ontario's urban population lived in permanent, often disabling, poverty with growing evidence that their condition was, if not worsening, not improving.[7]

For the eight thousand citizens of Owen Sound who, through personal, corporate, lodge and church subscriptions, dances and balls, raffles, and entertainments raised the capital to construct and operate their hospital, the immediate objects of their good works were the itinerant individuals and families who streamed through the lakeport on their way west to the prairie frontier of settlement between 1885 and 1905.[8] Meanwhile, since 1850 Hamilton's City Hospital, entirely funded and managed by its city council, had undergone three iterations as a "public necessity" – "not a fancy charity" – routinely expanding to accommodate ever larger numbers of indigent dependents who required a warrant from the mayor or a hospital commissioner to gain admission.[9] In Halifax, it was the medical profession who persuaded the city council, and subsequently the provincial government, to fund Halifax City Hospital (1859) and its successor, Victoria General Hospital (1887), as explicit medical charities for working-class patients.[10] A continent away, as the human flotsam and jetsam of the Cariboo gold rush accumulated in their settlement, the residents of New Westminster, the administrative seat of colonial British Columbia, founded a hospital in 1862 "mainly by the voluntary efforts of the Colonists for the reception of the indigent sick, irrespective of nationality, creed or colour." When the placer miners who had struck it rich failed to "contribute a portion of their gains ... for the relief of their sick or wounded fellow-colonists," the British Colonial Secretary was persuaded to fund the Royal Columbian Hospital as a facility for the whole colony.[11] By then the Toronto General and Montreal General hospitals had been in existence for nearly half a century, offering not only residential care but outpatient clinics for the urban poor and, eventually, providing the raw material for the education of medical students by the physicians and surgeons who comprised the hospitals' unpaid, honorary medical staffs. In these hospitals governors, life subscribers, and attending physicians wielded the power of free admission and treatment for deserving paupers. The working poor who could contribute to the cost of their hospitalization were encouraged to do so, and most hospitals maintained a few private rooms on a full cost-recovery basis to augment their income.[12] But as Appendix A illustrates, before 1900 income from patient fees represented a negligible proportion of annual hospital income in every jurisdiction. Where they existed, provincial government *per diem* grants for the care of indigent patients (Quebec, for example, provided none before 1921) and municipal *per diem* or annually negotiated grants for charity cases together comprised the principal component of the annual operating budgets of most late-nineteenth-century public hospitals. But neither public source was adequate, in itself, to defray the cost of patient maintenance and the upkeep or expansion of physical plants; and municipal funding was notoriously insecure and subject to the vicissitudes of local politics – so much so that Ontario's inspectors of hospitals openly discouraged the creation of municipally operated hospitals in preference to voluntary hospital associations whose success depended fundamentally on private philanthropy.[13] To whatever extent the best of these institutions eventually became models of late-Victorian hospital planning, development, and management, their medical, financial, and social viability were the products of the first great age of Canadian philanthropy in which the support and direction of the hospital reflected the private imperative of "doing good."[14]

Apart from their common purpose and sources of funding, these medical charities shared several other important characteristics: the nature of their clientele, their records of hospital morbidity, medical practice within the hospital, and hospital management structures. If poverty was the lowest common descriptor of hospital inmates, gender ran a close second. Charity patients were overwhelmingly male. In 1879, 95 per cent of the patients admitted to the Royal Columbian Hospital were men, as might be expected in a frontier community with a disproportionately male population. But at the same time, only 20 per cent of the yearly patients in the St Catharines hospital in in the long-settled Niagara peninsula were women. Male and female patients did not generally appear in even roughly equal proportions in Canada's general hospitals until the eve of the First World War, although a rapid rise in women's admissions was noticeable from the outset of hospital modernization after 1890.[15] Why this was the case is not clear; but when women's admissions began to accelerate, they were associated with significant increases, first, in gynaecological surgery and then in the preference for hospital births, principally among middle-class women. The Victorian hospital's reputation as a "warehouse of death"[16] undoubtedly made it repugnant to women of all classes, as did the close proximity of patients, many with infectious diseases, in the crowded public wards. Extant patient registers suggest, moreover, that among male patients young single men were overrepresented relative to other age groups, perhaps an indication of the dominant culture of ward life as well as the nature of indigence. For example, in 1900 the median age of adult male patients (those older than twelve years), who represented 60 per cent of all admissions in the Owen Sound General and Marine Hospital, was twenty-seven. A decade earlier in the St Catharines General and Marine Hospital, adult males, half of them under thirty, accounted for 70 per cent of all admissions. Whatever their age, 90 per cent of these men were labourers, as were the male inmates of the Toronto General Hospital in 1891, only 5 per cent of whom had occupations that did not require manual labour. Among the hospital's female inmates in 1891, only 25 per cent were categorized as wives, spinsters, and widows. The rest identified themselves as working women, most commonly (21%) household servants. Similarly, twenty-four of the twenty-eight female patients with occupations admitted to the St Catharines hospital in 1889 were domestic servants. This lends credence to a mid-century newspaper editor's opinion that one of the functions of Victorian public hospitals was to relieve "many respectable families ... of the expense and anxiety attendant on keeping sick servants in their houses."[17] Whatever the case may be, these hospitals clearly were one-class institutions populated by men and women whose incomes did not permit them to seek private medical care, whose familial situations made home care impossible, and whose periodic dependence on medical charity, a by-product of their marginal existences, probably characterized all aspects of their lives.[18]

What afflictions brought these patients to a hospital? Appendix B broadly describes patients admitted by disease classification in the late-nineteenth and early-twentieth centuries, relative to fairly recent statistics. Nineteenth-century hospital wards reflected the unreformed state of public health, the hazards of unregulated workplaces, the lifestyles of the working classes, and the transgressions of their masters.[19] Infectious, febrile, and parasitic diseases, and tuberculosis were the leading causes of admission, followed by injuries, poisonings, various forms of addiction, and genito-urinary diseases. Within this context, specific causes of admission were monotonously similar from one hospital to the next – typhoid fever, dysentery, and fractures were commonplace. So, too, were sexually transmitted diseases, alcoholism, rheumatism, and "debility," which seems to have been a generic label for unclassifiable admissions particularly, though not exclusively, among the elderly. Still, the unique hazards of servitude in Kingston, sea-faring in the Maritimes, mining in the Fraser Valley, and life in the teeming urban ghettos of Toronto and Montreal understandably produced a diverse, not monolithic, model of the nineteenth-century hospital.[20] Where the history of hospital morbidity coalesces is in the nature and duration of the care and treatment patients received.

In Ontario's late-Victorian hospitals, for example, patient stays averaged between 35 days (in 1880) and 25 days (in 1900), as they did in most Canadian hospitals. This reduction of nearly 30 per cent in two decades would seem to be evidence of a therapeutic environment changing for the better.[21] Some progress was indeed made in reducing the stays of certain patients, fever cases for example; but in institutions where it was not uncommon for elderly and chronically ill patients to remain in hospital for a year – in the extreme, five years and more[22] – the elimination of certain classes of patients or the arbitrary limitation of their length of stay also accounted for a reduction in the average duration of hospitalization.[23] As early as 1879 Inspector Langmuir noted that Ontario's hospitals could accommodate more needy patients and reduce the average length of hospital stays by refusing to admit patients with "the ordinary infirmities attendant upon old age," and "women who [were] … chiefly prostitutes and the mothers of illegitimate children," who were hospitalized four times longer (80 days) than "honest" working-class mothers who gave birth at home spent "lying-in."[24] [He might have had in mind the London City (later Victoria) Hospital, where domestic servants were commonly hidden away for three months to complete their "unacceptable pregnancies."[25]] Generally, given the inability of nineteenth-century medicine to intervene effectively in the course of most diseases and illnesses, patients lingered in hospital until they recovered, improved, or succumbed. The Hamilton City Hospital reported that in 1888, 38 per cent of patients treated were discharged as "cured"; but a similar number were simply discharged or died, and 20 per cent departed as "somewhat better" or "much improved," though not cured.[26]

Until the widespread acceptance of germ theory, of Lister's principles of antisepsis, and finally of asepsis, and without the advantage of a modern pharmacopoeia, hospital-based medicine could only relieve suffering with opiates, occasionally intervene surgically at last resort to save a life, and provide the necessities of life for the sick poor who had no other source of care. At the Toronto General, one of Canada's busiest and most progressive hospitals, in 1891 a mere 10 per cent of the patients admitted were subjected to surgery, and just 10 per cent of their number underwent invasive surgery. Only amputations were commonplace in a surgical regime where "the operative mortality from even the simplest procedures was so shocking that …[the] abdomen was never opened … Compound fractures rarely recovered. Strangulated hernia, if operated upon, usually led to death."[27] The death rate at the Hamilton City Hospital was 18 per cent, the maternal death rate for "robust country girls" admitted for childbirth was one in fourteen, and the infant mortality rate was 87/1000 live births.[28] For all patients, but in particular for surgical and maternity patients, the risk of cross-infection was simply too great, an "insurmountable barrier" to the use of hospitals by anyone except those unfortunate enough to be entirely dependent on medical charity or with no other source of care during illness.[29] Their need, and the provision of the clinical instructional material necessary for creating "a well-educated and properly-trained medical profession," were the limited purposes underlying the introduction of provincial grants to hospitals in Ontario in 1874.[30] For the remainder of the century, the best hope of improving the health of the population generally lay in public health reform.

That is not to say that nineteenth-century physicians and surgeons were either unprofessional or incompetent, or that hospital staff and management were not concerned with their patients' well-being. In most Victorian hospitals, attending physicians and surgeons either were appointed by governing boards from among the senior medical men in the city, as was the case at the Winnipeg General, or were local doctors who had volunteered to serve as attending physicians on weekly rotations, as they did in Owen Sound. With the exception of a resident House Surgeon who was paid a salary, attending physicians and surgeons volunteered their services and collected no fees from patients: they expected that voluntary hospital service would enhance their social standing in the community, and provide research and instructional opportunities for themselves and their students from the medical menagerie of the public wards. In this way, "charity held the hand of science."[31] Closed hospitals, which restricted medical practice to the board's appointed consultants and attending physicians, eventually came to be regarded by private practitioners, who were prohibited from following any of their patients into hospital, as unwarranted competition for patient recruitment and future income, as sources of indiscriminate political patronage, and as detriments to physician-patient relationships. Both the Winnipeg General and Hamilton City hospitals became embroiled in controversies over the issue of professional accessibility through the 1880s and 1890s, as appointed medical staff, private physicians, and boards increasingly contended for control of these hospitals. Board members vigorously defended the view that "the services of the members of the medical board being gratuitous, the exclusive privilege granted [of admitting and attending all patients, paying and free] should be confined to them"[32] In Hamilton, the war among the medical profession, city politicians, the press, and the public over the "profitable monopoly of hospital practice, so long held by a clique of physicians" went on for nearly a decade.[33] Both boards eventually relented, permitting all practitioners to admit their paying patients – and follow them – into the hospital. When this practice became commonplace, it was a significant concession to the redefinition of the hospital.[34] Meanwhile, governing boards provided indigent patients with the best care available within the limitations of their meagre budgets, the state of the medical arts, and their understanding of what the deserving poor deserved.

What they provided was a highly regulated environment where the patient's welfare was associated with deference, if not obedience, to authority. The Royal Columbian Hospital's rules for patients might have applied equally in the public wards of any Canadian general hospital before the Great War. Patients were required to "implicitly obey their Physicians and Nurses"; "keep themselves clean and orderly"; assist each other, and treat their fellow patients kindly; and "comport themselves decorously, quietly, and in an orderly manner." There were specific injunctions against smoking, inappropriate or abusive language, and bribing hospital employees. (The Owen Sound hospital's rules added loitering, whistling, playing cards, and wearing a hat or street clothes in bed as proscribed behaviour).[35] Failure to comply carried the threat of immediate expulsion, as exemplified by the fate of one fractious young woman who, "on a day you would not turn a dog out," was cast out of the Hamilton City Hospital "half naked, and the cabman was told to take her to the poorhouse."[36] She had complained that she had been served rotten eggs. Patients were encouraged, nevertheless, to report employees guilty of inattention, unkindness, or lassitude in the administration of food and medicine.[37] Enforcement of these regulations was the responsibility of medical superintendents and, more particularly, of matrons (later, lady superintendents) who supervised the cooks, laundry workers, porters, domestics, and a few minimally trained, more frequently untrained, nurses who comprised the hospitals' labour force before the widespread deployment of student nurses at the turn of the century. None of these employees, as historian Charles Rosenberg has pointed out, contributed to the pursuit of a defined medical regime or hospital experience associated with the patient's "biological reality."[38] Rather, they pursued the governors' social imperative to create a domestic environment characterized by order, harmony, cleanliness, and obedience[39] in which matron and physician, assisted by the household servants, provided material comfort to, and eased the suffering of, society's deserving medical dependants. Unlike the comfortable and well-ordered households of their sponsors, however, charity hospitals, like their inmates, existed on the margins of respectability. At a time when a fully employed skilled labourer's wages – nine dollars a week – allowed a family of five to just barely subsist on twenty-five cents per person per day, Ontario's general hospitals housed, fed, clothed, medicated, and ministered to their patients for about seventy cents per patient day, including the costs of wages, mortgages, building repairs, and fuel (Appendix A).[40] It seems unlikely that hospitalization anywhere in nineteenth-century Canada represented a pleasant relief from ordinary reality in any material sense.

Most Victorian hospitals were located either close to their principal client populations, on land unsuitable for other uses, or on isolated sites that withdrew the sick from the community – in any case, in the least environmentally friendly urban settings. Hamilton City Hospital was in the industrial east end where the city's highest mortality rates already obtained. The Winnipeg General was built on low-lying ground subject to flooding, the Vancouver City Hospital in an area associated with boarding houses and an unsavoury transient population. The Owen Sound General and Marine was just a short walk from the town's teeming waterfront and its most offensive public health problems. Foul odours, rats and other vermin, inadequate sanitation, and undependable heating and ventilating systems were commonplace in these institutions.[41] As for the internal culture of the hospital as experienced by patients and employees, the available evidence provides glimpses of a not always harmonious domestic commonwealth largely sustained by porridge, beef stew, tea, and black bread.[42]

An inquiry into the affairs of the Winnipeg General Hospital in 1880 was initiated on the basis of reports that the steward and his drinking companions had consumed the hospital's entire supply of medicinal liquor one Sunday afternoon, and that the male nurse had consummated an affair with the female cook during working hours in the hospital. A male patient admitted for treatment of a chronic kidney disease testified that the same steward had forced him to sleep on the floor even when a bed was available, and made him saw wood outdoors in inclement weather when he was "weak and poorly clad," and that the nurse "swore at and used abusive language" toward a female patient, and "used beastly language while the patients were eating and almost turned my stomach."[43] On the other hand, a daily roster of patients who were "often badly nourished, filthy ... fearful of medical treatment" and frequently violent, and who "submitted only resentfully to the wishes of the medical staff," undoubtedly tested the boundaries of hospital employees' humanitarianism.[44] Patients were also a source of public curiosity. It was not uncommon for a hundred visitors, most of whom had no reason to be there, to stroll the wards of the Winnipeg General Hospital on a Sunday afternoon, disturbing the patients whom they greatly outnumbered and annoying the staff, who proposed implementing admission by ticket.[45]

The marginal utility of their endeavours notwithstanding, two generations of enthusiastic lay governors sustained the voluntary Victorian-Canadian charitable hospital through good times and bad. Their purpose in creating and supporting these medical charities was aptly defined by the governors of the St Catharines General and Marine Hospital in 1870. "In this highly favoured land, the poor man, unless stricken down by disease or accident, is seldom compelled to mendicity, provided his habits are sober and industrious. The tie which unites the poor man to his richer neighbour ... should never in a healthy or Christian state of society be exchanged for a legal claim." That tie, "the holiest [duty] of man to man," was "spontaneous charity."[46] The Victorian general hospital was a social, not a medical, necessity that provided care as a privilege, not a right. As a surrogate for family and household, it offered a temporary refuge for the indigent, transient, and homeless population who required care as the result of injury, illness, or misadventure and who were unable to pay for medical and nursing services at any price. It was a fitting object of charity among middle-class Canadians equally as a personal moral imperative, as a civic responsibility of the rich toward the poor, and as an investment in social harmony. But as an agent of the healing arts, the nineteenth-century hospital became preserved in popular memory as a "chamber of horrors ... it [was] a misfortune for anyone to be admitted thereto."[47]

By the turn of the century, the Victorian general hospital was in the midst of a wholesale transformation. As late as 1890 the manager of the St Catharines General and Marine Hospital had regretted that "the excellent private wards of the hospital [were] not more taken advantage of at the small sum of $7.00 per week, for the use of room with board, midicine [sic], nurse's attendance and the services of the physician in charge *free* [was] exceedingly low and the patient [had] the privilege of employing any other physician at their [sic] own expense."[48] The manager's sole objective in promoting the use of the hospital by private paying patients was to make up the shortfall in the hospital's annual operating budget, which depended on government grants and charitable donations, in order to improve services to the hospital's principal population, its charity patients. A mere decade later, the editor of the *Dominion Medical Journal* observed what he identified as a significant "transition" of interest to his professional audience. "Originally the hospital was a charitable institution for the homeless poor. The advantages of medical treatment have become so marked of late years, however, that many prefer going to the hospital to being treated at home. They do not go to the hospital because it is a charitable institution for charitable reasons, but because of the improved conditions to be gained there."[49] By 1904, Ontario's inspector of hospitals, Dr Frederick Chamberlain was publicly complaining that the province's general hospitals were in danger of losing sight of "the original idea for which hospitals were established – the care of the sick poor": they now "devot[ed] more attention to the care of private patients who pay a goodly sum per week ... the tendency being towards an extravagant expenditure in providing rooms and fittings." Meanwhile, in order to accommodate more paying patients, the population of the public wards, Chamberlain observed, increasingly was being consigned to the least desirable spaces in hospitals where the quality of their care was deteriorating.[50] How did it happen that, in less than two decades, the general hospital shed its reputation as a warehouse of death for the indigent and working poor and began first to attract, then actively to court, the patronage of families and individuals who had once shunned the hospital and who were not only able, but now willing, to pay for hospitalization as their preferred source of health care? The answer is entwined in the cross-currents of social, demographic, and economic change that were transforming Canadian society between 1890 and 1920, and as complex as the undercurrents of scientific, technological, and educational development that were, at the same time, revising the definitions of disease and health and transforming the practice of medicine.

At the close of the nineteenth century, Canada was experiencing both a health crisis and a health-care crisis. The health crisis was the direct product of industrialization, urbanization, population growth – especially through immigration – and the insanitary conditions that prevailed as the result of inadequate and overcrowded housing, non-existent or ineffective sewage and garbage disposal, untreated, unprotected, and regularly contaminated municipal water systems and private wells, insufficient regulation of food and milk supplies, unsafe and overcrowded workplaces, and large concentrations of seasonally impoverished and malnourished working poor. In 1881 only one-quarter of Canada's 4.3 million people resided in urban places, of which nearly 80 per cent lived in cities, towns, and villages with fewer than 30,000 inhabitants. By 1921 Canada's population had doubled, 54 per cent of Canadians were now urban dwellers, and 42 per cent of them lived in cities of at least 100,000 people.[51] Winnipeg exemplified both the promise and the problem of urban development. Between 1881 and 1916 its population increased from 8,000 to 163,000 as Winnipeg became the focus of westward immigration, the western hub of a transcontinental transportation system, and the commercial centre of the new wheat economy of the prairies. But with this inexorable developmental process and its ensuing demographic pressures came public health problems that produced annual epidemics of environmentally induced contagion. One observer likened living conditions in Winnipeg's immigrant North End to those of a European village in the Middle Ages,[52] but he might have been describing the working-class districts of any Canadian city, among which Montreal's east end was the most notorious.[53]

In Winnipeg, and across Canada, the leading causes of death among Canadians between the ages of 15 and 50 in 1900 were tuberculosis, typhoid fever, respiratory disease, puerperal complications, and peritonitis. *Cholera infantum* (infant diarrhoea), tuberculosis, diphtheria, scarlet fever, whooping cough, and measles were the principal contributors to levels of child and infant mortality in Toronto and Montreal that we now associate with the underdeveloped Third World.[54] With the exception of peritonitis, the incidence of virtually all these diseases was exacerbated by urban poverty, and could be – eventually was – ameliorated either by public health reform or by improvements in standards of living. In the meantime, many Canadians were inclined to blame the improvident poor, especially the "teeming masses" of immigrants, for the crisis in public health. These "people who should never have been allowed to embark for this country," it was argued, represented not only the social but the unhealthy biological detritus of Europe and Asia which threatened Canadians with racial and moral degeneration and economic inefficiency.[55] From the 1880s until the mid-1920s, these immigrants, and their living conditions, became the focus of a diverse and intensive campaign of social, environmental, and moral reform intended, according to some historians, to realize a vision of human perfectibility manifested in the social and moral achievement of the Kingdom of Heaven on earth; and, according to others, to rein in the excesses of industrial capitalism and the dangerous working and immigrant classes through enforced conformity to the evangelical Christian social *mores* of the threatened middle classes.[56]

One of the first goals of the social reform movement was to improve public health in a concerted effort to eliminate the sources and the incidence of epidemic disease. As Appendix B illustrates, caring for the perennial victims of seasonal epidemics of air- and water-borne contagion became a major responsibility of community hospitals after 1890 and was one of the reasons for their rapid expansion. The problem among the urban working – and perhaps middle – classes was their inability to provide home care for sick and convalescent family members. Among working-class families, neither urban living conditions nor family economies were amenable to the prolonged nursing of the sick at home. Families of six or eight – sometimes augmented by unmarried boarders – crowded into one- or two-room tenement flats, were incapable of segregating the sick, especially the contagious sick, from the healthy, or of ministering to their needs when material survival depended on the collective contribution of all who could work to sustain the household's precarious income. A family quarantined by public health officials for six or eight weeks was effectively impoverished for the duration of the illness. Boarders – transient single working men and women – and large numbers of domestic servants whose employers would not maintain them when sick also represented a significant proportion of the urban population without family resources to call upon during illness.[57] These had traditionally been the users of the charity hospital, but by 1890 their numbers were greatly expanded, and they were more widely distributed throughout, and concentrated in, the nation's numerous emerging towns and cities. The need to provide these women and men with effective health care in the face of the mounting public health crisis was urgent – and not just medically. As Colin Howell has noted, for social progressives it was a short leap from the evidence of a diseased population requiring the best care that medicine had to offer to the apprehension of a "diseased social order that could be nursed back to health"[58] with the leadership provided, in each case, by appropriate experts in preventive social, moral, and scientific medicine.[59] By the end of the nineteenth century hospitals and their medical specialists, not the myriad quacks, charlatans, dispensers of folk remedies, and irregular practitioners – the traditional neighbourhood purveyors of "medicine" – now constituted the front line in the defence of public health.[60]

The palpable public health crisis among the urban poor explains the explosive growth of indigent hospital admissions and the need to expand hospital capacity at the end of the nineteenth century. The explanation for the appearance in hospitals after 1890 of a growing – soon to be dominant – clientele of paying middle-class patients is more complex. For example, the business cycle appears to have been partly responsible for the middle-class discovery of the hospital as an expedient alternative to professional home care. If medical journals and their correspondents are credible witnesses, it was during the economic panic of the mid 1890s, one of the century's most severe depressions, that large numbers of people who had formerly been able to afford surgeons, physicians, and special duty nurses for private medical care and treatment at home economized with hospitalization, which included a private room, board, nursing, and attendance by the best medical practitioners available, all for $8 to $12 a week, and without the stigma of being identified as, or having contact with, a charity patient. Other once prosperous victims of economic distress swallowed their pride and accepted hospital charity either as public ward patients or as out-patients.[61] With the return of better times, these individuals became an important new clientele of users who were able to pay not only for medical treatment but for recuperative care that reflected their standard of living, and were willing to pay because they were no longer terrified by the prospect of hospitalization, which from experience they now knew would do them no harm. This development seemed so "remarkable" to the Board of the Toronto General Hospital that it became the highlight of the hospital's 1905 Annual Report.

Up to within a comparatively recent period ... popular sentiment ... toward the hospital was one of timidity, rather than of confidence. It naturally followed that the demand for hospital accommodation was, comparatively speaking, limited and that the equipment and organization were relatively simple. Today all this is changed ... popular attitude toward the hospital has undergone a great transformation. In contrast with former times hospital aid is now sought for by rich and poor alike, not only for the graver, but for many of the minor ailments.[62]

Other hospitals replicated the Toronto General's experience. The limited supply of private rooms in Montreal's Royal Victoria Hospital was so much in demand by the 1890s that they had to be rationed among the attending medical staff and admission prioritized by medical urgency.[63] More generally, between 1885 and 1901 demand for hospitalization in Quebec led to a rapid expansion of hospital facilities – a 22 per cent increase in the number of institutions; by 1914 their wards were shared equally by medical indigents and the new class of paying patients.[64] In London, Ontario, when demand for private accommodation outstripped the Victoria Hospital's limited capacity in 1897, 20 per cent of the 140 beds already planned for new construction were summarily redefined as private rooms at the last minute.[65] Not surprisingly, the loss of their private patients and the associated income to hospitals angered physicians and surgeons, the majority of whom enjoyed no hospital privileges. The medical profession, general practitioners in particular, subsequently invested a great deal of emotional and political capital in establishing the principle that the removal of their patients from the home to the hospital should likewise do the physician no harm (see chapter 4).[66]

Nevertheless, as the twentieth century dawned there was compelling evidence that a new patient clientele prepared to purchase health from the hospital and hospital-based medical practitioners would lead the way to a new paradigm in the history of medicine. If, as knowledgeable observers commented, this change occurred in just fifteen years, "revolution" might be a better word than "transition" to describe the nature of this transformation. Evolution or revolution, it was tied not only to social, economic, and demographic change but, most importantly, to fundamental innovations in medical science which made hospitals safer places for the sick than home.

Several interrelated developments in medicine and health care converged in the 1890s to stimulate the re-invention of the hospital as a health-care facility for the whole population. The first of these was the advent of Listerism – *antisepsis*. In 1867 Joseph Lister, a Scottish surgeon, applied Pasteur's germ theory to the practice of surgery by experimenting with carbolic acid as a disinfectant for wounds and in the operating room. Lister's reports on the efficacy of his methods in reducing surgical deaths generated two decades of heated debate about the relative merits of antisepsis and general cleanliness as the best safeguards against hospital gangrene, pyaemia, septicaemia, and erysipelas, then the most common and deadly of hospital-induced infections. In the end, the new laboratory science of bacteriology confirmed the germ theory and its "preventive lessons" that initiated, after 1900, the era of "hygienic enlightenment" in everyday life.[67] Clinical experience ultimately produced the same result in the operating room and then throughout the hospital. *Asepsis* – a contagion-free environment – became the standard in hospitals in Europe and North America by the turn of the century.

Together, antisepsis and asepsis dramatically reduced surgical and general hospital mortality rates, rendering hospitals safer than home for surgery, and enabling previously fatal surgical intervention in acute illnesses, especially of the abdomen.[68] The Canadian proponents of antisepsis, led by Thomas Roddick of the Montreal General Hospital, had successfully proselytized their professional colleagues by 1890.[69] As one article in the *Canada Lancet* explained in 1884, it was not actually necessary to subscribe to the germ theory of putrefaction in order to practise antiseptic surgery. It was only necessary to appreciate the results that antisepsis and asepsis produced, wards in which "foul, purulent wounds are entirely out of date" and hospital infections "unheard-of."[70] One result of the physician's new "ability to cope with infective diseases" was that any general practitioner with access to an aseptic environment – a hospital – could "perform successfully many operations which at one time would only be attempted by surgeons of special skill and experience."[71]

A second development essential to the ascent of the modern general hospital was the introduction, by the end of the nineteenth century, of a skilled workforce of medical assistants – professional nurses, and more importantly their sisters-in-training, the student nurses of Canada's newly founded schools of nursing. The reforms promulgated in Britain after 1860 by Florence Nightingale and others to improve nurses' training, nursing standards, and hospital cleanliness eventually migrated to North America. St Catharines General and Marine Hospital established the first Canadian school of nursing, the Mack School, in 1874. A decade later there were still only three nursing schools in Ontario; but W.T. O'Reilly, the inspector of hospitals, was sufficiently impressed by their graduates' practical knowledge and standards of care that he urged hospitals throughout the province to initiate training schools in order to meet the inevitable demand for professional nurses on the part of hospitals, doctors, and private families.[72] Unlike their predecessors, poorly trained, uneducated, socially marginal nurses and orderlies whose "homely" care of the sick was, in retrospect, to be deprecated as a "painful experience" for doctor and patient alike,[73] a "well brought up class of Canadian women," observed the novelist Sara Jeanette Duncan in 1886, had begun to improve both the dignity and the rewards of nursing through professional training and achievement.[74]

The medical profession greeted this development with mixed feelings. On one hand, medical assistants with a rudimentary background in the basic sciences, anatomy, physiology, *materia medica*, hygiene, and toxicology, and with a practical grounding, from bedside experience, in patient care, might dramatically enhance the physician's effectiveness. Medical journals reported compelling evidence that professional nursing reduced patient mortality rates.[75] On the other, the "magnitude of the [doctors'] sacrifice" in allowing "the erection of nursing into a speciality" with its own "ornate system" of patient care seemed to amount to a "surrender [of] power ... which might be applied obstructively" to the physician's detriment.[76] The tangible threat posed by women as medical professionals was not limited to nurses. One Ontario government official warned that it was "a somewhat hazardous thing to engraft upon an imperfectly trained intellect too much technical knowledge ... There is a danger of training out the woman and the nurse, and leaving behind a mischievous woman doctor."[77] The debate over the appropriate medical role of the professional nurse, once launched, was never entirely resolved (and is still resurrected from time to time). By the end of the Victorian era, the consensus had emerged that nurses were skilled medical workers who, as subordinate handmaidens of doctors, brought not only their special training but feminine respectability and the innate nurturing instincts of women to a system of health care socially constructed along gendered lines of authority.[78]

In the end, it was not graduate nurses who were essential to the widespread distribution and efficient management of general hospitals, but pupil nurses who flocked to the often hastily conceived training schools that became the life-blood of cash-strapped hospitals trying to cope with a rapidly expanding population of both free and paying patients after 1890. The Vancouver General Hospital, newly opened in 1907, was typical. Its four graduate nurses supervised 35 students nurses who, during three years of training, were given room, board, $10 a month pocket money, and instruction in nursing science in return for twelve-hour shifts, six days a week with a patient load of at least twenty per shift. They became, in effect, the hospital's principal domestic servants with a broadly defined understanding of germ theory, aseptic procedures, patient care, medical record keeping, and deference to their superiors.[79] Even Vancouver's all-male city council thought this was an "outrageous" exploitation of "women's work" relative to the income and responsibilities of doctors. Defending the Vancouver General, the chair of the board of directors wrapped himself in the cloak of fiscal propriety: "We are tied down to the lowest [budgetary] notch," he said. "I suppose ... we have suffered in doing it."[80] The Vancouver General's reliance on this pool of cheap labour represented, however, the received wisdom of the hospital modernization movement. When the board of the Owen Sound General and Marine Hospital exhaustively investigated the merits of establishing a training school for nurses in 1900 for their fifty-bed institution, they were equally persuaded by the assurance of a dependable supply of inexpensive but dedicated and knowledgeable labour which reflected the limitations of the General and Marine's budget and the preferences of a growing clientele of demanding patients, and by the enhanced "standing and prestige" that would accrue to the hospital by the mere existence of the school.[81] Similarly, in Moncton, New Brunswick, before any plan to finance or operate the hospital proposed in 1895 was implemented, it was taken for granted that "the cheapest and best method of caring for the patients is by means of a training school for nurses."[82] By 1900, in short, the primary vehicle of efficient, cost-effective hospital care was the student nurse.

The medical efficacy of hospitalization was another matter. The age of heroic medicine – of bleeding, purging, blistering, and vomiting – had faded after 1850, gradually yielding to a new era of "scientific" medicine defined by greater diagnostic rigour, increased therapeutic utility, and the efficiency of medical specialization. In this transition, laboratory science and medical technology played critical roles. Bacteriology was a case in point. From its beginnings with the work of Pasteur and Koch in the 1860s, bacteriology had by the 1880s demonstrated the ability of laboratory science – basic science – not only to diagnose disease but, in conjunction with the emerging public health movement, to contain it. This, and similar demonstrations of the utility of "rational," disinterested, bench research spawned a new ideology of science rooted in the culture of the experimental laboratory and the dissemination of its new knowledge to an international fraternity of scientific investigators and practitioners.[83] This nascent research ideal, largely imported from Europe, especially Germany, was at once an implicit criticism of the supposedly clumsy empiricism of orthodox medical practice (based on the clinical observation of patients and the analysis of epidemiological evidence), and a direct challenge to the medical profession to consummate the marriage of applied medicine and laboratory science. The proponents of this union urged the profession in Canada and the United States to abandon medicine's traditional methods and its outdated didactic teaching for "the explanatory power ... and the prestige of technical knowledge *per se*," knowledge available not in the public wards of charity hospitals or in the overcrowded lecture halls of predominantly privately owned medical schools, but in the laboratories of the faculties of science and medicine that must eventually grace Canadian and American universities.[84]

Some historians of this movement have argued that the research ideal was "well-nigh irresistible" to medical educators in particular, and more generally to those among the medical profession who envisaged a new orthodoxy emerging from the marriage of science and medicine.[85] It would distance the practice of "scientific" medicine from both the outmoded art of the regular practitioner and from the eccentric practices of the homeopaths, naturopaths, charlatans, and quacks who cluttered the overcrowded market for medical services; it would discourage marginal students from entering the profession; and it would enhance the social prestige and cultural authority of licensed practitioners in their quest for medical hegemony.[86]

The rank and file of the Canadian medical profession nevertheless responded cautiously, sometimes virulently, to these overtures. As late as 1911 the *Canadian Medical Association Journal* was still grumbling that "made in Germany" had become the stamp "of excellence ... in practice" in Canada, whereas the country's best interests lay in "build[ing] up a Canadian medicine" characterized by the general abilities, at the bedside, of observant diagnosticians who, to be effective, need not rely on the "newer scientific attributes" of medical practice.[87] By 1911, however, this was tantamount to whistling past the graveyard of Victorian medicine, if only because the cachet of "scientific" medicine had already become firmly entrenched as the profession's visible hallmark of diagnostic and therapeutic optimism, if not superiority.[88] It was manifested, among other ways, by the proliferation of hospital laboratories. Some of these labs were primitive, but others, like the Hygienic Institute built in London, Ontario, in 1911, were state-of-the-art facilities to provide doctors and hospitals with the full range of laboratory diagnostic services[89] – and physicians became increasingly reliant on them. Following the appointment of Winnipeg General Hospital's first chemist in 1905, laboratory analysis of blood, urine, and tissue specimens simply became a routine occurrence for every patient admitted (see Appendix E), as physicians moved more confidently from a regime in which they had once treated patients to a regime in which they now treated diseases,[90] aided – and abetted – by the authority of basic science.

If physicians at first responded tentatively to the claims of laboratory science, they appear to have been less cautious about the promise of medical technology as the nineteenth century waned. This was perhaps, as one commentator has suggested, because technology, and its effects on patients, was susceptible to hands-on, empirical, trial-and-error experience by the individual practitioner in a way that pure research was not.[91] X-ray technology is the obvious example. By 1900 Roentgen's 1895 discovery of x-rays had led to the manufacture of a "static electrical machine" that was eventually used for the diagnosis of fractures, heart, kidney, and bladder diseases, and to treat, in conjunction with radium, various forms of skin and bone cancers. [92] This new technology quickly captured both popular and professional attention; but it took nearly two decades for its diagnostic capabilities and its dangers to be wholly appreciated. In the meantime, both private practitioners and hospitals acquired and used x-ray technology, if only as a public relations exercise that reinforced the "scientific" claims of modern medicine.[93] The Montreal General appointed its first "roentgenologist" in 1898. Two years later Toronto General Hospital installed an x-ray apparatus, as did the Winnipeg General.

Vancouver General acquired its machine in 1906 and reported a year later that it was in continuous use. Not to be outdone by their metropolitan rivals, smaller hospitals gradually purchased machines, usually at the urging of their medical staffs, or received them as gifts from progressive donors. Cornwall General installed an x-ray machine in 1908, the Owen Sound General and Marine in 1917.[94] The status of these early x-ray units as diagnostic and therapeutic tools can be inferred from the arrangements made for their operation. At the Vancouver General and the Montreal General, it was decided that the resident pharmacist/apothecary would operate the apparatus (at the Vancouver hospital, in consultation with the hospital electrician). In Owen Sound the unit was operated for four years by the local commercial photographer. Eventually, as the diagnostic potential of x-rays became better understood by the medical profession, and more importantly as the threat of laymen controlling a vital diagnostic and therapeutic process became evident, physicians purchased their own machines and learned to use them, while hospital medical staffs clamoured for physician control of institutional x-ray units.

The difficulty was that "roentgenology" or "skiagraphy" (radiology) was not yet a widely accepted field of professional education, and there were few centres where advanced training was available, none in North America before 1913.[95] Both the Vancouver General and the Owen Sound General and Marine were typical of hospitals that, after trying unsuccessfully to recruit a trained skiagrapher, sponsored a general practitioner for specialized study, who then returned as the resident radiologist, usually on a fee-sharing arrangement with the hospital.[96] To the editor of the Owen Sound *Sun Times*, the "miracle" of x-ray diagnostics and therapy was the daily revelation that "flesh and blood are subject to laws of which the race is so far completely ignorant."[97] To hospital boards the investment had a more practical attraction as a source of additional fees from patients once x-rays became commonplace. But even in the early days of radiography when fewer than 5 per cent of all Winnipeg General's patients were subjected to x-rays for any purpose, hospital surgeons confidently reported that their work was enhanced by the diagnostic capabilities of the technology. By 1915, 17 per cent of all patient visits resulted in a diagnostic x-ray; but it would take another decade for the proportion to increase to 50 per cent (see Appendix E). What is astonishing is that in 1915 twice as many Winnipeg General patients were given "electro-therapy" as received diagnostic x-rays, the equivalent of one of every three patient visits. As a result, by 1915 the X-ray Department was entirely self-supporting.[98] But the healing properties of x-rays – particularly in conjunction with radium – were no better understood than the dangers they posed to both patients and operators, a misapprehension that resulted in a sometimes reckless disregard for both, and exaggerated claims for the scope of their therapeutic utility.[99]

The claims and contributions of nursing science, laboratory science, and medical technology were all aspects of the growing complexity of medical science which at the turn of the century threatened to alter the time-tested relationship between allopathic practitioner and patient, replacing it with a battery of discrete tasks performed by experts in diagnosis, therapy, and patient care.[100] At the heart of this transformation was the advent of medical specialization, of which the appearance of radiology as a new branch by 1920 was just the most recent development. As early as the 1860s, North American physicians were attracted by the opportunities for post-graduate training in clinical specialties in Europe and the United Kingdom. By 1890 the American Medical Association had recognized ophthalmology, otology, neurology, gynaecology, dermatology, laryngology, surgery, and paediatrics as areas of specialization, and by 1914 there were 24 sub-disciplines. But the practice of specialized medicine, including clinical research, was initially restricted to large metropolitan hospitals affiliated with medical schools.[101] For example, among the 1,500 doctors licensed to practise medicine in predominantly agrarian Ontario in 1877, only one in ten had an education that exceeded basic licensing requirements, almost invariably qualifications in surgery or obstetrics (midwifery) that were acquired either at McGill (77%) or in the United Kingdom (17%).[102] Thirty years later, among the 45 per cent who had acquired additional formal qualifications, principally as Canadian-trained surgeons, there was a growing fraternity of ophthalmologists, gynaecologists, pathologists, and otolaryngologists, many with British and European post-graduate training.[103] Specialism, which claimed to produce better results than general medicine and therefore commanded higher fees,[104] alarmed general practitioners, who faced increased competition with the specialists for the wealthiest patients in an already overcrowded arena. "At any ... mansion in our large cities," one cynical observer noted in 1894, "you may see ... [the] eye doctor, the womb doctor, the skin doctor pass ... each other with a grimace or a growl."[105] A monopoly on the treatment of the well-to-do in their homes was one thing. A monopoly on the practice of hospital-based medicine was another.

As popular confidence in hospitalization dramatically increased at the end of the century, it was the specialists, as the providers of the hospitals' medical charity and as the instructors of medical students, who controlled medical practice in, and patient access to, both the public and the private wards of the hospitals, the site of the new "science" of medicine. Their hegemony was all the more alarming because specialism was not subject to objective accreditation in Canada until after 1945. Until then, "simply calling oneself a specialist was as valid a criterion as any" for limiting a practice.[106] For example, Gordon Fahrni, a former president of the Canadian Medical Association, recalled that he had tried general practice, obstetrics, gynaecology, and surgery, with a mere eight months' clinical experience before finally limiting his practice to surgery.[107] By 1900, in any event, it was already clear to Canadian general practitioners, the "camp followers of the army of science,"[108] that an alliance with the self-styled specialists to share and control hospital medical practice in their mutual interests was essential to their professional and economic survival. We will return to this issue in greater depth in chapter 4. What is of critical importance here is that the rise of medical specialism in Canada coincided with the substantial relocation of medical treatment from the patient's home and the physician's surgery to the hospital, and that this seems to have been a matter, equally, of cause and effect.

The growth of medical specialization at the Winnipeg General Hospital (Appendix D) serves to illustrate this interplay of demand and supply. In 1884 the WGH's voluntary medical staff consisted of six physicians, a surgeon, and two male midwives. By 1900 specialists in otolaryngology, pathology, and contagious diseases had been added, and the specialists outnumbered the generalists by nearly five to one. Over the next ten years, gynaecologists, orthopaedists, radiologists, and anaesthetists were recruited, followed, just before the war, by a paediatrician and two ophthalmologists. By 1914 the WGH's roster of appointed medical attendants was composed of thirty doctors – twenty-four specialists embracing eleven areas of clinical specialization. Winnipeg's explosive growth, and the presence of a proprietary medical school whose faculty held a monopoly on staff appointments at the WGH, made it attractive to a wide variety of medical practitioners, and the city's hospitals had little difficulty making highly qualified appointments. The same was true of Montreal where the MGH's roster of specialized sub-disciplines grew from 5 (ophthalmology, obstetrics/gynaecology, paediatrics, anaesthesiology, and roentgenology) in 1898 to 15 in 1920.[109] In Owen Sound, by contrast, the hospital's specialists tended to be homegrown. In 1914, the General and Marine Hospital's surgeons, otorhinolaryngologist, obstetrician, paediatrician, and internist – eight of the hospital's eleven attending physicians and surgeons – were local doctors who had completed undergraduate medical degrees at the University of Toronto, returned to general practice in their home town, and subsequently taken sabbaticals in England and Germany, with the hospital board's encouragement, to qualify as the G&M's resident specialists.[110]

However it was accomplished, the rapid expansion and diversification of hospital-centred medical specialization in both large and small general hospitals widened the range of diseases that doctors could treat, the effectiveness of their intervention, and the appeal of the hospital as the source of scientifically mitigated health. It also generated a wholesale restructuring of the hospital enterprise; a once simple dichotomy of medicine and surgery, it was rapidly reorganized around multiple services demanding expert direction and coordination to facilitate the growing complexity and sophistication – and to justify the cost – of the infrastructure now required to support hospital-based medical care. By 1914, the Winnipeg General Hospital was already organized into nine medical departments (Medicine, Surgery, Obstetrics, Gynaecology, Infectious Diseases, Eye/Ear/ Nose/Throat, Orthopaedics, Paediatrics, Out Doors/Dispensary) and four supporting departments (Electrical, Social Services, Pathology, Records). Even the records clerk's "painstaking" and "methodical" collection and collation of all the records pertaining to each patient's hospitalization and treatment (including autopsies, which the clerk was required to attend) had become an integral component of the new medical efficiency as social science, the domain of "men interested in statistics," was co-opted to investigate and track "the incidence and symptoms of disease."[111]

The convergence of these disparate, but related, developments in the hospital between 1890 and 1914 in the final analysis served principally to launch and sustain the emerging modern hospital's essential stock-in-trade, safe surgery. The *Canada Lancet* noted in 1906 that "practically no operative surgery is attempted in private houses. All such cases as require active surgical treatment had better betake themselves to a well-managed hospital."[112] The evidence from the records of individual hospitals confirms that in Canada, as in the United States, the advent of the new era of hospital-centred medicine was heralded by what has been described as an "astonishing" increase in the number of operations performed in hospitals.[113] Appendix A documents the experience between 1891 and 1930 of six Canadian hospitals whose surgical statistics generally follow the same pattern. At the turn of the century, surgical patients accounted for less than a third of admissions. On the eve of the Great War, surgical cases were approaching half of all admissions. No doubt because of the growing diversity of their medical services, in some larger hospitals like the Winnipeg General and the Toronto General patients admitted for surgery comprised a lower proportion of the annual patient population than in smaller institutions. But the rates of increase were dramatic everywhere. For example, between 1900 and 1914, annual admissions to the Winnipeg General Hospital increased 234 per cent but during the same period surgical admissions increased 327 per cent. Similarly, at the Toronto General Hospital between 1891 and 1905, while total annual admissions grew by less than 10 per cent, surgical cases grew by 155 per cent. During the first six years of the Vancouver General Hospital's existence (it opened in 1907) surgical admissions grew at twice the rate of all admissions. These rates were matched by the much smaller (and poorer) Owen Sound General and Marine Hospital at the same time. In fact, by 1910 Ontario's inspector of hospitals was convinced that small community hospitals everywhere in Ontario were outpacing their metropolitan sister institutions both in the quality of their surgical facilities and in the quantity of operations performed.[114] His observation begs the question of the nature of this epidemic of surgery.

Most of the surgery that was done in the name of medical innovation was, at least by modern standards, fairly commonplace. What was important, at the time, was that it was performed in hospitals with good results, and was relatively risk-free. We have already noted that in 1891, when just one-tenth of the Toronto General Hospital's patients had operations, only one in ten of those procedures involved invasive surgery. Twenty years later, at the Winnipeg General, the Vancouver General, and the Owen Sound General and Marine, appendectomies, herniotomies, adeno-tonsillectomies, hemorrhoidectomies, and a wide variety of gynaecological procedures filled the daily roster of hospital surgery, representing more than half of all operations performed. For example, at the Owen Sound General and Marine in 1915, one in four operations was an appendectomy, gynaecological cases one in five, herniotomies 16 per cent, and tonsillectomies 10 per cent. Generally, with the advent of safer abdominal surgery, diseases of the digestive system became the most common cause of hospitalization until they were supplanted by childbirth in the 1940s (see Appendix B). To all intents and purposes, the new model hospital was first of all the surgeon's workshop.

It was to this newly medicalized hospital, more particularly into the hands of the specialist and the surgeon, that the middle classes voluntarilty surrendered themselves in ever larger numbers after 1890 for the scientific diagnosis and mitigation of their acute diseases. Together, paying patients and scientific medicine demanded, defined – and finally erected – the capstone of this medical transformation and the popular interest that followed in its wake, a hospital edifice that was an appropriate site for the practice of medical science and for the treatment and recuperative care of the discriminating middle-class patient. The Victorian hospital, frequently situated out of sight in the least desirable areas of the city, with its spartan accommodation, vermin, rank odours, limited facilities, and almshouse – or at least boarding-house – environment, may have served the needs of the "rather tough lot of men" and the indigent incurables who used its custodial services, and the purposes of the citizens who maintained the charity.[115] It could never become a monument to "the union of science, art, business skill, and charity" that inspired "hospitals' appeal to the imagination of all classes"[116] in the first decade of the twentieth century. What was required was "a perfect hospital, perfect in general scheme, perfect in all subsidiary arrangements and conveniences and perfect in details and equipment."[117]

The introductory (1912) issue of *The Hospital World*, Canada's first journal for hospital professionals, effusively reported that the recently reconstructed Toronto General Hospital met these criteria. It simply seemed to "possess everything that is regarded as necessary": "battleship" linoleum floors, rubber-wheeled equipment, silent call bells, and a silent internal telephone system, all to muffle offending noise; scrubbable wall surfaces decorated in comforting pastels; vitreous china fixtures in terrazzo-tiled bathrooms; sterilized chilled water in every ward's drinking fountains; twelve state-of-the-art operating suites; a self-contained 1,850 horsepower electrical generating plant; a massive incinerator to dispose of all hospital waste; and private accommodations for nurses and nursing students.[118] The crowning *sine qua non*, however, was the 150-bed, $400,000, segregated private patients' "pavilion," where guests lived *en suite* in outside, humidified rooms flooded with sunlight in the daytime, indirectly lit at night, with private telephones and diet kitchens. Mahogany, old ivory, or oak panelling accented the walls. Persian area rugs covered the hardwood floors. "The impression conveyed ... is that of a large residential hotel possessing every comfort and luxury."[119] The charge for a three-room suite with balcony, including board, services of domestic staff and nurses, medicines, surgical dressings, and the use of operating rooms, was $100 per week. One hundred and twenty miles north of Toronto, Owen Sound, "a progressive town ... [in an] age of progress," reconstructed its hospital at the same time for about one tenth of the Toronto General's outlay, but the content was familiar: new operating suites; the best surgical equipment available; diet kitchens, dispensaries, and tiled bathroom and lavatory facilities on every floor; a nurses' residence; elevators; and, of course, ten new donor-funded *en suite* private rooms with fireplaces, "extravagant" furnishings, and first-class service, "everything required," said the board chair, "to safe-guard life."[120]

But whose lives? The Winnipeg General Hospital was repeatedly criticized after 1890 for compromising its enviable reputation as a provider of medical charity to the poor by succumbing to the lure of the marketplace for differentiated health care, as evidenced by the board's preference for expanding private and semi-private ward capacity at the expense of cheap or free public ward accommodation. The board's defence was that the "treatment of private patients tends to elevate the standards of a hospital, adds to its efficiency and supplies a very essential element in the training of the nurse, who is later to take care of this class of patients in their own home ... While the semi-private wards supply these advantages to a more limited extent, they place the resources of the hospital within the means of the less fortunate who ... would not care to become patients in the charity wards ... Further, if a hospital [is] supported to a considerable extent by public funds and voluntary contributions ... it is unfair to withhold [its] advantages from its supporters because they are able and willing to pay for them."[121]

The arguments that upper- and middle-class patients elevated the culture of the hospital, that their wealth should not be a barrier to hospitalization, and that preferential, segregated treatment in the hospital was socially, if not medically, essential to them, were somewhat disingenuous even in 1908. Demand for hospital-based medical care expanded exponentially among all sectors of the population after 1890. The extent to which patients ultimately were pushed into hospitals by doctors as a matter of convenience or medical judgment, were pulled into hospitals by the promise of effective scientific mediation in their illnesses, or were simply compelled to seek hospitalization because their social and economic circumstances left them no alternative, is unquantifiable. What is certain is that between 1890 and 1910, as the result of this demand, hospitals became at least two-tiered institutions shared by their rapidly expanding patient population of medical indigents seeking free treatment and by a new clientele of users prepared to build community hospitals and then pay for hospitalization appropriate to their station in life and clearly distinct, if not segregated, from the facilities normally available to indigents. Both groups of users were seeking health, not hospitality. Their presence and their expectations permanently changed the scope, the purpose, and the political economy of the general hospital. The hospitals' traditional sources of income – private donations and government grants – scarcely provided for the marginal maintenance of their charity patients. Now trustees were confronted not only with the task of underwriting the hospital's historical, and rapidly proliferating, social obligations, but of providing a costly, differentiated environment for its new middle-class users, and, as well, funding its seemingly insatiable quest for "money to keep up with the latest developments" in medical science.[122] In response, hospital boards and managers, supported by the medical profession, seized the day, seasoned their traditional altruism with a large helping of current business theory, embraced their new clientele, and blatantly remade the hospital to please the new paying consumer, whose self-interest in purchasing the advantages of good health would sustain, henceforward, the hospital's social and scientific missions.

In effect, doctors, board members, and hospital managers transformed the hospital into a fitting place for the middle class to overcome its fears of hospitalization, especially the social stigma attached to the public wards, and to reap the benefits of scientific medicine and hospital professionalism at prices that subsidized the cost of providing hospital-based scientific medicine to the entire community. They accomplished this by replicating institutionally the social structures of their communities through the hospital's tiered system of private, semi-private, and public wards with their graded standards of care, amenities conducive to convalescence, degrees of privacy, restrictions on individual behaviour, and choice of medical attendants – all determined by the simple dichotomy between paying and indigent patients, and by the level of paid hospital services the patient could afford. Differentiated, socially segregated, and expensive health care for the middle class, based on its ability and willingness to pay for it, became the engine that would drive and sustain the community hospital as the preferred site for the active scientific treatment of disease among all social classes.

Both in broad outline and in many of its essential details, the new system of hospital-based community health care was largely in place by 1910, just a decade after the first signals of a paradigm transformation had caught widespread public and professional attention. The new model hospital was a place where fear had been supplanted by hope, passive care by active treatment, diagnostic empiricism by medical technology and laboratory science, social homogeneity by social exclusiveness, and, not least of all, public charity by personal choice and responsibility for the quality of care received. Science had set the stage. Social change had defined the cast. Unrelenting popular demand, fed by the promise of the script, determined the investment required and the eventual tariff to be charged. Looking ahead from the vantage point of 1912 to the advent of the next millennium, the president of the Ontario Hospital Association saw an unlimited horizon for the hospital's new mission: "Thousands of hospitals have been erected on this continent during the last few years, and many more are in the course of erection. The end is not yet. The closing years of the century upon which we have entered will be marked by an enormous increase in the number of institutions for the care of the sick ... This will necessitate the educating of the people...into more liberal support of hospitals ... Economy and efficiency shall be our watchwords."[123] Others were less sanguine about the future implications of the events that had been set in motion, especially the promise of affordable scientific health care. "Since there is no possibility that we shall ever return to former Hospital standards, nor is it desirable that we should," warned the superintendent of the Winnipeg General in 1918, "those who are expecting the cost of operating Hospitals ... to greatly diminish ... are probably doomed to disappointment."[124]

2 A Factory for the Production of Health

As the demand for hospitalization escalated, boards of established hospitals scrambled to provide greater patient accessibility. Communities without public hospitals struggled to acquire them. In both cases the pressures were similar. Medical specialism in general, and surgery in particular, sources of the new hospitalism, required up-to-date facilities, equipment, diagnostic services, and standards of care consistent with their therapeutic mission. The middle and upper classes, whose newly discovered willingness to enter hospital when sick had launched the revolution, and whose ability to pay for care and treatment had largely financed it, demanded, as one hospital's publicity put it, "All the Comforts of Home Without the Errors of Love."[1] As the price of their on-going financial support, provincial governments continued to insist on the primacy of the hospital's historical role as a charity providing medical assistance to the sick poor, and on the demonstrable commitment of the public and of municipal governments to the hospitals' humanitarian work. Lay governors and directors, by turns overwhelmed and indefatigable in their quest to satisfy governments, the medical profession, their paying patients, their community patrons, and the recipients of their charity, adopted the catch phrases of the era of "scientific" industrial management as the rationale for their response to these often conflicting priorities. They insisted that the hospital was now primarily a business, not a charity, a factory whose product was health at a price all but the indigent could afford; that their preferred patients were, first, those who could be cured and, second, those who paid for treatment and care; that patients who could not pay should be discouraged from using a disproportionate share of the hospital's resources derived from the fees of paying patients; and that the object of managerial and medical efficiency was the enhancement of the hospital's scientific, not its social, mission. In 1910 this goal seemed achievable. Two decades later, it had begun to slip away as the continuing demand for the hospital's social and medical services, and the concomitant escalation of hospital-based medicine's production costs, threatened to deprive all but the very rich and the very poor of its promise.

When Dr Helen MacMurchy,[2] Ontario's inspector of hospitals, drafted her report on provincial hospital activities in 1916, what most impressed her was the pace, the quantity, and the modernity of the hospital construction and institutional infrastructure improvements taking place everywhere in the province in spite of the constraints on financial and human resources imposed by the war in Europe. Some of the most discernible changes were more numerous and improved private wards, laboratories, steam laundries and steam heat, power plants, elevators, indirect lighting, maternity and paediatrics wards, diet kitchens, nurses' residences, refrigeration plants, sun rooms, roof gardens, silent call bells, telephone systems, incinerators, lecture rooms, sterilizers, fire-proofing, and x-ray units.[3] Had she been able to cast a broader net, or had she revised her list just a few years later, MacMurchy might have added motorized ambulances, parking lots, visitors' cafeterias, outpatient clinics and emergency wards, medical libraries, and physiotherapy units. These were the amenities that defined modernization for new and expanding hospitals alike. With them came a vastly enlarged roster of essential personnel – electricians, plumbers, stationary engineers, carpenters, cleaners, switchboard operators, lab technicians, specialized nurses, physiotherapists, dietitians, social workers, admitting clerks, records managers, and housekeepers – all of whom were the responsibility of an emerging bureaucracy of supervisors, bookkeepers, office managers, and especially hospital superintendents who administered the ballooning operating budgets of these increasingly complex institutions.

Between 1891 and 1920, for example, the Winnipeg General Hospital's annual patient population rose by 1600 per cent, but its operating budget expanded by more than 2,500 per cent, encompassing twenty-one major categories of expenditures, of which salaries were the greatest, compared with just six in 1891 when food was the principal object of expense. Hospital construction costs that had been $200 per bed in 1890 escalated to as much as $5,000 a bed by the end of the 1920s. Between 1900 and 1925 the cost of x-ray units increased a hundredfold.[4] The trend toward costs being associated with complexity rather than with simple productivity, as measured by admissions or separations, was evident early in the process. In 1905 the board of the Toronto General Hospital noted, in defence of its soaring budget demands, that if hospitals only had to contend with "the routine care of the sick" they would be very economical to operate; but their new responsibility to "add to the general stock of medical knowledge" through the active treatment of acutely ill patients explained why hospital-based health care was destined to be complex and costly.[5] Hindsight confirmed the prediction. Looking back in 1928 over three decades of hospital development, the editor of *The Canadian Hospital* marvelled at the billion-dollar-a-year "truly giant [North American] industry [that had] grown completely beyond old methods and old viewpoints ," beyond even public understanding of, and appreciation for, what the hospital had become. Regrettably, he noted, popular sentiment now seemed out of "harmony" with hospital practices.[6] Yet it was precisely in the name of social "harmony" that the largely voluntary boards of new and established hospitals responded as they did to the conflicting interests that contended for primacy in the emerging institution for the scientific treatment and prevention of disease.

The government of Manitoba noted with satisfaction in 1903 that the boards of the province's public hospitals were "composed of the best and most capable and responsible persons in the community." [7] The comment might have applied to most community hospitals, large and small, as Harrisons and Lemons in Owen Sound, Flavelles in Toronto, Pratts in Hamilton, Motts and Persses in Winnipeg, Purdys and Sumners in Moncton, and their counterparts throughout Canada provided board leadership and the influence necessary to encourage the participation – and the charity – of their peers. "Responsible persons" meant, of course, men, especially businessmen. Women generally were excluded from being directors and trustees in the age of maternal feminism. Their public activities were deemed to be most appropriate when their community involvement reflected woman's domestic and maternal disposition for the material and moral nurturing of her family. Women's/Ladies Hospital Auxiliaries/Societies/Aids, in which the wives and daughters of trustees played prominent roles, became the less-than-equal partners of male boards with particular responsibilities for hospital housekeeping matters and *matériel*, raising funds for linen, crockery, ward furnishings, and, during major capital campaigns, for funding the construction of private wards, especially for maternity and paediatrics patients. Occasionally, determined women cast off this role. Promoting public and official support for the proposed Moncton hospital, and organizing its funding, was largely the work of a few forceful women.[8] Unhappy with the condition of the Owen Sound General and Marine Hospital and with the evident inability of its all-male Board to implement financial and construction plans for modernization, the Ladies' Hospital Aid in 1909 withdrew its essential support from the hospital until three seats were reserved for its members.[9] The ensuing capital campaign was an unqualified success. The Ontario Hospital Association had forty-five affiliated Hospital Aids in 1930 and calculated that, since its founding twenty-five years earlier, its ten oldest auxiliaries had raised about $1.5 million.[10] In the meantime, female hospital voluntarism had also changed; volunteers acquired greater direct responsibility for patient welfare through their closer affiliation with emerging hospital social service departments. For example, by 1920 the Women's Hospital Society of the Winnipeg General Hospital was effectively funding and managing the hospital's Convalescent Home.[11] At the Toronto General Hospital in the 1920s, volunteer committees made layettes for newborns, sold patients' occupational therapy handiwork, provided advice to new mothers, transported patients, supplied free hospital-leaving clothing for indigents, and operated a special meal service for diabetics.[12]

The male trustees' principal function was straightforward enough. Voluntary public general hospitals were incorporated under provincial legislation as charitable trusts authorized to conduct business and to receive government capital and operating grants. They functioned under the direction of boards of trustees elected by and responsible to the trust's membership, which consisted of life and annual members who subscribed nominal fees to the support of the hospital. Membership, board membership in particular, carried with it the responsibility of meeting the hospital's annual fiscal obligations without incurring deficits, and securing the institution's debts.[13] Though paved with the volunteers' good intentions, the road to fiscal equilibrium was difficult to navigate – even hazardous – given the rate at which hospitals were built and regularly expanded to meet demand. On two separate occasions between 1900 and 1914, long before the era of board liability, the individual members of Winnipeg General Hospital's board secured the hospital's mortgaged bank debt with personal notes because the city, or the province, or Winnipeg ratepayers, failed to support the hospital's financial plans.[14] By 1930, when the hospital's assets were valued at nearly $2 million, about 25 per cent of that value, conservatively estimated, was the direct result of board fund-raising activities. This work had a dual objective:

accessibility and modernization. If accessibility had been merely a matter of supply and demand, trustees' problems might have been limited to assuring simple bed capacity. The appearance of an entirely new clientele of discriminating middle- and upper-class patients willing and able to patronize the hospital with premium fees in return for a differentiated level of care, however, radically altered the concept, and the costs, of hospital construction and service; but so did the determination of the medical profession to renew the hospital as the primary site for scientific medical practice based on "the ideals of specialization and technical competence."[15] Those who could pay for the best that hospital medical care had to offer demanded it. Those who aspired to provide the best hospital care claimed the professional's right to define and implement it. Implicitly, a board's job was to serve both and in so doing to ensure that the hospital's traditional clientele, the poor and the destitute, who were far more numerous than their more comfortable neighbours, also reaped the benefits of incremental improvement. Indeed, governments insisted on it.

Whether provincial governments traditionally had subsidized the maintenance of indigent patients, as in Ontario, or every bed, as was the case in British Columbia, government support was always conditional, and never sufficient. This was by design, not accident. In Ontario, the official viewpoint was that community ownership of hospitals was something akin to a patriotic duty, and that by making individuals philanthropically responsible for sustaining some significant portion of the hospital's work, especially its charitable obligations, "Our Hospital" would evoke the same proprietary emotions as flag and country.[16] In Manitoba, the type of hospital considered to be "most desirable in a democracy" was the "mixed" hospital in which those who could not pay and those who could contribute only modestly toward their hospitalization should benefit as much as patients who could afford the full cost of "privacy ... and refinement"; hence the need for appropriately "mixed" hospital revenues – government grants, charitable subscriptions, and scaled patient fees.[17] When the government of Quebec belatedly instituted formula-based provincial hospital subsidies in 1921, its legislation made hospital boards and municipalities equal partners with the province in funding indigent hospitalization. Innovative taxes on hotel and restaurant meals, and an amusement tax (including taxes on gambling and wagering) provided the province's and the municipalities' shares; but hospital boards were left to their own devices to find the remaining third of the cost of treating indigents, on which receipt of the provincial grant depended.[18] Whatever the argument, notwithstanding their enthusiasm for the redefined community hospital, provincial governments continued to insist on the primacy of hospitals' historical mission as agents of public and private philanthropy for the provision of medical charity to the poor. Government maintenance grants, where they existed, were therefore set below the actual daily costs of caring for indigent patients (Quebec's legislation arbitrarily fixed the *per diem* rate that hospitals could charge municipalities for indigent care), and in return for accepting those grants, hospitals usually were prohibited from refusing admission to any patients regardless of their medical condition or ability to pay.

Above all, provincial governments insisted that medical indigents were a municipal, not a provincial, responsibility, and that municipalities should contribute significantly to their support. This often left hospitals to negotiate appropriate financial arrangements with the diverse rural and suburban municipalities whose citizens increasingly used urban hospitals. The Vancouver General Hospital had to negotiate with five suburban municipalities for indigent grants, while in Ontario the provincial *per diem* for indigents after 1912 was contingent on at least matching municipal grants.[19] The ineluctable arithmetic of these arrangements, in any event, was that the sick poor and those who could contribute only minimally to their own hospitalization continued to be hospitals' largest clientele [see Appendix F(3)], while the assured revenue for their maintenance and treatment was always, deliberately, less than the cost of providing it. In this way, Ontario's Inspector Bruce Smith explained in 1913, "the rich help the poor, and everyone is encouraged to contribute according to their means. The result is that the total cost is so distributed that the hospital cannot be regarded as a burden to any community."[20]

This was not to be the experience of the local businessmen who served as voluntary hospital governors, directors, and trustees, nor, ultimately, of patients. In the early stages of hospital transformation the mixed model of funding may have worked reasonably well, given community enthusiasm for hospital building. The legislature of Manitoba was told in 1903 that hospital boards were so adept at commanding "the most generous sympathy and support" that the province's hospitals "are all apparently on 'easy street'."[21] The Owen Sound General and Marine was probably typical of hospitals in smaller communities at the time. Annual "Hospital Sundays" when the collections from the town's churches were assigned to the hospital, tag days, donations of goods and services by local merchants and industries, the subscriptions of life governors, bequests from grateful patients, fund-raising activities organized by the Ladies' Auxiliary or service clubs – linen showers, concerts, teas, bake sales, balls – and the construction and furnishing of wards by companies, churches, lodges, and benevolent societies in return for the right to nominate patients for free care and treatment – all contributed, in the heady early days of community hospital boosterism, to the bottom line of deficit-free financial stability. The hospital even maintained its own vegetable garden, laying hens, and a cow to reduce the cost of food.[22]

Charitable contributions, however, soon ceased to be a significant factor in hospitals' annual budgets. Bricks and mortar, major equipment, and dedicated wards continued to attract corporate and personal gifts and became the focus of major capital campaigns as hospitals were again and again forced to expand. But in Ontario, as Appendix F(1) illustrates, patient fees by 1905 were already the principal and fastest growing source of hospital operating income, and as they grew in importance between 1905 and 1915, hospital charity rapidly dropped away as a significant source of revenue, a signal that the paying user would tolerate increased levels of either voluntary or involuntary (in the form of inflated hospital fees) contributions to the hospital, but not both. Voluntary contributions to Quebec's hospitals followed the same downward trajectory [see Appendix F(2)] in the wake of the provincial government's newly imposed taxes that supported indigent hospitalization after 1920. In any event, the investment required to sustain accessibility for all, to enhance infrastructure, and to further medical science very quickly outdistanced the historical boundaries of private social altruism and the limitations of the public purse. Someone had to pay. The patient was the obvious candidate. The challenge for boards was to persuade every patient able to pay to accept fee structures that reflected, not the actual cost of his or her hospitalization, but the income requirements necessary to sustain both the hospital's scientific and humanitarian missions, the twin sources of its "voracious and constant appetite for capital."[23]

It took twenty-five years to perfect the rationale that guided volunteer boards' more or less common response to the challenge of hospital funding. It was neatly synthesized by the secretary-treasurer of the board of the Lethbridge, Alberta, hospital in 1926: "The hospital has a very necessary service ... to sell ... and the recipient must pay .... To retain the highest ideal of hospital service, I believe ... in a separation of the professional and business departments ... the one demanding what is necessary to maintain the ideal, and the other endeavouring ... to satisfy the demand. Real co-operative business administration ... can do much to curtail expenditure and not interfere ... with service."[24]

Hospitals were no longer charities. They were now, according to their medical and lay proponents, industries. Specifically, hospitals were "factories [whose] product is health."[25] Their annual reports were their "production sheets."[26] The "business organization of a hospital [came] nearest to being perfect when it most nearly [approached] the organization of a business."[27] The task of ideal board members – "successful, enthusiastic, broad-minded citizen[s]"[28] – was to pursue industrial standards of "efficiency and economy" in order to assure the hospital's shareholders – patients, doctors, governments, donors, and communities – that each interest group received a real return for its continued investment in the hospital's mission, that no segment of society was unjustly encumbered or disadvantaged, relative to other stakeholders, by the new economics of hospital-based medical care, and, if they were, that it was the justifiable price of both fiduciary and social responsibility. If boards had a hidden agenda in all of this, it was that governments, as the guarantors of indigent hospitalization, might be persuaded by the businesslike efficiency produced by "the science of modern hospital management"[29] to reward hospitals with the full costs of indigent care, thereby tempering the hospital's fees for paying patients, warding off debt, and increasing the income available to hospitals for medical innovation.

The hospital-as-factory metaphor and the invocation of "efficiency" as the yardstick of the hospital's success reflect the widespread influence of Taylorism, the movement launched in the United States by the popularity of the ideas of Frederick Taylor. An engineer, Taylor had begun in 1895 to disseminate his theory of scientific industrial management; it was based principally on the use of time-and-motion studies to reduce the manufacturing process to a set of discrete, cost-efficient tasks and thereby enhance worker productivity and company profits. Taylor's goal was the "maximum prosperity" for employer and employee through the development of the "state of maximum efficiency" appropriate for each plant, and each task within the plant. This required that management impose "*enforced* standardization of methods, *enforced* ... working conditions, and *enforced* co-operation" among workers (the italics are Taylor's). It also required that employees change their mindset and behave as winners, not "quitters," in the interest of the mutual prosperity of workers and owners generated by increased productivity, increased profits, and higher wages. On a loftier plane, Taylor argued that the public had a right – greater even than the right of capital to a living profit and of labour to a living wage – to enjoy the lowest possible prices and a concomitant higher standard of living. It was this third party right, Taylor insisted, the people's right, that ultimately would force "efficiency" on capital and labour in the interests of maintaining social harmony and social justice.[30] Progressive reformers across North America seized on Taylor's concept of efficiency as a panacea for many of industrial society's specific ills, and as a vehicle for middle-class social control over the apparent excesses of industrial capitalism. In the larger context of social theory and organization, "efficient and good came [close] to meaning the same thing," the moral prerequisites for social harmony based, not on the ideal of equality, but on the idea of effectively (that is, scientifically and objectively) managing and controlling social relationships. "Social efficiency" promised social harmony through the enforced restraint of self-interest.[31] What better place than the community general hospital to apply the gospel of social harmony achievable through the correlated efficiencies of scientific business management and scientific medicine in the interests of effective and affordable health for all?

The analogy between the hospital and the factory as a complex unit of social and economic productivity sustained equally by scientific management and scientific medicine was more than mere rhetoric. In a recently industrialized society, it seemed appropriate to apply an industrial model to hospital organization and medical practice. It offered an effective rationale for the new objectives of health care and the infrastructures required to achieve them.[32] Even the critics of the modernizing hospital resorted to the language of the shop floor. One general practitioner complained, for example, of the "seamy side" of medical specialization – "the presumption of special knowledge without special ... experience" – that was now concentrated in the wards and laboratories of public hospitals; the physician had "degenerat[ed] into a factory piece worker," never understanding the whole patient or the whole process.[33] The goal of medical education was succinctly expressed as the process of preparing young doctors for assimilation by the "hospital machine."[34] The factory floor was now an assemblage of diverse medical, paramedical, and support personnel concentrated in a single location, organized as a co-ordinated team to deliver economically efficient, medically effective diagnostic, therapeutic, and convalescent services in a way that distinguished them from the old (and, implicitly, wasteful and now redundant) order.[35] Just as the modern factory had replaced home production, and the modern school curriculum had supplanted the family's instructional function, the hospital had superseded the home, even among the rich, as the "sick-room" of the community by virtue of the "the team-work of the ... physician, surgeon, pathologist, radiologist, nurses, dietitian, [and the] apparatus, planning, orderliness, [and] quiet" that made the new hospital a model of modern "social administration."[36]

Whether public general hospitals were capable of achieving scientific and social efficiency, effectiveness, and economy through managerial and medical diligence was another matter. Volunteer trustees were not "efficiency experts." Hospital management structures, which in Canada changed very little between 1870 and 1940, were inappropriate for achieving a high degree of business efficiency. The nature of hospital productivity, wellness, was not amenable to objective cost-benefit analysis.[37] Before the era of professional hospital administrators bearing degrees in management science, accounting, or public administration, there were essentially two models of hospital management structures, both hangovers from the Victorian charitable enterprise. The Vancouver General Hospital typified the most complex model. There, from 1906 until 1930, management of the hospital was divided among three administrators, each independently accountable to a different committee of the board and, ultimately, to the board chairman. The managing secretary was the equivalent of a modern vice-president (finance and physical plant), responsible for the hospital's accounts, records, buildings and grounds, and the employees associated with those activities. The medical superintendent oversaw all of the hospital's medical activities, medical staff (except nurses), medical facilities (operating suites, diagnostic service departments) and equipment, admissions, and hospital hygiene. All female staff (including student nurses and graduate nurses) reported to the lady superintendent, who was responsible for the kitchen, laundry, housekeeping, and nursing departments, for the nurse training school, and for the male orderlies. Of these three managers, only the lady superintendent appears to have exercised independent budget supervision without the direct approval of the board for her expenditures. The managing secretary, however, was charged with ensuring that the other two managers received, understood, and implemented board policies, directives, and decisions. Lines of authority were diffused; individual administrators negotiated their areas' financial requirements directly with the board, and they protected their administrative independence, as far as possible, from board interference.

By contrast, at the Owen Sound General and Marine Hospital, which was typical of smaller hospitals across Canada, from 1893 until 1939 the entire hospital was managed by one individual, the lady superintendent, an experienced graduate nurse. The (paid) secretary-treasurer of the board oversaw the accounts, while the chairman of the medical staff (a rotating position) dealt directly with the board on

non-monetary medical issues.[38] But the daily operations of the hospital and the work of all its employees except the medical staff were the
lady superintendent's responsibility. In both models, effective control
of the hospital's operating budget and the management decisions
related to it rested with boards and their committees of citizen
volunteers. Ontario's hospital inspectorate, while praising the "self-
sacrificing devotional zeal" of local hospital boards, advised them not
to "dictate regarding the internal management of an institution."[39]
The very nature of the enterprise, however, especially its tenuous
funding within the context of lay trusteeship of a community
resource, seemed to demand micro-management, often reactively and
belatedly in response to the most recent crisis, or opportunity, that
confronted trustees. Only in 1922, a quarter century after the creation
of a lay board, was the superintendent of the Hamilton City Hospital,
for example, permitted to manage his operating budget without daily
item-by-item spending authorization from the board chair.[40]

This concentration of decision-making in the hands of voluntary
hospital boards frequently thwarted doctors' interests in directing, if
not controlling, institutional priorities. "In what other line of life," the
editor of the *Western Canada Medical Journal* demanded in 1913, "are
outsiders [that is, non-professionals] allowed to decide vital questions" because they are "merely philanthropically interested," while
doctors, whose professional reputations defined the hospital, were
denied representation on most hospital boards?[41] The Manitoba
Commission on Public Welfare was just as adamant that there was
"no necessity for medical men having a hand in the administration of
a hospital" because partisan trustees tended toward narrowness of
vision.[42] That is to say, they were considered to be self-serving. At the
same time, boards were dependent on the good will of local medical
associations to sustain the flow of paying patients to their hospitals,
to provide philanthropic medical care to indigent patients, and to
promote the hospital's attractions to potential new practitioners. In
short, doctors were boards' only direct link to the medical marketplace, just as hospital privileges had become the key to preferment
and success among doctors.[43] As a result, even if doctors largely
failed in their bid to control hospitals directly, this mutual dependence, together with the profession's medical and scientific authority, usually sustained, for all practical purposes, a symbiotic relationship in which boards and doctors, most of whom were not hospital
employees, could find common ground in order to promote the hospitals' medical reputation. Lady superintendents and managers were
more clearly the board's servants, employed at its pleasure and
bearing the brunt of its displeasure, or the ire of the doctors, when

medical or financial efficiency was compromised. When the medical staff at the Owen Sound General and Marine Hospital complained in 1909 that "the efficiency of the work done in the hospital [was] sacrificed to cheapness" by the "inefficient" lady superintendent, for whom they professed the highest "personal regard," she lost her job – essentially for carrying out the board's instructions.[44]

It was within this organizational, philosophical, and political context that hospital boards, between 1905 and 1920, set about transforming the once-charitable enterprise into a business. The factors over which boards could exercise some control – income, costs, and accessibility – were limited and interrelated. The immediate priority was to maximize income in order to finance accessibility and modernization. The key to success was to encourage physicians to hospitalize their paying patients. Some boards moved quickly to end their bitter twenty-year debate with the medical profession over the relative merits of "closed" or "open" hospitals. Under the Victorian system of appointed voluntary medical staffs, honorary or visiting physicians and surgeons treated the poor free of charge, but in return they claimed exclusive right to treat any private, paying patient referred to the hospital.[45] With the advent of popular interest in hospitalization, especially among well-to-do patients, and amidst fierce competition for business within a burgeoning medical profession, the "closed" hospital infuriated physicians who were deprived of hospital appointments and denied hospital privileges They regarded the practice as a direct assault on their professional and financial well-being and as an unfair advantage for honorary staff in the recruitment of new paying patients. For example, in Winnipeg in 1904 there were one hundred licensed medical practitioners, of whom only seventeen were appointed as attending physicians at the General Hospital. It was claimed that "social, financial, and political ... expediency" determined who would receive these lucrative appointments,[46] which carried with them the right to admit patients to hospital and to treat exclusively all patients except those admitted to private wards. It seems less clear that patients cared as passionately about being treated by their family physicians while in hospital. Initially, one of the attractions of hospital care was the paying patient's choice of the "free" attendance of staff physicians and surgeons usually included in room charges. The *Canada Lancet* argued on behalf of the medical profession that it should be "laid down as a sound principle that a hospital should not furnish free attendance for any patient[s]" except paupers.[47] Heeding the advice, boards began to grant all licensed physicians the privilege of having their paying patients admitted to hospital and following the patient there as the attending physician, collecting fees for both office- and hospital-based services. It would take much longer for hospitals to recognize the right of every patient, paying or free, to be attended by the physician of his or her choice. Charity patients remained the responsibility of the appointed staff in large urban hospitals;[48] and in smaller community hospitals local physicians attended indigent patients on a *rota* system. Wherever it was implemented, the new dispensation was intended to ensure a steady flow of paying patients, especially private ward patients, through the hospital.

Hospital capacity, especially for private patients, was continually expanded, or adjusted, to stay abreast of demand and to enhance income. Major expansions, such as that of the Toronto General in 1912, provided the obvious opportunity for most hospitals to add significant new private patient capacity. Between phases of new construction, boards also routinely renovated to expand private wards. By removing some non-essential activity from the hospital and squeezing more beds into already crowded public wards they could increase private patient capacity and still meet their mounting obligations to indigents. Nurses' accommodations were especially vulnerable. Hamilton City Hospital, for example, moved all of its nurses into renovated working-class houses in order to convert the nurses' hospital accommodations into private wards; the additional revenues made the trade-off financially attractive. The Vancouver General Hospital, faced with the prospect of either restricting admissions of private and semi-private patients to accommodate more indigents, or greatly increasing the number of beds in existing public wards, chose the latter course. The public wards became so overcrowded and disagreeable that they were a subject of a formal public inquiry into the management of the hospital. But much was at stake. When Winnipeg General temporarily converted several private wards to public in 1912 in response to a crisis in indigent admissions, the hospital experienced a dramatic reduction in essential revenues.[49] Privacy, or some semblance of it, was what the paying public demanded. Some hospitals even opened "semi-public" wards in order to enhance the range of choices available to patients who resisted public ward accommodation but were only able to afford a modest degree of differentiated care. "This intermediate accommodation is very largely in demand," the Winnipeg General's administration reported in 1911, "and ... absolutely necessary. [W]ere [it] not available, many patients unable to afford the more expensive private room would be forced to take advantage of the public wards."[50] The hospital's medical staff angrily opposed carving "semi-public" wards out of the public wards so that "patients of moderate means" unable to afford semi-private care could still feel differentiated from indigents. To restrain fee increases that threatened to deny respectable patients access at least to semi-private beds, the staff proposed retrenchment – fewer administrators, heavier patient loads for nurses and orderlies in the public wards, and restrictions on the availability of diagnostic services for indigents.[51]

The patient demand for differentiated care that drove this privacy imperative was not necessarily what it seemed to be. Canada in the first decade of the twentieth century had a relatively small population. Sixty per cent of families enjoyed only a marginal, subsistence-level existence. Six hundred dollars was the maximum annual wage a fully employed factory hand (or an operating room head nurse) could expect, or $1,000 in the case of a highly skilled craftsman (or a medical superintendent), before the Great War. Consequently, the proportion of the population who could actually afford three weeks' private ward hospitalization at $7 a week in 1902, or $24 a week in 1915 ($21 for semi-private), plus the costs of a personal attending physician and private duty nurses, must have been very limited.[52] Why, then, did the demand for differentiated care outside the public wards continue unabated for nearly three decades?

First, the stigma of the Victorian public ward persisted, and was magnified by the actions of boards eager to accommodate more private and semi-private patients. Not only were public wards becoming increasingly overcrowded as the result of hospital admissions priorities and a burgeoning urban population, but in hospitals such as the Vancouver General they were also associated with racial discrimination, and with the segregation of chronic, unmanageable, and medically "dirty" (that is, dying and untreatable) indigents of all races. Even at the 1912 rate of a dollar a day for maintenance and treatment, most respectable citizens did not want to share public ward accommodation with these cases.[53] A second factor was the growing population of female patients. As more women were hospitalized first for gynaecological procedures and then for childbirth (women comprised 57% of all Toronto General Hospital admissions by 1925), privacy was their preference.[54] Third, physicians and surgeons undoubtedly influenced patient choices both directly and indirectly. As early as 1903 the *Canada Lancet* urged the member institutions of the newly established Ontario Hospital Association to refuse public ward admission and free medical attendance to any patient who appeared able to afford at least semi-private care and the services of a personal physician. Two years later the Toronto General Hospital implemented such a rule, removing patients' freedom of choice.[55] In the final analysis, large numbers of patients undoubtedly requested private or semi-private accommodation simply to secure what the hospitals were promising – the best care available in an environment superior to, and safer than, home. Even therapeutic powers were ascribed to the higher-priced single rooms. "[T]here is practically no type of disease or illness," advised the editor of the *Canadian Hospital*, "that cannot be treated to better advantage [in] a private room."[56] Patients simply demanded private accommodation whether they could afford it or not. Many never intended to pay, or otherwise defaulted on their hospital accounts after discharge. The price the hospital paid for posing as "the best hotel in the county" was outstanding hotel bills, an unacceptable loss of essential revenue.

In short order, "the business of the business" became rigorous control of admissions so as to avoid post-discharge debt collection from a growing population of defaulters. Screening patients before admission to determine their ability to pay private ward charges, requiring prepayment or other guarantees of financial reliability before admission, and forcefully evicting them for non-payment became commonplace. Early in the transforming process, hospitals large and small were forced to resort to the services of collection agencies to recover unpaid maintenance fees, a task made all the more difficult by the transient nature of city and town populations.[57] Forced to adopt more aggressive tactics, Hamilton City Hospital first denied former private patients with overdue accounts re-admission anywhere in the hospital until they paid up. When this policy failed, the board implemented weekly account settlement in advance for all paying patients. Private patients failing to comply were immediately transferred to the public wards.[58] Vancouver General Hospital, after experiencing account delinquencies approaching sixty per cent, refused to admit patients to private or semi-private wards unless they, too, paid weekly, in advance, on threat of removal to the public ward. Alternatively, the VGH would accept a reliable third-party guarantor for the whole account. A story that VGH's admitting clerks had searched a dead patient's pockets for his delinquent fees was apocryphal; but the complaint of a woman already prepped for a radical mastectomy who was pursued into the operating room by clerks demanding payment guarantees was not.[59] Faced with too many patients who "ask for more than they can afford," VGH was forced to screen – heartlessly in patients' opinions, and before any treatment was rendered – every patient seeking differentiated care, in order to restrict accessibility to its revenue-generating private and semi-private wards to patients who could and would pay.[60] With physicians determined to root out what they saw as abuse of the public wards by allegedly prosperous patients seeking free medical care, and boards determined to thwart the aspirations to private care of impoverished freeloaders, patients might have wondered just who the voluntary general hospital was meant to serve.

Hospital authorities had no doubts on this score. Hospital wards were intended for those patients, paying and indigent alike, who would benefit most from active medical intervention in their acute diseases. But an equitable distribution of hospitals' therapeutic benefits among all medically deserving patients could only be supported by an unequal distribution of their income requirements. Income from paying patients had to offset the cost of indigent maintenance. The combination of too many free patients hospitalized for too long and too few paying patients (or inappropriate user fees) was a recipe for financial disaster; hence hospitals' basic operating premise: every patient who could pay, should pay, according to his or her means and preferences, some of the costs, the whole cost, or more than the actual cost of hospitalization. The bed the patient occupied – free public, paying public, semi-public, semi-private, or private – determined the income that would or should be derived from individual patients to support the costs of maintaining all patients. The more indigents the hospital was obliged to admit for free care and treatment, the more income it had to derive from paying patients either through higher fees or greater numbers. There were limits to both. Consequently, malingering, incurable, chronically ill, essentially custodial, or worse, trivial, indigent cases were unwelcome. They occupied beds required by acute cases, inflated the average duration of patient stays (an important measure of efficiency), and caused fee increases that might alienate paying patients. The alternative to costly hospital expansions to accommodate the indigent and the private wards necessary to pay for them was to discourage and limit indigent hospitalization. Hospitals inevitably became preoccupied with the political economy of the public wards.

Hospital boards and medical staffs took seriously their responsibility for the sick poor, even if they sometimes lapsed into the archaic terminology of the Poor Laws to distinguish between "provident" and "improvident" recipients of medical charity.[61] What increasingly preoccupied them as they wrestled with the new medical and financial environment was the apparent gulf between the hospital's mandate as the dispenser of scientifically appropriate treatment to cases most likely to benefit from aggressive therapeutic intervention, and the out-dated custodial function that continued to characterize the work of the indigent wards. The board of the Toronto General Hospital complained in 1916, for example, that its most pressing problems were the indigent tubercular, insane, syphilitic, and chronically ill adults, and sick orphaned street children, whose collective "medico-social" care consumed too many of the hospital's limited resources.[62] Other hospitals would have added infective patients, homeless elderly persons, alcoholics, long-stay convalescent patients, and indigents admitted for diagnosis simply because they could not afford to visit a private practitioner.[63] These patients occupied much-needed acute care beds in the public wards, contributed to their over-crowding, and appeared to be one significant reason for their continuing social and medical stigma. They also negatively influenced hospitals' reputation for medical efficiency, as measured by the average duration of patient stays, annual hospital separations, and costs per patient day, indicators that hospitals relentlessly collected and cited as evidence of their efficiency. For all of these reasons, boards sought to divest themselves of responsibility for this social warehousing, but without much success.

The Commission of Inquiry into the management of the Vancouver General Hospital in 1912 heard a lengthy rehearsal of the hospital's problems arising from the care of elderly, deranged, and chronically ill patients and recommended to the government that hospitalization should be restricted to patients who could benefit from the "special medical treatment" that only a hospital could provide.[64] This was an unlikely development in any political constituency at a time when alternative care facilities for the incurable, the chronically ill, and the elderly were negligible. In the same year, the government of Ontario made the admission of any sick person for any reason an absolute prerequisite for continued hospital funding because, it explained, the "public will not support ... discrimination" on the basis of hospital-centred medical priorities.[65] Caught between political intransigence and their necessarily austere financial plans, hospital boards sought other avenues for removing indigents from hospital beds.

This dilemma was compounded by the ongoing social and public health crises arising from the swelling population of the urban, largely immigrant, working poor who were the principal victims of environmentally induced epidemic disease, and whose relationship with professional medicine was, at best, tangential. Among social reformers, improving the health of the urban poor was the highest priority. For public hospitals, the immense logistical and financial implications of underwriting the medical consequences of public health reform were daunting. It was a task tailor-made for the efficiency movement: to address the health of the urban poor through preventive medicine within the context of the more general goal of minimizing indigent hospitalization, in an effort to reduce hospitals' liability for the direct costs of indigent health care and at the same time free more hospital resources for acute care.[66] Social reformers, medical schools, and beleaguered hospital officials rediscovered the outpatient clinic, which had been common (as a dispensary) in the Victorian charitable hospital, and they redefined it. The Winnipeg General Hospital provided a model for other Canadian hospitals. Its outpatient clinic, established in 1887, had grown steadily, keeping pace with overall public usage of the hospital until 1903. Faced with the hospital's inability to meet the demand for surgical beds and private accommodation, with a severe budget crisis and unprecedented demand for free care as the result of massive European immigration into the city, the board decided to build a new outpatient department. The facility was provided with a separate medical staff, and its clientele was restricted to persons who demonstrably could not afford private consultations and did not require hospitalization for their illnesses.[67] As Appendix E indicates, the service grew by leaps and bounds thereafter. By 1914 the outpatient clinics, representing all of the hospital's medical services, including dentistry, and largely staffed by students from the Manitoba Medical College,[68] were treating twice as many patients annually as the in-patient wards. The Vancouver General Hospital, which had treated a total of 2,800 outpatients between 1904 and 1914, adopted a similar strategy and treated 2,400 outpatients in 1915 alone, the first year of operation for the new facility whose first priority was non-paying patients.[69] When combined with the resources of an aggressive social services department, hospital outreach proved to be a powerful tool of preventive medicine and health education, and an effective measure for restraining the demand for hospital admissions among the working poor.

The first Canadian university degree program in social service was implemented in 1914 at the University of Toronto,[70] but there were few professional social workers even in the 1920s. Large metropolitan hospitals nevertheless were quick to see the advantages of trained caseworkers (public health nurses when no social workers were available) assisting inner-city indigent patients to identify their legitimate medical needs in relation to hospital services and resources. At the Toronto General Hospital, medical social work focused on assessing indigent and chronically ill patients in order to reduce admissions and help "clear the wards" for acute cases. Caseworkers' responsibilities included arranging alternative sources of care until patients became self-supporting, visiting patients' homes to ensure that doctors' instructions were carried out, communicating with other social agencies interested in the patient's welfare, and educating nurses about the social problems of indigent patients.[71] The first hospital social service department to be established in Canada, the Winnipeg General's, worked extensively, with the aid of interpreters and female volunteers, among the Central European immigrant families of Winnipeg's North End, offering them "at least one friend" in the system. Through the education of wives and mothers in particular, the social workers hoped to promote the appropriate use of the hospital's resources, especially its outpatient clinics, in order to reduce unnecessary hospitalization.[72]

Small community hospitals with neither the resources nor the volume of traffic to warrant outpatient or social service departments no doubt continued to rely on the traditional charity of local physicians to treat the indigent walking wounded in their surgeries and keep malingerers out of hospital; but with no relief from the obligation to admit all sick persons, even when hospitals were taxed to capacity, administrators were sometimes forced to take extraordinary measures to cope with their responsibilities. At the height of one such crisis the board of the Owen Sound General and Marine Hospital contracted with private citizens to take convalescing indigent patients into their homes in order to free much-needed hospital beds.[73] Larger hospitals like the Vancouver General and the Winnipeg General eventually maintained separate convalescent annexes – re-inventions of the Victorian charity hospital – for these purposes. In the absence of other community-based social care facilities, long-stay elderly patients were a particular problem, in some cases prompting boards to assume legal guardianship as a way to access patients' assets for maintenance costs when there was no alternative to their hospitalization.[74] This Malthusian approach to the related problems of overcrowding and under funding attracted criticism from both governments and the public; but in the context of the "build it and they will come" environment in which they operated, boards found themselves trapped between the Scylla of sickness, irrespective of class, and the Charybdis of potential consumer resistance among paying patients to perpetual fee increases driven principally by rates of indigent hospitalization. "[We] cannot run the hospital on air, hot or cold," lamented one official. "We have to get money somehow or another."[75]

In the final analysis, the essential source of this necessary income was the paying patient. As Appendix A illustrates, among virtually all of the hospitals referenced in this study, between 1900 and 1910 patient fees and "other income" (principally voluntary donations, legacies, and interest on endowments) provided roughly two-thirds of annual hospital operating income. More significantly, from about 1910 onward, patient fees alone began their steady climb from their first plateau, about half of all operating revenues, to become the primary source of institutional funding, and in the case of many individual hospitals up to 80 per cent. Large and small institutions alike followed the same pattern. Patient fees accounted for 74 per cent of the Montreal General's income in 1925 compared to just 28 per cent two decades earlier.[76] At the Winnipeg General Hospital (see Appendix E) patient fees represented 49 per cent of operating revenues in 1910, two-thirds in 1920, and over 80 per cent in 1930. More to the point, WGH revenues from private and semi-private ward patients rose from less than 25 per cent of income in 1910 to nearly 70 per cent in 1920. At the much smaller Cornwall General Hospital, where charity patients made up 50 per cent of the annual patient population in 1900, by 1911 two-thirds of the patients admitted paid for their care, and of these, 68 per cent elected to pay for private ward service.[77] Through their fees they paid for their own care, subsidized indigent care, and sustained the increasingly complex infrastructure of services needed by all patients. Thus, while hospital operating costs per patient day increased 180 per cent in Ontario between 1910 and 1930, charges to paying patients for their maintenance grew by more than 300 per cent (see Appendix N). In short, by the outbreak of the Great War, the interdependence of hospitals, medical science, social medicine, and affluent patients was firmly entrenched in Canada. Perhaps not surprisingly, the first casualty of the new hospital economics was the voluntary medical charity of the middle class, as public hospitals routinely introduced higher and increasingly varied charges for their products in order to generate revenues.

Separate fees for discrete medical services proved to be a lucrative source of new income. Operating room charges were among the first, and were quickly followed by fees for diagnostic and therapeutic x-rays (commonly split between the hospital and the radiographer), laboratory fees, ambulance charges, and room and board charges for private duty nurses, all paid by the patient, all geared to full cost recovery by the hospital. At the Winnipeg General by 1922, these extra charges inflated revenues from paying patients by 54 per cent, and the hospital's annual income by 12 per cent.[78] More questionable was the growing practice among hospitals, especially when faced with financial distress, of sending their student nurses out to patients' homes as private duty nurses and retaining all of the fees as hospital income. The Canadian Society for Superintendents of Training Schools for Student Nurses publicly condemned the action as "absolutely wrong and blameworthy," and of no educational value to the student nurse whose unsupervised work outside the hospital carried potential legal liability. "To make the thing more glaring," the society complained, "the hospital boasts of the money its pupil nurses have earned."[79] Only slightly less galling to potential nursing recruits was the decision of some hospitals not to pay pupil nurses on the pretext that paid training attracted an "undesirable class" of applicants. "No mention is made of the savings to hospitals, which must be very great," huffed a correspondent of The *Canadian Nurse*. "There is no class of men who would submit, even for a large salary, to such long hours as the average nurse in training."[80]

The degree to which hospitals had become dependent on student nurses as an inexhaustible source of cheap labour was underscored when the Ontario government passed the *Ontario Nurse Registration Act* in 1922. A new Division of Nurse Registration assumed responsibility for the regulation, standardization, and inspection of nursing schools, enforcing rules on admissions' qualifications, curricula, hours of work, and working conditions. The effect was an immediate employment crisis in Ontario hospitals. Those who could not meet the new standards faced the loss of their student nurses; the others saw a significant reduction in student nurses' services and higher wages for registered graduate nurses to replace lost student labour, the source of much of the hospitals' economic "efficiency."[81]

The culmination of the efficiency movement among hospitals, and the very epitome of Taylorism, was the hospital standardization initiative undertaken by the American College of Surgeons (ACS) at the end of World War One.[82] Determined to make hospitals fitting venues for the teaching and practice of scientific medicine, particularly specialized medicine, the college, beginning in 1918, undertook a survey of all North American hospitals with at least one hundred beds. On the basis of the survey, the ACS developed an accreditation program that required conforming hospitals to maintain a minimum standard of medical services, professional behaviour, and organizational structure consistent with the best practices so far developed, including the lessons learned from mobilizing allied army medical services during the Great War.[83] The basic components of hospital standardization were defined as: the organization of the medical staff into services appropriate for the complexity of the hospital; at least monthly meetings of the medical staff to review formally all hospital deaths and to assign responsibility in cases of suspected medical and surgical impropriety; adherence to the highest professional ethics; the maintenance of at least minimal on-site pathological laboratories and x-ray units; round-the-clock availability of a resident anaesthetist; and the production of complete, archived, clinical records for each patient, from pre-operative diagnoses through detailed reports of each operation to the rationalization of predischarge examinations with all of the intervening paperwork.[84] Accreditation eventually affected a hospital's right to serve as a teaching hospital, recruit interns, and maintain a nursing school. In 1918 just 13 per cent of the continent's largest hospitals met this test of medical efficiency; by 1920 about 50 per cent.[85]

Prompted by Dr Malcolm MacEachern, the medical superintendent of the Vancouver General Hospital (who would soon become director of hospital activities for the American College of Physicians), the Canadian Medical Association formally endorsed hospital standardization in 1921. "Every sick person is a waste, a non-producer, a liability while being treated ," MacEachern explained. The patient's return to health, "the one hundred percent" dividend of the "factory" whose "product is health," should be attributable, he argued, solely to the medical efficiency of the hospital as defined by the objective standards of professional practice adopted and enforced by the medical profession.[86] Hospitals as disparate as the Owen Sound General and Marine and the Vancouver General embraced standardization and were successful in acquiring accreditation. Surprisingly, public awareness of the standardization program was high. The superintendent of the Royal Columbian Hospital in New Westminster was "astounded" that the ballroom of the Hotel Vancouver "was full to overflowing" for a public presentation on hospital standards by a representative of the ACS.[87] The movement received a mixed reaction, however, from general practitioners and some hospital boards. Resistance among physicians arose especially to what they regarded as the onerous record-keeping requirements of the standardization program, responsibilities they deemed better suited to residents and interns and their indigent patients than to busy independent practitioners and their private patients.[88] Notwithstanding MacEachern's claim that all of the 150 physicians and surgeons with privileges at the Vancouver General had "heartily endorsed and adopted" this rigorous new regime, the College of Surgeons warned him that his overzealous pursuit of perfection, especially in medical record-keeping, was at least partly responsible for discouraging compliance among Canadian doctors by obscuring, with relentless detail, the purpose of what was intended to be "a simple matter."[89] Nevertheless, standardization and routinization in the name of scientific objectivity and therapeutic efficiency represented, finally, the medicalization of the hospital's mission. Now, highest priority for the deployment of hospital resources would be assigned to needs associated with the practice of scientific medicine as determined by the medical profession.[90] Henceforward, the hospital's "authority" and efficiency would flow from its successes in the dispassionate engagement between science and disease. No other priorities were acceptable in a "standard hospital."

There was, however, both less – and more – to the model of the modern hospital as an efficient, standardized "recovery factory"[91] than its proponents claimed. For one thing, throughout this phase of hospital development there were enormous disparities in medical "efficiency" between large and small hospitals. Thirty years after the advent of standardization, for every major metropolitan hospital that boasted all of the accoutrements of a health sciences centre there were still five small hospitals with fewer than fifty beds and few, if any, of the hallmarks of diagnostic, therapeutic, or recuperative innovations embraced by the ideal of the "health factory."[92] The argument that the cost of standardization was negligible and could be covered by "a small daily overhead"[93] charge to patients was clearly lost on the boards of those community hospitals that could not support an in-house pathologist, radiologist, or anaesthetist and were therefore consigned to second-class status and denied accreditation.[94] In addition, much of the "science" associated with the "standard" hospital was the product of a growing hospital workforce of medical technicians and paramedical personnel who were often inadequately trained and poorly remunerated, or whose professional expertise went unrecognized in a hierarchical system of scientific authority in which only physicians were permitted to interpret the results of diagnostic tests. Most of these workers were women, commonly graduate nurses who were either expected to be factotums, especially in small hospitals, or were able to find hospital employment only by adapting their skills to non-nursing tasks as office workers, as laboratory or x-ray technicians, and frequently as anaesthetists.[95] Nor were these workers alone as faceless and professionally marginalized members of the factory/hospital's "team" of health care experts. To a greater or lesser extent, depending on doctors' familiarity with (or fear of) the "scientific" content of their work, dieticians and physiotherapists, whose qualifications did not acquire the same professional cachet even as nursing until after World War Two, were usually relegated to largely invisible supporting roles. Dietitians begged for greater recognition as contributors to the hospital's medical function, especially in preventive medicine; because of their university degrees (and, from the mid-1920s, their role in the treatment of diabetes) they were more successful than the minimally trained physiotherapists – practitioners of heat, light, and massage therapy, and "remedial gymnastics" – who began to appear in the 1920s.[96] Together with the hospital's complement of student nurses, these workers collectively constituted the health factory's medically, scientifically, and socially essential shop-floor workforce whose principal attribute was its status as *"maternage mal salarié,"* underpaid gendered labour that contributed equally to the hospital's medical and economic efficiencies.[97] When their search for professional accreditation eventually converged with wartime labour shortages, hospital labour costs sky-rocketed.[98]

Another source of the health factory's "efficiency" was the unpaid labour of medical students. The hospital standardization initiative was in large measure the medical profession's belated response to evidence of unacceptably low standards of medical education in North America that had been compiled by an American educator, Abraham Flexner, in 1910. Commissioned by the Carnegie Foundation for the Advancement of Teaching, Flexner's survey of medical schools was a scathing indictment of the training provided, in particular, by small, proprietary medical schools. He weighed their didactic instructional methods and traditional curricula against his preferred model: university-centred faculties of medicine allied with state-of-the-art modern hospitals that sustained programs of instruction rooted equally in basic laboratory science and in extensive practical experience gained in the hospital's dispensaries, wards, and clinical laboratories.[99] Flexner's conclusions were often too hasty; he determined, for example, after a mere thirty-minute tour of its facilities, that the Faculty of Medicine at Laval University's Montreal campus was firmly mired in the nineteenth century.[100] (More generally he concluded that only three of Canada's eight medical schools – McGill, University of Toronto, and Manitoba Medical College – approached excellence.)[101] In any event, after the Great War, the Council on Medical Education of the American Medical Association rewrote its curricular expectations with particular reference to the provision of hospital clerkships and internships as preferred components of undergraduate medical education. Among its other objectives, the hospital standardization movement was intended to create, for these instructional purposes, uniform minimum standards for hospitals that either were directly affiliated with faculties of medicine or accepted their interns.

In the 1920s, consequently, compulsory clerkships and internships constituting a fifth year of undergraduate medical education became more common among Canadian faculties of medicine. The University of Manitoba Faculty of Medicine instituted its compulsory internships in 1923 (and immediately earned an "A" rating from the AMA); by the end of the decade it had 50 interns a year, distributed among nine different hospitals in four provinces and the state of Minnesota.[102] The Université de Montréal implemented its internship program in 1927 in the belief that the direct observation of the sick and the diagnosis of their diseases was now an essential component of medical education; but the faculty took this step in spite of the evidence that the interns' actual experience would likely reflect, and be subordinated to, the priorities of their hospital hosts, not pedagogical objectives.[103] In some hospitals the interns rotated through all of the services. In others they were limited to the outpatient dispensary. Other hospitals turned over their public wards and outpatient departments, or substantial segments of them, to university medical faculties for their exclusive use as teaching facilities. Unsalaried (by the hospital) university medical faculty and unpaid interns shouldered the hospital's burden of indigent patient care, even as families and family physicians worried about the psychological effects on patients of being depersonalized, in the first instance, as "clinical material."[104] But Flexner's prescription was clear: this was the only way to ensure that the medical student became assimilated into the culture of the health factory.[105]

By the mid-1920s, the modern Canadian public general hospital, though still a work in progress, had been largely defined, at least in terms of its clientele, medical mission and authority, management structures, institutional culture, resource base, and financial constraints. Even the catalogue of complaints and criticisms derived from patients' close encounters with hospital-centred heath care was already well developed (see chapter 6). The re-invention of the general hospital, for better and for worse, had been accomplished essentially by community volunteers in response to popular, professional, and political pressure to create a new "public utility"[106] that would distribute the benefits of scientific medicine to all segments of society through the interaction of private philanthropy, public finance, and individual consumerism. Hospitals accepted the challenge on the assumption that demonstrable success in sustaining an institution characterized by social utility, medical indispensability, fiscal responsibility, and administrative efficiency would continue to find favour with patients, philanthropists, communities, and governments. Their on-going support would satisfy, in turn, the hospital's appetite for perpetual, and expensive, renewal driven by consumer demand and medical progress. In the process, voluntary boards had achieved some notable successes – and suffered at least one nagging failure – in their promotion of the factory whose product was health.

Appendix J brings together some data on hospital usage and capacity in Ontario. It seems clear that by the mid-1920s in Ontario, hospital boards had successfully met the challenge of patient demand. As annual admissions climbed from fewer than 15 per thousand of population in 1900 to about 60 per thousand in 1930, expansion (beds per thousand of population) and innovation – outpatient departments for example – kept pace with demand, at least in the longer term. This allowed hospitals to operate within their capacity, which, at an average annual rate of 60 per cent, represented full usage on a seasonally adjusted basis. Cataclysmic events – the Great War, the Spanish Influenza epidemic of 1919 – sorely tested hospitals' physical and medical capacities as, cyclically, did more predictable local public health emergencies such as outbreaks of typhoid, diphtheria, or scarlet fever. Moreover, notwithstanding their perennial complaint about their obligation to house long-stay incurables and its effects on their productivity, hospitals made steady progress in the successful management of their patients. More rapid patient turnover translated into a more efficient response to demand in the form of more admissions. Patient stays that had typically averaged five weeks in the Victorian charity hospital had been reduced by 40 per cent by 1905, and by 1928 averaged about two weeks. (Appendix H examines this change, as recorded in the patient registers of the Owen Sound General and Marine, in greater detail.) What is evident is that the greatest strides in patient management were made precisely in those areas of acute treatment and care that had first generated widespread popular interest and trust in the hospital as the "surgeon's workshop." Diseases of the digestive system, genito-urinary disorders, fractures, and the injuries of accident victims (now much increased due to the automobile) were most susceptible to the surgical skills around which the hospital's medical resources and services were structured. Successful intervention was reflected not only by shorter stays but also by surgical death rates that were lower than hospital mortality generally (see chapter 6).

Within this context, the general hospital, once predominantly the refuge of younger single men, now counted growing numbers of women and children among its clientele.[107] As the evidence of the changing distribution of patients among the hospital's medical services suggests (see Appendix I), by the 1920s the fastest-growing areas of hospital service were otolaryngology, gynaecology, obstetrics, and maternity. The era of routine childhood tonsillectomies had arrived, as had the paediatrician. Children, who represented about 15 per cent of Winnipeg General patients in 1902, comprised nearly 25 per cent of all WGH admissions by the mid-1920s; and by 1930 women, children, and infants together constituted two-thirds of all its admitted patients.[108] The growing presence of women was due in part to the prewar increase in surgical procedures for gynaecological disorders. By the 1920s, prenatal care and parturition were becoming important reasons for the hospitalization of women. Canada had one of the most unenviable records of infant and maternal mortality in the

Western world between 1900 and 1930. Maternal mortality averaged 5.6 per 1,000 live births in 1926; it ranged from 7.6 in Saskatchewan to 4.6 in Nova Scotia.[109] Infant mortality rates were bleaker still, 103 per 1,000 live births in English Canada, 163 in Quebec in 1920.[110] The problem of infant and child mortality was generally perceived to be the responsibility of the public health movement, particularly as it was concerned with environmental factors and the education of expectant mothers.[111] Maternal welfare, on the other hand, had passed, under professional compulsion, from midwives to licensed physicians and obstetricians for whom the hospital, not the home, had become the preferred place for medical attendance at births. At the same time, partly owing to the influence of female volunteers, and as yet another way to recruit paying patients, hospitals had begun to promote hospitalization for childbirth by constructing attractive maternity wards where mothers could escape domestic responsibility for a time. It is not clear whether women elected hospital births as a consequence of more affluent circumstances in the early 1920s, or in response to their physicians' concern for their medical well-being. What is certain is that the trend toward hospital births accelerated dramatically in Canada between 1920 and 1940. In Ontario (see Appendix G), and in British Columbia (with the second highest provincial rate of maternal mortality), the pattern was well established in the 1920s.[112] But it is also the case that, in spite of the concerns of medical specialists and their zealous attempts to identify and remedy the sources of maternal mortality, the hospitalization and medicalization of childbirth made no significant improvement in the maternal death rate until after the Second World War.[113] A leading Canadian expert concluded that physicians and obstetricians should "set aside the question of educating the public" in these matters until they had educated themselves in the shortcomings of their science.[114]

The inevitable limitations of medical science aside, between 1900 and 1920 voluntary hospital boards across Canada had been remarkably successful, for the most part, in launching and sustaining a new model of effective community health care intended to be accessible to all according to their needs and means. Across Canada, there were nearly 600 community general hospitals, one for approximately every 18,000 people, with an average daily capacity of 3–4 acute care beds per thousand of population. This was not yet a health-care *system*, even in the limited context of contemporary attempts at standardization. Cottage hospitals in frontier areas, general hospitals in small towns and cities, taxpayer-supported municipal hospitals in the west, Red Cross hospitals in the north, metropolitan teaching hospitals, and even a few specialized hospitals for women and children all represented significant variations in the quest for accessibility, for effective medical intervention, and, increasingly, for preventive medicine through outpatient clinics and social service departments. They were not created equal, and the major metropolitan hospitals set the standards that their medical satellites envied and attempted to emulate. The Winnipeg General Hospital thought that one of its most important assets was the Canadian Pacific Railway, because it funnelled paying patients from communities all along its main line – from Port Arthur in the east to Calgary in the west – into Winnipeg, in their search for treatment superior to that available in their own communities.[115] And paying patients were the key to success, everywhere, as measured by the imperative, "in these days of advanced surgical and medical science ... to keep abreast of the times [and] provide all that is best and latest in methods of treatment."[116]

It has been argued that patients were "happy to pay for the privilege" of hospitalization that produced health.[117] But there were many more Canadians who could not pay for health than there were who could. The most visible legacy of the hospital efficiency movement between 1900 and 1930 was the two- or even three-tiered structure of patient care that emerged in the name of social utility, financial necessity, and institutional priorities dictated equally by scientific and humanitarian imperatives. The hospital physically, socially, and even medically segregated the rich, the working poor, and the indigent – and determined the quality of their hospital experience – on the basis of their ability (or inability) to pay.[118] Arguably, everyone benefited according to his or her means and needs as the last vestiges of the once charitable, one-class Victorian hospital gave way to the health factory whose productive potential was underpinned by a tacit social contract between the hospital and its new middle-class patients. They would assume much of the burden of indigent care and medical progress in return for businesslike hospital financial and social accountability, medical utility, and, above all, levels of privacy and comfort for themselves that symbolized their status as consumers, not objects, of scientific medicine. By the early 1920s, however, there was growing evidence that the ability, and willingness, of these middle-class patients to pay for hospital-based health care in their communities was neither limitless nor a foregone conclusion. There were disturbing signs of open resistance, debates about alternative strategies for financing community health care, growing concerns for the plight of the medically disadvantaged, and new social and economic challenges for the public general hospital.

The general hospital that acquired its defining characteristics between 1900 and 1920 was essentially the work of volunteers determined to mediate successfully among the self-interested priorities of patients, the medical profession, governments, philanthropists, and social classes in order to create and sustain a socially useful, scientifically progressive, financially viable centre of acute health care for their communities. These volunteers combined social commitment, hard work, and an understanding of local needs and opportunities with contemporary philosophies of scientific management to promote an efficient, effective, and economical service within complex hospital medical and administrative structures, and rapidly escalating capital and operating costs. Through innovation, regulation, and direct intervention, community hospital boards managed, in good times and bad, to accommodate the consumer demand that attended the apparent promise of scientific health care for all, especially safe surgery, in an institutional setting. But this was accomplished by replicating in the hospital the familiar social structures of the community. Differentiated care, in segregated wards, at rates scaled to the patient's ability to pay separated the indigent from the patient of moderate means, and both from the rich. In this way, the unequal taxation of the hospital's patients helped to sustain a more equitable distribution of its benefits as long as public policy continued to require a philanthropic contribution from the rich to the hospitalization of the poor. But both as a social and as an economic strategy, taxation of the hospital's affluent patients to maintain its medico-social dependants had already run its course by the mid-1920s.

3 For "Patients of Moderate Means"

The hospital standardization movement in the early 1920s was the culmination of a quarter century of intense institutional development driven by the interplay of patient demand, scientific and technological innovation, professional self-interest, and social utilitarianism. Standardization was intended to signal the triumph of scientific health care – and the demise of the Victorian charitable hospital – by giving accredited hospitals an objectively verifiable stamp of approval for their organizational efficiency, professional accountability, and medical authority. What remained unresolved was the question of how to sustain, and more widely disseminate, the new standard in the face of the growing dependence of health, in terms of both accessibility and quality of care, on wealth. The vital issues were: first, how to contain the soaring costs of postwar hospital-centred community health care in order to retain the essential patronage of paying patients; second, how to define and maintain accessibility for all on the basis of legitimate need in a decade of growing fiscal insecurity and social dislocation; and, finally, how to protect hospitals' scientific mandate, defined by the momentum of therapeutic utility, from what were perceived to be the regressive effects of a resurgence of social medicine in the aftermath of World War One.

The bellwether employed by hospital authorities, the medical profession, bureaucrats, and politicians to monitor hospitals' success in dealing with these issues was the so-called "patient of moderate means," the "patient of average income ... who under ordinary conditions meets the full family and community responsibility, but finds

hospital treatment a heavy financial burden ... and is too independent to accept charity."[1] The continued patronage of these users paying for acute care for themselves and their families was a sign of
institutional health, whereas a decline in their numbers, absolutely
or as a proportion of all admissions, spelled impending trouble. By
definition, hospitals no longer affordable to the patient of moderate
means, whose fees represented the difference between annual
reports being written in black or red ink, would revert to the status
of warehouses for the indigent. Thus, amid growing concerns for the
medical welfare of the "average" patient in the 1920s, hospital
authorities and governments began to canvass alternate schemes for
funding public hospitals. The wholesale disappearance of paying
patients from hospitals in the 1930s, threatening the return to the
Victorian charitable hospital, raised political and social alarms that
led to a national reappraisal of health care. In the 1940s, when the
"average" patient reappeared in force with the help of voluntary
health insurance, the inability of general hospitals to cope with the
renewed demand after a decade of retrenchment, and the widening
gulf between the health-care expectations of insured and uninsured
families in a new paradigm of therapeutic innovation, hastened the
advent of state medicine.

Public hospitals emerged from the Great War with a distinguished
record of service to the civilian population and to the troops at the
front. Hospitals were the source of the medical personnel whose surgical and nursing skills stanched the wounds of the allied armies. In
Manitoba, for example, a third of the medical profession and half of
the registered medical students volunteered for active duty.[2] Across
Canada hospitals coped with reduced staffs and the higher costs
associated with wartime price controls and shortages, especially of
food and fuel. At the Winnipeg General, in 1917 alone the hospital's
costs per patient day increased 42 per cent, and between 1914 and
1917 *per diem* patient maintenance costs at the Owen Sound General
and Marine shot up 53 per cent. Meanwhile, charitable donations had
dropped off sharply as contributors redirected their support to war-
related charities.[3] There was no concomitant let-up in patient care,
however, as local hospitals provided medical services to recruits
training at nearby military encampments and to returned soldiers
requiring rehabilitation. The Vancouver General Hospital, for example, raised by public subscription three-fifths of the costs of a military
annex that opened in 1917, and cared for 10,000 servicemen in just
two years.[4] When war was followed immediately by a major public
health crisis, the Spanish Influenza epidemic of 1918–19, hospitals

again stepped into the breach, clearing their wards to accommodate the most serious cases of the new plague. In Owen Sound, where high school teachers were recruited to care for the sick, 20 per cent of the population was afflicted with the "flu" and one percent of its victims, mostly young adults, died.[5] By 1919, after five years of belt-tightening to cope with the special circumstances created by the war, and with hospitals' medical reputation further enhanced by their recent extraordinary service, hospital authorities welcomed the return to normality, anticipating a much-needed peace dividend – relief from the inflationary pressures attributable to wartime exigencies, and the resumption of unrestrained medical consumerism by paying patients.

The dividend failed to materialize. Between 1914 and 1930 the Canadian Cost of Living Index increased 50 per cent, as did the Consumer Price Index. But the index of Canadian hospital public ward charges doubled, as hospital operating costs spiralled upward.[6] More specific evidence of the rapid inflation of hospital costs in general, and the cost to patients in particular, can be gleaned from the historical statistics for Ontario general hospitals (see Appendix N).[7] In Ontario between 1915 and 1930, the index of hospital costs per patient day rose 135 per cent, and was matched by increases in hospital income per patient day. But whereas the index of daily charges to paying patients had lagged behind hospital costs and income before 1914, thereafter the increase in daily patient charges exceeded increases in the other indices by a wide margin. Between 1915 and 1930 the index of daily patient charges rose 225 per cent. Half of this inflation was the result of wartime conditions and the rest was due to rising rates through the 1920s. In short, hospital costs continued to rise, and the balance between costs and income was sustained by the ever more burdensome fees of paying patients.

What most alarmed hospital authorities was a significant postwar resurgence in the number of patients claiming indigent admission to general hospitals and a coincidental decline in the proportion of patients paying the full rate of hospitalization. Between 1920 and 1926 the percentage of patient-stay days subsidized by the government of Ontario grew from 45 per cent to 57 per cent annually, the highest rate of indigent hospitalization since 1915.[8] Other constituencies reported similar problems. The Winnipeg General Hospital's managers complained throughout the 1920s about its expanding population of the chronically ill, incurable, and indigent who, they argued, needlessly occupied acute-care beds at great cost to the hospital in terms of both money and labour.[9] At the Vancouver General Hospital, surgical waiting lists of 150 and serious overcrowding in the public wards were chronic conditions throughout the 1920s, the result of accelerated postwar urban population growth, and also of larger numbers of unemployed transients and long-stay patients with no other source of medical or convalescent care.[10] In Quebec throughout the 1920s, two-thirds of all hospital patients required some form of subsidization, as the socioeconomic victims of the war, postwar epidemics of influenza and venereal disease, demobilization and unemployment, old age, and rural depopulation sought the charity of the hospitals [see Appendix F(3)].[11] These institutional events were symptoms of more generalized social and demographic phenomena occurring in Canadian society.

The Great War was almost immediately followed by an economic depression that lasted until 1925. It created a massive national employment crisis, exacerbated by 600,000 demobilized soldiers re-entering the workforce, with unemployment rates frequently in excess of 10 per cent. Transience became a way of life for the unemployed. Federal, provincial, and municipal authorities scrambled to assign responsibility for temporary unemployment and poor relief, which was usually limited to married men with families. This crisis was intensified by rural depopulation, as farm mechanization and the lure of urban life hastened the drift to the cities of families and individuals which had begun before the Great War.[12] To this social dislocation there was added, in the 1920s, a new element in Canada's historical demographic patterns. Before the war, about 4.5 per cent of the population had reached the age of 65. Throughout the 1920s, 1930s, and 1940s the proportion of elderly persons among the Canadian population increased by about one per cent per decade.[13] With the decline of traditional family support systems for the elderly, the widespread social and economic distress of the early 1920s, and the absence of adequate alternative public or private geriatric and chronic-care facilities, the looming problem of long-term care of the aged poor was first experienced by the public general hospitals, adding to their concerns about the visible growth and persistence of medical indigence.

Whatever the cause, hospital authorities insisted that they could no longer cope either financially or logistically with the burden of underfunded indigent care, which forced them again and again to raise their charges to paying patients in order to support ever larger numbers of the sick, often elderly, poor. The editor of the *Canadian Medical Association Journal* summarized the concern of doctors and hospital officials:

All who are interested in hospital work realize that at the present the financial problem is a serious one and that a vigorous ... campaign is essential to save the situation. The time is past when support for the care of the sick poor can be obtained through funds raised from private philanthropy. Not only are modern hospitals expensive beyond anything formerly conceived of ... but the high cost of living and [the recently introduced] income tax absorb much of the money formerly available for charitable purposes. On the other hand, the increase of poverty and unemployment and the influx of a new ... immigrant population ... create a greatly increased number of indigent sick demanding care.[14]

Moreover, hospitals insisted, many of these new medical indigents had once been paying patients. Now, if not forced out of the hospital entirely, "haunted by the spectre of 'the cost,'"[15] they had been driven into the free wards, thereby closing the circle of medical pauperization.[16] What was required was a political solution to the problem of indigent care. The hospitals' preference was full government subsidization of the cost of indigent treatment and care in order to keep hospitalization affordable for the average paying patient. Thus, in the spring of 1921 the British Columbia Hospital Association formally petitioned its provincial government to institute a provincial hospital tax on incomes that would sustain the full cost of hospitals' social and medical responsibilities.[17] In the wake of the crisis, the Ontario Hospital Association estimated that 27 per cent of its member hospitals' annual revenues from paying patients was being used to support the care of indigents, incurables, and the chronically ill,[18] the source of their rapidly accumulating operating losses and escalating patient fees. Not persuaded by hospitals' accounting principles, the Ontario government made its own calculations and concluded that the actual shortfall in the hospitals' annual operating income by 1928 was a mere 4.5 per cent ($397,000) on total annual operating revenues of nearly $8.9 million, 72 per cent of which represented patient fees. Eliminating this arguably modest underfunding would require either a 15 per cent increase in annual provincial and municipal grants, which the government opposed, or a further 6 per cent increase in patient fees, to which hospitals objected. The government chose to believe, however, that by virtue of their non-operating income, Ontario hospitals in fact enjoyed a yearly surplus of 5 per cent.[19]

In Quebec, patient fees had peaked as a proportion of total hospital income in the 1920s and levelled off for the next two decades at half the contribution made by patients in Ontario [Appendix F(2)], perhaps because patients requiring some form of subsidy represented a much higher proportion of the patient population [see Appendix F(3)]. In spite of the Quebec government's new initiative to fund indigent hospitalization through amusement taxes, however, there were still perennial income shortfalls. They appear to have been made up at first from unattributed "other" income secured by hospital boards [see Appendix F(2)], especially loans, guaranteed by the Quebec government, which amounted to nearly $3 million in 1925, and rose to $12 million on the eve of the depression.[20] In time, however, Quebec's major public hospitals followed the same path as Ontario's, and by the end of World War Two their paying patients contributed nearly 70 per cent of their total income.[21] In short, hospitals everywhere had few choices. They either had to increase patient fees amid signs of an incipient revolt among consumers, who publicly denounced "exorbitant" hospital charges and privately resisted renewed attempts to reinvigorate voluntary individual hospital philanthropy as a moral and social obligation, or they had to acquire unacceptable debt loads.[22]

Doctors were no less alarmed than hospital administrators at the trend of events. Having linked their fortunes to hospital-based practices, and having experienced a significant postwar increase in their standards of living,[23] physicians feared that hospital fees would become a serious deterrent to the necessary hospitalization of their paying patients. Worse, the possibility that their paying patients would inflate the already growing population seeking free treatment in the public wards and dispensaries in order to avoid both hospital and doctors' fees was unthinkable. It was in response to these fears that the Montreal General Hospital undertook a two-year study of the social and economic circumstances of its indigent dispensary patients and reported, in 1928, that the number of outpatients abusing its charity and cheating doctors of their fees was statistically negligible.[24] The Canadian Medical Association (CMA) nevertheless chose to identify undeserving indigents as the main threat to hospitals' financial stability, and railed against the "blank cheque" by which those "who cannot, or will not, or do not pay" for hospitalization "may draw upon the resources of the community," particularly at the expense of paying patients. Government policies that taxed "the ordinary sick citizen" through exorbitant hospital fees used to support the improvident were tantamount, said the doctors, to "robb[ing] the rich to relieve the distresses of the poor." The result, hospitals "for the poor and the rich, but impossible for all between," was unacceptable to middle-class Canadians.[25] The editor of the Toronto *Globe and Mail* agreed. He could appreciate that provincial governments were "chary of further expenditures on health," but wondered why "a most desirable class of citizens ... the 'white collar' class," was being abandoned, through inadequate indigent funding, to face alone the insurmountable costs of illness at the risk of their health and of "the standard of efficiency of the whole community."[26] One possible remedy, ventured the CMA *Journal* in 1927, "might be ... some general plan of more or less compulsory personal insurance under state auspices" that Canadians paid when they were well so that doctors and hospitals could be paid when they were sick.[27] This was not official CMA policy. Neither was it an entirely new idea.

During and immediately following the Great War there was a brief flurry of public and professional interest in national health insurance schemes stimulated by the implementation of Britain's *National Insurance Act* (1911), by the incontrovertible need for massive public health reform, and by the social idealism generated by the success of Canada's national war effort.[28] Much of this debate took place in academic and professional journals; but the government of British Columbia, prompted by the province's unacceptably high maternal and infant mortality and by rapidly rising rates and costs of hospitalization, appointed a commission of inquiry in 1919 to examine the question of state health insurance. The Health Insurance Commission's report, submitted in 1921, concluded that there was both a health and a health-care crisis in postwar British Columbia that was not limited to infant and maternal welfare.[29] The healthfulness of the male population they judged by the results of military medical assessments of men who had volunteered or had been conscripted for service during the war. One-quarter of British Columbian recruits were considered medically unfit to serve in any capacity, and a similar number were unfit for combat.[30] The province and the nation, the commissioners concluded, were ignoring at their peril "the vital necessity of a healthy womanhood and manhood to the well-being of the country," in particular its "industrial development which in turn is the keystone to national achievement."[31]

The remedy, the commissioners argued, was a health insurance scheme that would ensure workers and their families access to "efficient medical services" without jeopardizing "the financial requirements of the home."[32] The commission's investigations revealed that among B.C.'s most highly-skilled workers in the forest, mining, manufacturing, and transportation industries, the vicissitudes of seasonal unemployment kept potential annual incomes of $1,500 at real levels of between $1,000–$1,200. This was barely adequate for "the present cost of food, clothing, shelter and the ... necessities of life," leaving no margin for wages lost through sickness, or for saving to pay for medical care.[33] The commissioners estimated that at least half the province's families fell into this category. Their economic circumstances, compounded by their greater propensity for illness and injury due to their poverty and the nature of their employment, forced them into medical indigence and a reliance on the good will of physicians and the mercy of hospitals where they formed the growing underclass of patients – 60 per cent of the Vancouver General's annual admissions who were unable to pay for care at any price.[34] A fortunate minority of workers' families, about 5 per cent, were protected by some form of medical insurance through friendly societies, fraternal orders, or employer-sponsored contracts with physicians and hospitals. Their experience led the commissioners to recommend a provincial scheme of compulsory health insurance for all British Columbians with annual family incomes of less than $3,000, as well as a maternity payment of $35 to every new mother whose labour had been attended by a licensed physician or qualified nurse. The commission was convinced that these measures would significantly reduce rates of infant and maternal mortality, and arrest the medical pauperization of working families. They would also cut back the volume of medical philanthropy dispensed by harried physicians, and end hospitals' need to rely on "tag days" and funding "drives" as essential sources of income in the face of political indifference to the health of working people.[35] The commissioners added, no doubt for political consumption, the dire warning that the "bolsheviks of today ... sprang from the homes of the poor, the handicapped, the sick, and the scantily educated."[36]

The British Columbia Medical Association saw much that was "academically" defensible in some future scheme of comprehensive compulsory health insurance, but did not support the B.C. Hospital Association's call for a special hospital tax on incomes. The doctors' preferred a greater public investment in hospital infrastructure to accelerate the pace of hospital standardization, particularly through the expansion of diagnostic services.[37] In short, the doctors' priority was the enhancement of the physicians' workshop through the employment of more specialists and the acquisition of more technology. With the sharp economic upturn that sustained a half decade of prosperity between 1925 and 1929, Canadian doctors lost interest in issues of health insurance and state medicine altogether.[38] For the remainder of the decade, hospitals in British Columbia, as in the rest of Canada, struggled with rising costs, recurrent deficits, a "begrudged and belittling indigent hospital service," and the "economic waste" of a re-emergent custodial function[39] at the expense of the patient of moderate means. Then the economy plunged into depression, leaving hospitals to face the continuing loss of their tourist class passengers, a vast increase in steerage, with only first class passengers to keep the great ship afloat.[40] That the poor were blamed for hijacking the modern hospital in the 1920s was an indication of how far removed the community health centre, its medical missionaries, and their administrative acolytes were from the ideals of the recently interred Victorian general hospital.[41]

The social and economic roller coaster of the 1920s was a dress rehearsal for the "dirty" 'thirties which were ushered in, in Canada, by the collapse of the international wheat market and the bottoming-out of wheat prices at $0.32 a bushel, the lowest price ever. By 1932 total farm income in Saskatchewan was just 20 per cent of what it had been in 1925 and, as the depression enveloped commerce and industry, 26 per cent of the national workforce was unemployed. With the disruption of farming, commerce, manufacturing, and employment, total government revenues declined by 47 per cent from their pre-depression peak, while the demand for unemployment relief surged. Across the country, one in five families survived on relief. For 53 of the 84 months between May 1932 and April 1939, governments at all levels in Canada provided direct relief to more than a million individuals. Relief disbursements by governments from 1931 until 1937 totalled $713 million. Half this amount came from the federal government, but before 1936 it had ruthlessly shifted the burden of relief to the provinces who, in turn, passed their responsibilities to municipalities still carrying debt loads acquired during the 'twenties. By 1933, Manitoba, having already spent $8 million on relief, was essentially bankrupt; British Columbia, with the highest unemployment rate in Canada and in the process of being stripped of one-third of its federal relief funding, was on the verge of default.[42] As dependants of provincial and municipal governments specifically with respect to their legal and moral obligations for medical relief to the sick poor, Canada's public general hospitals were quickly caught up in the political, social, and economic upheavals of the Great Depression.

For hospitals, the major consequences of the depression flowed from the social dislocation associated with massive unemployment, reduced family incomes, homelessness, the rise in demand for medical relief, and the increased incidence of diseases and illnesses attributed to the decline of personal health among impoverished Canadians – all within the context of rapidly diminishing provincial and municipal government tolerance for additional claims on their relief budgets. Unless it was absolutely necessary, people avoided hospitalization, especially for surgery. In particular, the clientele of private and semi-private ward patients shrank significantly. Hospital revenues declined as well (or at least failed to grow), but not only from reduced admissions. The hospital bills of "paying" patients simply became uncollectable and had to be written off as bad debts.

Meanwhile, the volume of free service provided in outpatient departments rose dramatically. So did the demand for free and partially subsidized public-ward inpatient accommodation that was accompanied by longer hospital stays as the rigours of the "shabby and humiliating ... half life ... accepted as the only real alternative to starvation"[43] began to take their toll on Canadians of all ages, but especially the elderly. Helpless to augment income, specifically through higher patient fees, faced with a rapid resurgence of indigent admissions, and lacking additional government support (in some cases, through municipal inability to pay for medical relief), hospitals slashed expenditures where possible, and accumulated deficits. Some closed their doors permanently. In Saskatchewan, by the time the depression had run its course, thirty-three local hospitals had been forced to shut down.[44] For the rest, a decade of retrenchment left them incapable of responding appropriately to the next crisis that awaited them after 1939.

The impact of the depression on Manitoba's hospitals was immediate (see Appendix L). In the first year, the cost of indigent hospitalization increased more than sixfold at least partly as the result of the growing phenomenon of homelessness. Transients accounted for 3 per cent of all indigent patients in 1930, prompting the government to amend the *Hospital Aid Act* to make municipality of residence the test of responsibility for the costs of indigent hospitalization. By 1933 that burden, borne principally by municipalities and hospitals, exceeded $1.5 million annually. To offset some of the effects of this legislation, the government also reduced municipal per diem liability by 15 per cent (and the provincial grant by 20 per cent), and authorized local medical health officers to control indigent admissions through hospitalization warrants, or to remove from hospitals indigents no longer requiring acute care or treatment. But there was no respite in view. Although total admissions declined between 1929 and 1934, as did the annual total number of patient-days accumulated by provincial hospitals, by 1934 public ward patients – almost all of whom represented some charge against the public purse – accounted for 84 per cent of all admissions and 88 per cent of patient-stay days. In 1936, private and semi-private ward patients comprised just 16 per cent of all admissions, an intolerable loss of operating income. In fact, between 1929 and 1935, total hospital operating income in Manitoba was reduced by 15 per cent, a loss only partially mitigated by hospitals' ability to reduce expenditures, in the same period, by about 6 per cent.[45] Winnipeg hospitals were especially hard hit by the economics of medical relief.

A survey of its patients conducted by Winnipeg General Hospital in 1931 revealed that 60 per cent of its employable inpatients, and 81 per cent of its outpatients, were unemployed. This undoubtedly explains why, between 1929 and 1934, annual inpatient admissions fell by 12 per cent, as did the number of operations performed annually, while outpatient visits increased by nearly 85 per cent. There was a corresponding increase in the number of patients seeking free inpatient services, particularly chronically ill and incurable patients requiring custodial care. Notwithstanding the hospital's attempted economies, which included abolishing student nurses' allowances and shutting down the outpatient department for six months in 1933, the hospital's accumulated deficit by 1935 had reached $174,000, 26 per cent of its annual operating budget. A major source of the problem was the loss of private patients' fees, which had once comprised more than half of WGH's annual income and which, by 1935, contributed less than 30 per cent of the operating budget (see Appendix L).[46] Moreover, in the midst of this turmoil, from July until December 1933, Winnipeg doctors, through their strike action, effectively closed down the city's hospitals to all indigents receiving provincial or municipal relief until the provincial government guaranteed doctors a payment of 50 per cent of the Manitoba Medical Association's scheduled consultation fee for each indigent treated in hospital by a member physician.[47] Frustrated hospital authorities confessed that "it was utterly impossible to maintain the balance" between their legal and their humanitarian responsibilities in the face of so much distress.[48]

British Columbia hospitals fared no better (Appendix K). Hospital admissions increased, but not as rapidly as total patient-stay days. Public wards were filled to capacity with patients unable to pay, while private and semi-private beds went begging for occupants. Revenues received from, or on behalf of, patients appeared to remain stable, but the reality of uncollectable accounts was simply buried in the footnotes of annual reports. Prohibited by law from using federal unemployment relief funds for medical relief, the province provided inadequate medical relief grants to municipalities in what even the provincial health officer characterized as a "paternalistic" fashion.[49] Finally, in 1935, the province's new Liberal government led by T.D. Patullo promised to implement for British Columbians a "little New Deal" that would include a provincial scheme of comprehensive health insurance not unlike the program recommended by the 1919 Commission of Inquiry. The legislation was passed in 1937 but was never proclaimed because of the hostile opposition of the British Columbia Medical Association, who attacked the act's failure to address the issue of full compensation for doctors for the treatment of indigents in their surgeries.[50] The only legacy of the "new deal" for hospitals was higher staff complements and wage bills resulting from minimum wage and hours of work legislation that applied to nurses, nursing students, and nurses' aides.

In New Westminster, the Royal Columbian Hospital (see Appendix K) was inundated by indigent patients, but was soon without the resources to deal with them. In 1931, 54 per cent of its billed patient charges were uncollectable; in 1932, 65 per cent. By 1933 the staff had agreed to a 10 per cent wage reduction (already poorly paid student nurses were exempt) which lasted until 1935, but to help with greater workloads the hospital was able to recruit six unemployed graduate nurses at the bargain rate of $20 a month plus room, board, and laundry.[51] The nurses hoped in this way, they said, to "gain additional experience."[52] Meanwhile, the superintendent was authorized to negotiate the price of hospital care with individual patients, thirty of whom in 1935 worked off hospital bills of $2,622 with 920 collective days of labour as painters, carpenters, electricians, plasterers, mechanics, and maids.[53] Fifteen kilometres to the west, the Vancouver General Hospital was similarly besieged from 1929 until 1937 by patients seeking free or partially subsidized care and treatment. While patient fees declined to just 25 per cent of revenues, surgical procedures were reduced by 45 per cent, and the private pavilion was half empty, public ward patients overflowed into the corridors, and outpatient consultations increased fivefold.[54] To make matters worse, after quarrelling with the VGH board for four years over physician responsibility for free medical care in the outpatient clinic, Vancouver physicians in 1933 withdrew their services for eight months from indigent outpatients supported by unemployment relief funds until the city and the hospital agreed to partial compensation for each consultation.[55] As late as 1937 this agreement still left at least 12,000 Vancouverites, mostly elderly men and women on federal old age and military pensions, and veterans' allowances, ineligible for medical relief and entirely dependent on the philanthropy of doctors and hospitals.[56]

At the onset of the depression in Ontario, hospitals had some reason to hope that they might be protected from further erosion of their financial situation. In 1930 the Ontario Royal Commission on Public Welfare submitted its much-anticipated report.[57] Using data nearly two years out of date, the commission contradicted the government's earlier analysis, documenting a pre-depression shortfall in hospital income of $1.65 million annually. The "great middle class of self-respecting people" who perceived hospitalization as a "desperate blow" financially, the commission concluded, should not be expected to pay for themselves and pay again to support indigent patients.[58] Consequently, in the commissioners' opinion, all charity patients "should be accepted completely as a public charge."[59] When discussing the report with the Ontario Hospital Association, one of the commissioners noted that the existing system made "invidious distinctions" among patients based solely on their ability to pay. He went further than his colleagues to suggest that "the State will be faced before long with the question of giving every citizen the right to minimum hospital care at state expense."[60] The immediate realities of the depression dictated otherwise. When a new *Hospitals Act* was proclaimed in Ontario a year later, its principal features were a clause prohibiting the "needless duplication" of hospital services in communities with existing facilities, and another binding municipalities to provincially determined regulations and costs for the support of indigents.[61] By 1934 the Ontario Department of Health conceded that "pay patients [could] no longer pay," municipalities found it "difficult to raise their statutory contributions in face of shrinking revenues," and "the stream of bequests and donations" had dried up, while demand for hospitals' services was "ever-increasing." "Who shall say what the next ... stage of their transition shall be?"[62]

In fact, the Ontario Department of Health monitored the "transition" very closely for the next six years and at the end of the decade published a five-volume *post mortem*.[63] Among other consequences for hospitals, by 1935 revenues had declined a further 13 per cent, only partly offset by a reduction in operating costs of about 10 per cent overall, or roughly 15 per cent per bed. At the same time, gross receipts from self-pay patients plummeted 25 per cent. In 1936 nearly 40 per cent of all the patients discharged by hospitals in Ontario's six largest cities were indigents, representing 70 per cent of all the indigents receiving care in Ontario general hospitals that year. Wholly or partially subsidized patients typically accounted for 43 per cent of the annual population of Ontario hospitals, but consumed 56 per cent of all days of care provided. In 1934, 28 per cent of the cost of that care was borne by municipalities, 11 per cent by the provincial government, and the remainder from patient revenues.[64] The recipients of this care represented a significant variation on the indigent population of the Victorian charitable hospital who had been primarily young, single men. Medical indigents in depression Ontario tended to be older men and women, disproportionately elderly and unable to receive convalescent care at home, who suffered principally from cardiovascular and respiratory diseases and diseases of the digestive tract. Indigent patients collectively accounted for 37 per cent of total days of care in 1936, but for two-thirds of total days of care and treatment for cardiovascular illnesses. Overall, indigents were found to have been hospitalized more frequently and required longer stays than younger self-pay patients because, the survey noted, a larger proportion of indigent than self-pay patients tended to be chronically ill and to exhibit a "weak psychological stimulus for recovery."[65] The authors concluded that in view of the new evidence of the impact of an aging population on hospitals – followed closely by the growing propensity for hospital births – the rates and the costs of hospitalization, driven by public demand, would inevitably increase in bad times or good.

Notwithstanding the survey's conclusion that medical indigents were principally a problem for hospitals in large cities, in both Cornwall and Kingston as late as 1937 the number of patients who received free hospitalization was the equivalent of 2 per cent of the population.[66] In Owen Sound (see Appendix M) where, by the winter of 1933–34, 17 per cent of the population was on relief, welfare recipients represented 20 per cent of all admissions to the General and Marine Hospital. The largest diagnostic category of admissions was "ill-defined," a clear indication that indigents were being hospitalized principally for social and economic reasons. Meanwhile hospital income from paying patients had declined by half over the preceding three years, while charges to local municipalities for medical relief had increased by two-thirds. Owen Sound was already spending half of its welfare budget on medical relief when the hospital, reeling from its inability to collect the accounts of self-pay patients, insisted that the city council pay the full cost of indigent care. In desperation, the local welfare board halted all indigent hospital admissions unless a warrant was specifically issued by the mayor, excluded pregnant women on relief from giving birth in the hospital, and prohibited the hospital and its doctors from ordering diagnostic tests or prescription medicines, except in emergency circumstances, for any indigent patient.[67] The threatened loss of the hospital's nurse training school, and the labour supply it represented, because there was not enough money to adequately staff the program, was a blow the General and Marine could not have survived. Yet survive it did; but with an accrued deficit equal, by 1937, to one-third of its annual income, a similar amount in uncollectable accounts, and an equipment inventory that had not been upgraded since 1929.[68] With the return of better times, the board of trustees petitioned the city council for funds to undo the damage wrought by the depression. The board president was surprised to be repudiated with the admonition that, in the public's view, the community hospital had become a "medical centre" operated for the benefit of physicians and surgeons practising medicine that only the rich or the indigent could afford. For everyone else, "sickness [was] an expensive luxury."[69]

The criticism was slightly, but not wholly, wide of the mark. In the thirty years preceding the Great Depression public general hospitals had consciously defined themselves as medical workshops specializing in the scientific treatment of acutely ill patients. The ability of a significant minority, if not the majority, of these patients to pay the full cost of medical services largely accounted for hospitals' capacity both to achieve and advance their scientific potential, and to meet the social obligations of an institution whose community base and partial public funding required that it should be accessible to all, regardless of ability to pay. The effect of the depression was to reverse the course of the hospitals' recent historical development. Inflated charges for both care and treatment, and a declining standard of living, drove self-pay patients out of the hospitals, thereby vastly increasing hospitals' social and custodial responsibilities. The income lost by the withdrawal of paying patients could not be replaced by governments, especially municipal councils tottering on the verge of fiscal default. As hospitals had been predicting for a decade, their financial house of cards and the structures of medical care that it supported fell down.

But after thirty years of exposure to hospitals' claims that they were an indispensable public utility providing essential scientific and humanitarian services to their communities, the public was unable, in the aftermath of this crisis, to reconcile hospitals' altruistic self-image with the frequently grudging response to human need on the part of hospitals and physicians alike during the depression. The League for Social Reconstruction summarized the conundrum in its 1935 publication *Social Planning for Canada*. Canada's medical personnel and facilities had been demonstrably underemployed and underutilized while "men, women and children needing [their] services" went untreated merely because "the industry that is equipped to provide them cannot *sell* its goods." The "bankruptcy of the existing system" was self-evident.[70] What was to be done?

The outbreak of war in Europe in 1939, then in the Pacific, further exacerbated the grave condition of hospitals. The enlistment of physicians, nurses, and interns in the Canadian armed forces, coupled with the availability of better-paying jobs for women in war-related industries than as student or graduate nurses, severely limited the pool of medical professionals for civilian employment.[71] As essential industries subject to the regulation of the War Time Prices and Trade Board, hospital employment practices, purchasing power, and rate structures were also restricted, increasing operating costs and reducing income[72] These developments coincided with a significant renewal of demand for hospitalization throughout the 1940s. As Appendices K–L illustrate, greater utilization – more accurately, growing inaccessibility – was a theme common to every jurisdiction throughout the 1940s. For example, in Ontario where hospital admissions stagnated during the depression and hospitals operated well below capacity, between 1941 and 1948 annual admissions rose by two-thirds. By the end of the decade, based on immediate need and anticipated near-term usage, the province had a projected shortage of 10,000 acute-care beds.[73] In Manitoba from 1941 onward, the Winnipeg General Hospital had a perpetual waiting list for admission which reached 450 in 1946. By 1951 the hospital's surgeons had estimated that they required at least four additional operating suites to cope with the backlog of essential and elective surgery.[74] Throughout the province by 1944, hospitals were accommodating 7 per cent more beds than their approved capacity; but outside Winnipeg and Brandon the majority of local hospitals did not provide the range of diagnostic services essential for the appropriate treatment of patients – hence the additional pressures on large urban hospitals.[75] In British Columbia, the superintendent of Vancouver General Hospital reported as early as 1940 that the hospital could no longer afford the luxury of allowing patients three to five days to recover from surgery before they were discharged. Now patients were "up in a chair one day and discharged the next" with "new patients ... admitted before the beds are even cool." He guessed that "some of the patients going out are about as ill as those entering."[76] Nationally, between 1932 and 1945 the number of beds in Canadian public general hospitals increased by only 35 per cent, while admissions rose by nearly 110 per cent, and then doubled in the next fifteen years.[77]

This resurgence of hospitalization had several sources. First, the depression rate of medical indigence continued, only partially abated, into the 1940s. For example, in Quebec in 1951 the costs of indigent hospitalization accounted for nearly 25 per cent of all hospital expenditures (while government subsidization met only half of these costs at a time when hospital operating costs generally had tripled since 1938).[78] Among the large numbers of people still seeking medical relief, elderly, chronically ill patients with no other sources of support and refuge were the most visible. They at least were now recognized as a social problem clearly requiring a solution other than hospitalization in the longer term.[79] Whatever their individual circumstances, even with the return of better times medical indigents, in Manitoba for example, continued to account for between a quarter and one third of all admissions, and for nearly half of all days of care.[80] A more recent circumstance was the popularity among women and their physicians for hospital births. Prior to the depression, only a third of all births in Ontario took place in a hospital. By 1941 the proportion of hospital births had risen to two-thirds, and by 1946 to 80 per cent. In 1947, 27 per cent of all patients discharged from Ontario's public general hospitals were women admitted for child-birth or complications of pregnancy.[81] As with the beginning of life, after 1940 the end of life too moved from home to hospital. Before 1930 fewer than one in five deaths in Ontario occurred in a hospital. By the mid-1940s that proportion had risen to about 40 per cent,[82] a shift that recent scholarship has attributed as much to the limited availability of women's home-based labour in the 1930s and 1940s as to the growing medicalization of society.[83] More generally, hospital morbidity patterns reflected significant changes in the reasons for, and the rates of, hospitalization associated with certain diseases. Between 1938 and 1947 hospitals in Ontario witnessed a jump not only in admissions for childbirth, but for diseases of the respiratory and circulatory systems, and more days of care attributed to cancer patients. Consequently, whereas in 1938 childbirth, accidents, cancer, and diseases of the circulatory, respiratory, digestive, and genito-urinary systems – the leading causes of admission for acute treatment – had accounted for 70 per cent of all discharges and deaths, by 1947 degenerative and lifestyle diseases represented 82 per cent of all dis-charges and deaths.[84] Wartime conditions also contributed to greater hospital use because of the higher occurrence of industrial accidents and limitations on home care due to the widespread employment of women in war-related occupations.[85] Following the war, population growth alone – immigration and the baby boom – accounted for slightly more than a third of the continuing growth in admissions.[86] Finally, the advent of private hospital and medical insurance schemes significantly increased hospital admissions, especially for the white collar class, whose threatened medical impoverishment had exer-cised doctors, hospital administrators, and newspaper editors before the depression, and whose desertion of the hospitals – or hospital bills – during the thirties seemed to account, in turn, for the hospitals' subsequent financial woes.

In 1937 a mere seven hundred Canadians participated in medical insurance plans.[87] Frustrated equally by governments' refusal to increase indigent per diems to contain the fees of self-pay patients, and by the political failure of provincially sponsored health insurance schemes (for example in Alberta and British Columbia), and deter-mined to regain the confidence of their paying clientele, provincial hospital associations agreed in the dying days of the depression to protect their own interests by creating a hospital-sponsored not-for-profit group hospital insurance plan. Using the Blue Cross model (and name) borrowed from American hospitals,[88] and underwritten by each provincial hospital association as Associated Medical Services, Blue Cross plans were made available through employers. The plans commonly provided a choice of standard or semi-private ward care, full coverage for most diagnostic services and other "extras," coverage for dependants and for childbirth, free choice of hospital and physician, and up to twenty-one days of hospital care annually. Subscribers could upgrade their accommodation by paying the differential costs. As George Stephens, the president of the Canadian Hospital Council, explained, this was "not state medicine." Rather, it was a measure aimed at the "middle third" of employed Canadians who should not have to accept medical charity at public expense but whose annual incomes did not permit them to save for medical emergencies. Blue Cross would promote their "security, independence, [and] self respect and [an] improvement in community morale."[89] Other commercial and private plans followed. Without an employer contribution to premiums, these schemes could be prohibitively expensive; but as a means of orderly budgeting for sickness in the face of the spiralling costs of hospitalization, they were swiftly embraced by middle-income Canadians, and by their employers who were willing to pay for them.[90]

Nationwide, following the implementation of the Ontario, Manitoba, and British Columbia plans in 1940–41, the participation rate grew from 35,000 to 1.5 million subscribers by 1951.[91] By 1948 one of every four patients admitted to a hospital in Ontario carried some form of hospitalization insurance. At its apogee in 1956 (on the eve of the national *Hospital Insurance and Diagnostic Services Act*) the voluntary hospital care insurance movement embraced 45 per cent of all Canadians; they were far more likely (by 50%) to seek hospitalization than uninsured groups in the population.[92] Appendix O illustrates the effect of this transition on Ontario's public general hospitals. Patients with hospital insurance were also more inclined to opt for semi-private or private ward care (their premiums entitled them to standard ward care), and they did not linger in hospital any longer than cost-conscious self-pay private and semi-private ward patients. Their impact on hospital finances was remarkable. By 1957 self-pay patients, on whom hospitals had depended for most of their income before 1930, accounted for less than 30 per cent of hospital income. Voluntary hospital insurance schemes provided nearly an equal proportion (27%), and governments contributed about 40 per cent.[93]

Moreover, since hospitals' "extra" charges for operating and delivery room usage, anaesthesia, dressings, drugs, laboratory tests, and physiotherapy and diagnostic radiological services were covered by Blue Cross – charges that could inflate patients' bills by 50 per cent and had contributed to the growing backlog of uncollectable accounts in the 1930s[94] – hospitals were doubly rewarded for their entry into the field of health insurance. Guaranteed payment, full private and semi-private wards, and rapid patient turnover had been hospitals' quest since their flirtation with Taylorism thirty years earlier.

In spite of the astonishing increases in hospital revenues and expenditures (267% between 1942 and 1951, nearly 275% between 1945 and 1954)[95] as war gave way to peacetime reconstruction, and as more Canadians acquired prepaid health insurance, it was abundantly clear that voluntary community hospitals still could not cope with the costs of doing business within the traditional system of hospital funding in the face of the new demands being made upon them. The principal sources of the mounting total national hospital expenditures – physical capacity to accommodate the volume of care required, the changing scope of hospital morbidity, and the acquisition of trained personnel, technology, and specialized facilities to sustain the quality of care that the postwar revolution in diagnostics and therapeutics made possible – were quite beyond the resources of the community hospital. In a country where the highest rates of hospital usage typically occurred in mid-sized cities and towns whose women, children, aged, and poor were the primary users of hospital services, it was simply no longer possible – or desirable – to contemplate maintaining a minimum acceptable standard of hospital-centred health care for all, based on the finite limitations of local public and private resources. In particular, the ability of perpetually increasing user fees to fund both medical science and medical need was exhausted. By 1951 Canadian families were already spending 2.5 per cent ($373.8 million) of their annual disposable personal income on health care, one quarter of it on prepaid health insurance plans, a similar proportion on direct payments to physicians, 20 per cent on drugs and medications, and about 17 per cent in direct payments to hospitals. The poorest families (with less than $1500 annual income), who comprised a third of the population, accounted, however, for less than one fifth (17.3%) of this expenditure. The most affluent quarter of the population (with incomes in excess of $2,999) was responsible for nearly 40% of it, while middle-income families' share of these expenditures was roughly proportionate to their representation among the total population (41%).[96] That there was still "an

inverse relationship between income and sickness and a direct relationship between income and volume of health care received"[97] was
incontrovertible. That the cost of redressing that relationship could
no longer be borne involuntarily by the sick alone, or cooperatively
by a single community, also seemed to many Canadians to be incontrovertible by the 1950s, when each new therapeutic advance made
by international medical science redefined not only the promise, but
the cost, of life.[98]

The situation in Manitoba, where health-care services were studied
repetitively between 1940 and 1950 by citizens' groups, external consultants, and government officials,[99] illustrates the complexity that
now characterized the problem of hospital-centred health care, and
the depth of popular and official concern. Among other issues, the
unequal distribution, both quantitatively and qualitatively, of hospital and physicians' services between rural and urban Manitobans
represented the most significant problem of accessibility. By 1942
more than 500 focus groups sponsored by the Manitoba Federation of
Agriculture (MFA) were enquiring into the need to provide rural and
small town Manitobans with the same access to quality health care
that the citizens of Winnipeg enjoyed. Although thirty communities
outside Winnipeg had hospital facilities, more than two-thirds of the
province's hospital beds were in Winnipeg, which had 40 per cent of
the population. These rural and small-town hospitals lacked professional administrators, comprehensive diagnostic facilities, pharmacies, reliable equipment, and, most important, an adequate complement of qualified medical professionals. Physicians could not be
attracted to communities with non-existent, or antiquated, hospital
facilities. These hospitals had lost their most qualified nurses during
the depression and could not compete successfully, in terms of
salaries, accommodations, and challenging work, for replacements in
the wartime labour market. Meanwhile, the loss of income during the
thirties had robbed farm families of their limited ability to pay for
hospitalization or medical care, and after the depression farm
incomes did not recover sufficiently to improve the situation. Reluctant to accept charity, farm families let illnesses go untreated to their
own detriment and that of the whole population. This, however, was
a trait that rural dwellers shared with the urban working class. In
1936 more than 80 per cent of Manitoban wage earners, urban and
rural, had annual incomes under $1,450, considerably less than the
amount a family needed to bear the cost of normal medical expenses
in a system where "the manner in which an individual obtains medical care is determined practically by his ability to pay."[100] As a result,
more than a third of Manitobans were potential medical indigents

even though about half of that group were self-supporting and "self-respecting" in every way except for medical contingencies.

The response of Manitoba hospitals to the continued growth of demand for their services combined with the declining ability of Manitobans to pay the full cost of care and treatment was to economize ruthlessly, in particular to pare costs as far as possible, in order to match income from basic indigent hospitalization rates. In this way, provincial and municipal *per diem* subsidies would largely carry hospitals' operating budgets. Indeed, it became clear that many small hospitals were conspiring with municipal governments, physicians, and individual patients to keep free beds filled in order to collect the guaranteed provincial grant while municipalities subsequently and surreptitiously recovered their contribution from the discharged patient. But it was a vicious circle. Government officials and private consultants estimated that combined municipal and provincial grant income still left hospitals with a deficit of $1.80 to $3.00 per patient day to be recovered from other sources, principally from paying patients, whose numbers had dwindled to about 50 per cent of all patients by war's end. Without adequate resources to modernize and remain attractive to medical professionals, with a declining clientele of paying patients, and with mounting debts in spite of their economies, Manitoba's small community general hospitals were in danger of regressing to a state of medical irrelevance. The advent of Associated Medical Services of Manitoba (Blue Cross), moreover, essentially benefited employed city-dwellers and urban hospitals: farmers could not afford the premiums, even if they had been eligible to subscribe. The only common theme running through all of the documentation accumulated during the decade was the conclusion that, for all of the reasons cited above, Manitoba hospitals and physicians were generous to a fault in making public ward hospitalization at public (municipal and provincial) expense available for the asking in order to accommodate the health-care needs of their fellow citizens.

This was not what Manitobans wanted. It was time, the MFA focus groups reported, to "establish the principle of collective responsibility for individual health or individual sickness" and to recognize that "there must be a limit" to individual liability and a concomitant acceptance of community responsibility for the costs of health and health care in a modern system of integrated, public, health services.[101]

By 1940, this proposition, its ramifications, and its social consequences had already been discussed off and on for thirty years, principally by hospital authorities and medical professionals. Their analyses were usually interpreted as Cassandrian hand-wringing to justify off-loading the unwelcome charitable obligations of general hospitals and doctors on the public purse in order to pursue the ideal of elitist medicine conveyed by the image of the hospital as a highly efficient medical technocracy. But as the social and economic realities of the depression were first experienced by an entire generation of Canadians and then became indelibly etched in their mindset, the human costs of an unresponsive health-care system, or, perhaps more accurately, the absence of a health-care system capable of responding to a national health crisis, began to attract the attention of social theorists, social activists, civil servants, politicians, and governments. The social-democratic League for Social Reconstruction, some of whose members had immediate, expert knowledge of the medical relief problems in Ontario and British Columbia,[102] re-emphasized the inequalities of health care, especially access to hospitalization, in its blueprint for social reform, *Social Planning for Canada*. The issue achieved greater visibility, however, when it was addressed by the *Report of the Royal Commission on Dominion-Provincial Relations*. The Rowell-Sirois Commission, which was established in 1937 and reported in 1940, accepted that "the health activities of governments are ... only beginning" and that a rapid increase in public expenditures for preventive medicine, medical research, and health insurance was inevitable. Acknowledging that constitutional jurisdiction and "regional differences ... militate[d] against an acceptable national scheme" of health insurance, the commissioners argued that through federal-provincial cooperation provinces should be encouraged and helped to create mechanisms for the universal provision of medical and hospital services without fearing the fiscal consequences.[103]

This recommendation subsequently became central to Prime Minister Mackenzie King's vision of postwar social reconstruction. More accurately, perhaps, it became one of the flags around which Ottawa's new breed of influential civil servants committed to social reform through state intervention to bring about "a marriage of the utilitarian and liberal ideals of individual happiness" could rally.[104] Their careful nurturing of this, and other, social security initiatives led in time to the creation of the House of Commons' Special Committee on Social Security and its expert advisory committees such as the Advisory Committee on Health Insurance (the Heagerty Committee) to plan for postwar reconstruction. The Special Committee's work was completed in 1944. The arguments heard by these committees in support of national health insurance were summarized in a report, *Social Security for Canada*, researched and written by Professor

Leonard Marsh, McGill University, who had become Canada's leading expert on unemployment and medical relief during the depression. Marsh argued that the general case for national health insurance
was simply basic human need for adequate medical care and the
irrefutable evidence that "most family incomes, excepting only those
at the highest levels, are insufficient to meet the costs of continuous
or serious illness."[105] He emphasized, however, the "special case" to
be made on behalf of the "average wage-earner" (i.e., the "patient of
moderate means") who, in every Canadian jurisdiction, was "'unable
to provide adequate medical care for himself and for his family' if left
to his own resources."[106] Health insurance could not be limited, consequently, to the assistance of the poor. Its benefits had to extend,
whatever the cost, "to the largest possible population," and coverage
must be comprehensive, including the services of physicians, specialists, and nurses, hospitalization, drugs, diagnostic facilities, and
convalescent care.[107] Finally, Marsh argued, premiums should be
based on income, not equity, with governments assisting or assuming
the premiums of the poor. The resultant scheme would save lives,
reduce the cost of other social services, improve efficiency, and
eliminate destitution. To that end, the Heagerty Committee actually
drafted the legislation required to implement a national scheme of
compulsory and contributory health insurance through federal-
provincial cooperation.[108]

The work of the Commons Special Committee on Social Security
and its sub-committees was watched, and abetted, by the Canadian
Medical Association (see chapter 4), by the Catholic Hospital Association, and by the Canadian Hospital Council representing provincial
hospital associations. In his oral presentation to the Special Committee on Social Security Dr Harvey Agnew, executive director of the
Council, focused his remarks on the necessity of preserving, within
any scheme of national health insurance, the historical uniqueness
and autonomy of Canada's voluntary community public general hospitals. Their work, he insisted, required coordinated planning, fair
remuneration, and standardized facilities quantitatively and qualitatively adequate for their medical mission. It did not require central-
ized management, direction, or control. In return for its support of
the proposed plan, the Council's minimum conditions were the continued right of voluntary hospital boards to determine the nature of,
and qualifications for, physicians' hospital privileges, the right of
patients to select their own physicians, the right of insured persons to
choose private or semi-private ward accommodation at premium
rates for supplementary payments, the patient's right to the privacy
of his or her clinical records, and retention of the hospitals' charitable

status and voluntary management.[109] In a detailed separate statement enumerating the terms and conditions of public hospitals' participation in a national health insurance plan, the Hospital Council went further, insisting on the right of voluntary boards to continue to make all necessary rules and regulations, as well as management decisions, for the governance of patients and the administration of their hospitals without interference from health insurance bureaucracies. Hospitals also proposed to exempt from any legislation the "extra" services that accounted for a significant proportion of their current and future revenues from patients – x-rays, electrocardiograms, radium treatments, oxygen therapy, anaesthetists' services, and certain types of physiotherapy.[110] If these conditions seemed self-serving, they were at least consistent with voluntary hospitals' historical experience. What hospitals wanted was what they had always wanted: to be relieved of the costs of treating indigents and, consequently, to relieve their preferred clientele, the middle class, of the high costs of differentiated care. At the same time, they wanted to maintain their ability to respond to the demand for accessibility appropriate for all classes and for continuous therapeutic improvement by tapping all available sources of income, charitable, private, and public. Their goal, in short, was to use a national health insurance scheme to protect and enhance their individual strengths and eliminate the weaknesses that had evolved out of forty years of getting by on the uncertain wages of a private enterprise hiding behind the skirts of medical philanthropy (or, perhaps, vice versa) and paying a high price for the resulting confusion.

As it happened, the work of both the committee and the council was for nought, at least in the short term. In spite of the fact that three out of four Canadians supported national health insurance,[111] when Prime Minister Mackenzie King presented his "Green Book" of national social security proposals to a federal-provincial conference in 1945, he encountered a chorus of dissent. Provincial concerns about constitutional authority and fear of a federal tax grab, growing consternation within the Canadian Medical Association, which had unreservedly endorsed the original plan, and vocal opposition from the business community provided the prime minister with convenient excuses – while publicly citing constitutional uncertainty – to set aside the program for postwar reconstruction, which he now found too expensive and politically risky.[112] When Ottawa next broached the subject of federal financing for national health care initiatives, at the 1948 federal-provincial conference, it was in the form of a program of National Health Grants to support a broad range of activities related to the eventual implementation of provincial health insurance programs that included hospital construction, health-care planning, public health programs, and support for professional training and education. But it would be another decade before the provinces, led by Ontario, put health insurance back on the federal-provincial agenda as a provincial initiative and responsibility to be funded, nevertheless, primarily through generous transfer payments from the federal government.

What had transpired, in the meantime, was, first, an impressive array of research; for example, the multi-volume *Report of the Ontario Health Survey Committee* (1951) and the *Canadian Sickness Survey* (1951), which had documented, chapter and verse, the crisis that all knowledgeable observers had witnessed or predicted over the preceding decade, and that an entire generation of patients had experienced first-hand. Equally important was the example set by Saskatchewan, where T.C. Douglas's CCF government – elected in 1944 as the first avowedly socialist government in North American history – deliberately seized upon health care as the public issue most suitable for a "demonstration of what a socialist government can do for the people."[113] Douglas (who was both premier and minister of public health) appointed Henry Sigerist, an internationally respected historian of medicine, as a one-man commission to survey the province's health needs. Following a whirlwind three-week provincial tour in the autumn of 1944, Sigerist produced his brief report in just one week. In it, he cited unaffordable health care in the cities and non-existent facilities and personnel in rural Saskatchewan as evidence of the demonstrable need for the gradual introduction of publicly funded health care and a vastly enhanced health-care infrastructure beginning with 1,500 additional hospital beds, fully equipped district health centres, and inducements for doctors and nurses to locate and stay in Saskatchewan.[114] Popular opinion was already galvanized in support of a dramatic political response, not least of all through the lobbying of the State Hospital and Medical League that boasted a membership of 5,000. The result was the implementation of the contributory Saskatchewan Hospital Services Plan on 1 January 1947. Under the aegis of the plan, hospital construction in Saskatchewan expanded at three times the national rate, bed capacity at four times the national average, usage more than twice the national rate, and the annual rate of hospitalization by 26 per cent. Local hospital boards retained their autonomy, medical indigence disappeared along with hospital deficits, and rural hospitals proliferated. More instructively, doctors prospered under the system in which the elimination of hospital bills promoted more frequent visits to physicians (and, as a result, employment for doctors), and physicians' incomes that soon became the highest in Canada.[115] Finally, as Doug Owram has convincingly demonstrated, after 1945 the generation of Canadians who had survived the depredations of depression and war yearned for the domestic stability, personal fulfilment, material comfort, and respectability that had been denied them for fifteen years.[116] Implementing the long-delayed promises of the welfare state was a necessary antidote to the tenuousness of their new-found prosperity and their persistent anxieties about an uncertain future.

The federal *Hospital Insurance and Diagnostic Services Act* (Bill 320) was enacted 1 May 1957, and the stage was set for the next iteration of the Canadian public general hospital, two decades after British Columbia had attempted to implement the first contributory, compulsory, one-tiered universal health insurance plan in North America.[117]

The public hospital's route from Victorian charnel house to state-funded primary community health-care centre was strewn with the casualties of the institution's long march: financial stability, paying patients, medical indigents, municipal governments, private philanthropy, the chronically ill, hospital employees and, in the end, popular confidence. The flaw in the optimistic premise that launched the post-Victorian hospital was the assumption that health was a commodity whose value made it marketable among the Canadian middle and upper classes at prices they could and would pay, even if those prices were unrelated to the actual cost of their own care and treatment. Because of hospitals' continuing legal, financial, and humanitarian obligations to their original clientele, the medically indigent, every paying patient's hospital bill was inflated, in effect, by an involuntary contribution to the hospital's philanthropic responsibilities, which were inadequately financed, as a matter of social policy, by provincial and municipal governments in the belief that personal and/or community charity toward the deserving poor was a fundamental social and moral obligation of respectable citizens. But the formula whereby equitable access by all users to the hospital's inestimable therapeutic promises, regardless of their ability to pay, depended on the deep pockets of paying patients inevitably broke down under the pressure of unrelenting demand for hospitalization and the costs of medical innovation. It took a social and economic catastrophe – the depression – to expose this unworkable premise, in particular the limited tolerance of middle-class consumers, to the hard light of day; but long before 1930 the consequences of burdening a local community's affluent sick with the perpetually inflated costs of treating every person whose illness required or deserved the care of the science-driven "factory whose product was health" had already become apparent. In the 1920s, indigent patients were resented, the hospital's custodial function was denied, institutional efficiency became synonymous with parsimony, and paying patients were cultivated for their ability to pay rather than their need for hospitalization. Medical efficacy had became synonymous with the high-priced skills of specialists and with diagnostic innovations that distinguished institutional medicine from the now-discounted arts of the general practitioner; and the line between the socially responsive and the medically conservative hospital had become more visible as hospitals pursued their preferred new identity as centres for the treatment of diseases, not individuals. They were only marginally successful as "health factories" in the very best of times; but even minor perturbations in local, regional, and national economies made their quest tenuous. Major crises portended complete social, medical, and financial collapse. The eventual solution had been anticipated almost from the advent of the modern hospital. It took half a century of trial by fire, and the threatened medical disenfranchisement of the fragile Canadian middle class, to bring about its implementation.

4 Camp Followers of the Army of Science

The emergence and subsequent development of the modern Canadian hospital were influenced by many forces, not least of which were the interactions of governors, administrators, doctors, nurses, and patients whose respective experiences reflected evolving hospital culture. The role of the medical profession, as it pursued its own path from its status as a marginalized trade in the nineteenth century to being respected as a profession at the leading edge of basic and applied science by the middle of the twentieth century, was particularly critical. General hospitals began to develop their modern form when "scientific" medicine, the political and economic interests of the medical profession, and the growing predisposition of the sick toward hospitalization converged at the end of the nineteenth century, propelling the former hospice for paupers and transients into a new mode as the essential source – for all – of medical intervention in acute illnesses. Having first made hospitals safe for patients, science then made them more medically effective through advances in diagnostics and therapeutics, especially surgery. But popularly acclaimed hospital-centred scientific medicine initially divided an overcrowded and under-employed medical profession into two camps: the elite specialists, who historically had enjoyed honorary hospital appointments and the privileges they entailed, and their more numerous colleagues in general practice, who were denied access to hospital facilities and were threatened, consequently, with a loss of both income and prestige when their patients' preference for hospital over home care materialized.

The result was a twenty-year struggle by general practitioners to secure the right to participate fully in hospital-centred medical care. Their first objective was to be allowed to follow their paying patients into hospitals, and treat them there without the intermediation of appointed medical staff. An equally important goal was to convince patients, hospital administration, and attending medical staff that hospital charity wards should be reserved for patients who demonstrably deserved doctors' and hospitals' medical philanthropy and should be closed to patients who were able to pay for medical care and whose admission as indigents cheated family doctors of a fee. Once they had succeeded in gaining hospital privileges and defining the limits and conditions of medical philanthropy, rank-and-file doctors inevitably turned their attention to the hospital's medical and political cultures, in particular to the issue of physician control of its medical priorities, organization, and efficiency, and of its policies that affected doctor-patient relationships, the independence of physicians as medical practitioners, and their success as independent entrepreneurs. The doctors' ideal was "medical democracy," the concept of collegial governance inherent in the ideology of professional *laissez-faire,* that is, freedom from the intervention of any authority except their peer group in determining and exercising their institutional rights, privileges, and obligations. This was the political counterpart to the idea of the hospital as a group or "team" practice; but the concept of medical democracy did not extend beyond the principal players on the medical team.

The ideal was short-lived in any event. In the best of times, beginning just on the eve of World War One, the new symbiotic relationship among hospitals, patients, and the medical profession sustained what Jacques Bernier describes as the "belle époque" of Canadian medicine characterized by the hegemony, authority, and autonomy of a medical profession united in the pursuit of a common agenda.[1] By the end of the Great Depression, however, the relationship was already filled with tension. Etiology-driven admissions and treatment priorities had given way to the unwelcome realities of social (some thought socialist) medicine as hospitals curtailed practitioners' privileges in order to achieve essential economies and limit institutional liability, and as a new wave of hospital-centred medical elitism began to encroach on the golden age of general practice.

To understand the interaction of doctors and hospitals after 1890, it is helpful briefly to review the history of the medical profession in Canada in the last half of the nineteenth century. An essential starting place is R.D. Gidney and W.P.J. Millar's analysis of the "liberal" professions in their seminal work *Professional Gentlemen: The Professions in Nineteenth-Century Ontario*.[2] Like their counterparts in Victorian England, barristers, clergymen, and physicians in colonial British North America enjoyed the status of "gentlemen" in spite of their lack of inherited wealth and their need to earn a living in the marketplace. According to Gidney and Millar, these were men who, because of their liberal education, their contribution to "the larger social good," and their "independence" – moral and intellectual – from the rank and file of ordinary people, constituted an "aristocracy of education," or at least a restricted meritocracy essential to the development of the colony. Consequently, their status was protected by the state, by legislation that made them self-governing and self-regulating in terms of the control of professional education, licensing, and the enforcement of ethical standards. An act of the provincial legislature incorporating the College of Physicians and Surgeons of Ontario in 1869 (Quebec's College was created in 1847 and other provinces enacted similar legislation in due course) was the culmination of a quarter-century of political manoeuvring to make the medical profession an autonomous community, a "state within a state."[3] It was also the beginning of an equally lengthy campaign to rid the medical marketplace of the myriad pretenders to medical legitimacy and to protect and promote the material and political interests of so-called "regular" practitioners.

The problem was that for most of the latter half of the nineteenth century medicine was an overcrowded "profession" in Canada. "Regular" practitioners, men (and very few women before 1900) educated at a traditional medical school, in a specialist hospital, or as apprentices to licensed practitioners, competed for patients with so-called irregulars, a category that included homeopaths, eclectics, and botanics (herb or "root" doctors), as well as midwives, surgeon-apothecaries, and a limitless stream of faith healers, "wise women," purveyors of folk medicine, and "quacks" mostly peddling patent medicines.[4] Moreover, the therapeutics of the irregulars and the charlatans were at least as popular – sometimes more so – as the "self-confident" trial-and-error empiricism[5] of regular practitioners, which might result in bleeding, blistering, purging, the administration of life-threatening and addictive drugs such as laudanum and calomel, and, as a last resort, high-risk surgery, treatments associated with the era of "heroic" medicine that had reached its apogee in the 1850s. Thereafter, heroic therapy gradually faded, eventually to be replaced by "scientific" medicine.[6] In the interim, "the medical profession ... did not enjoy a large measure of public confidence ... People were sceptical of physicians ... suspicious of medical students ... easily diverted by ... sects which did not employ bitter medicines and debilitating measures ... and were greatly disturbed by ... the seeming indifference [of medical men] to the welfare of actual sufferers from disease."[7] As if to endorse the public's apparent preference for some forms of alternative medicine, Ontario's legislators accorded homeopaths and eclectics the same privileged status as regular practitioners.

What was worse for the practitioners of orthodox medicine was that they were divided against themselves. The "schoolmen" – physicians and surgeons whose medical faculty appointments, research activities, and honorary consultancies in the major charitable hospitals provided professional status that translated into social prestige and comfortable livings[8] – did not have the same pragmatic agenda as the more numerous and economically besieged urban general practitioners; and both were as remote from the concerns of the country physicians who toiled on the back concessions as they were from the emerging clinical science of European medicine. Professional disunity was blamed for orthodox medicine's low visibility and waning prestige. "We as a class have hitherto displayed too little of that *esprit de corps* so necessary to the advancement of any body of workers," the editor of the *Canada Lancet* complained in 1883. "Let us turn over a new leaf, or ... take one from the koran of our sister professions,"[9] law and the ministry.

The "new leaf," in the long term, was the legal exclusion from medical practice of all but the graduates of accredited medical schools. This was not accomplished nationally until 1912, after the profession had finally consolidated its claims to be recognized as the sole purveyor of "scientific" medicine.[10] In the short term, the physicians' goal was to restrict entry to the profession by limiting the numbers of students admitted to medical schools so as to reduce the resultant pool of licensed practitioners. This, it was argued, would end overcrowding in the profession, improve competence, lessen competition for patients, and increase doctors' standard of living. Beginning in the mid-1880s, the Ontario Medical Board, with the support of the profession, began to raise the qualifications of candidates for provincial licensing examinations by redefining the premedical educational requirements for medical school applicants and raising examination fees.[11] This strategy alienated both the proprietary medical schools, who resented the loss of essential student fees, and the public, who resisted the formation of an elitist professional monopoly over personal health-care services. The Patrons of Industry, a populist international farmers' movement organized to challenge the protectionist impulses of capital and labour that they claimed resulted in restrictive practices disadvantageous to the farmer as both producer and

consumer, singled out the medical profession as one of the worst
examples of the abuses of entrenched privilege. Even country doctors
were denied membership in the Patrons, who demanded free trade in
medical practice to reduce the costs of health care, and easier access
to medical education to encourage the social and economic mobility
of farm children. When the Patrons captured 20 per cent of Ontario's
legislative seats in 1894, they used their brief ascendancy to force the
provincial government to acknowledge popular resentment of the
regular practitioners' claims to exclusivity and to roll back some of
the protections the profession had gained in the preceding decade.[12]
Populist sentiment also had the effect of further dividing the profession against itself as the proprietary medical schools, the eclectics and
the homeopaths, and the rank and file of distressed regular practitioners vied for public support over the accessibility and content of
medical education and the terms and conditions of medical licensing
and practice.

Regular practitioners defended their monopolistic objectives similarly on the basis of the presumed social, as well as professional, arguments for exclusivity. "We firmly believe that medicine is a calling, not
a trade; that the tradesman and business man may, with entire propri-
ety, adopt methods that would degrade the physician."[13] Restricted
and selective entry into the "calling" was highly desirable in order to
sustain not only the medical, but also the social, integrity of the profession. "[We] are not aware that poor men or poor men's sons make
better doctors than rich men's sons, and on the contrary are of the opinion that the entrance into the profession of the sons of wealthy people
will be a positive benefit by bringing into the fold a more liberally educated and independent set of men."[14] Their contribution to society was
not to be confused "by some writer whose brain was as heavily leaded
as the type in which his effusions appeared" with the work of farmers,
mechanics, or labourers, or even the "non-productive callings – such as
lawyers, preachers, middlemen, and salaried officials." The highest
form of productivity, the contribution of the "over-worked doctor," lay
"in raising from the sick bed and prolonging the life" of some member
of the other classes.[15] Nevertheless, in Ontario in the mid-1890s the legislature rolled back the profession's hard-won higher matriculation
and licensing standards, and, although the regular practitioners could
provide comforting statistical evidence that the number of medical
graduates had declined between 1888 and 1904, other evidence – the
geographical mobility of doctors, for example – suggests that medicine, in urban Canada at least, remained an overcrowded business
composed principally of underemployed general practitioners desperately seeking some competitive advantage.[16]

The engine of exclusivity finally appeared in the form of "scientific" medicine, the marriage of basic laboratory science and applied medicine that occurred in the closing decades of the nineteenth century and was consummated by 1920. The "research ideal," epitomized by startling advances in microbiology, chemistry, and bacteriology, conferred a new legitimacy on orthodox medicine in several ways. It associated medical education with a degree of scientific rigour that competing sects could not claim. It created diagnostic tools and therapeutic advances – serums and anti-toxins, for example – that enhanced the regular practitioner's effectiveness. It provided the theoretical and practical modalities that defined the scope and the success of the public health movement, which in turn propelled orthodox medicine and its gentlemen practitioners into the forefront of progressive social and moral reform between 1885 and 1920. The research ideal also encouraged the development of medical specialization with its implications of diagnostic and therapeutic superiority. Above all, it turned the hospital – the specialists' preserve – into the site of advanced diagnostic services and the latest medical technologies, the safest place for the successful invasive treatment of acute disease, and the source of a supporting cast of experts in specific diseases, patient care, and patient services – all to enhance the physician's art and skill.[17]

Some historians of this transition urge caution in interpreting the new scientific imperative as the great legitimator of medical orthodoxy and its ultimate triumph in the marketplace over alternative medicine. There is simply too much evidence, they argue, that ordinary practitioners mistrusted the ideology of "rational" science, clung tenaciously to their time-tested empirical diagnostic techniques, and adopted a sometimes cavalier trial-and-error approach to new methods and therapies, co-opting what was immediately practicable and rejecting or ignoring the "science" behind the application. What attracted the clinicians, according to this argument, was the prestige of being associated with the "culture" of science, not scientific inquiry per se.[18] Nevertheless, as Gidney and Millar, among others, conclude, regular practitioners were the ultimate beneficiaries of the popular response to "scientific" medicine. Orthodox medicine's progress toward a less threatening, popularly acceptable, therapeutic regime can be gauged, for example, by the evidence on childbirth in Ontario where, by the end of the nineteenth century, the traditional midwife-assisted home birth had been almost wholly supplanted by physician-attended births, as women placed their confidence, and their own and their infants' lives, in the hands of licensed practitioners. But the Ontario Medical Association's relentless lobbying against midwifery also contributed to its disappearance as an occupation.[19] Similarly, in rural Quebec by the first decade of the twentieth century, the historical sway of faith healers, folk medicine, and irregular practitioners was giving way to the authority of the knowledgeable and competent general practitioner whose willingness to accommodate a union of science and tradition was soon translated into dominance of the medical marketplace, social prestige, and economic success.[20] At the same time, however, it was the impossibly difficult midwifery qualifying exams supervised by the Quebec College of Physicians and Surgeons that were largely responsible for the rapid demise of "sages-femmes" after 1891.[21] But nowhere was the death of therapeutic sectarianism and the triumph of orthodoxy at the end of the nineteenth century revealed more boldly than in the surging popularity of voluntary hospitalization for the investigation, treatment, and cure of disease by the specialized and technical science of medicine.

If the medical profession selectively co-opted the elements of science and technology that enhanced the appeal, if not the practice, of applied medicine after 1890, it seemed that nothing short of the outright appropriation of the hospital would suffice for the economic security and professional authority of rank-and-file general practitioners, as the empirical evidence of patient preference for the "progressive specialization" associated with the hospital revolution mounted. Rapidly waning competition from irregular practitioners and quacks was just as rapidly superseded by growing competition between specialists and generalists for medical dominance. [22]

Whether or not the medical profession was generally overcrowded and underemployed in turn-of-the-century Canada, there was no question that in the larger cities and towns a rapidly expanding population of medical practitioners struggled to attract the confidence – and the fees – of a similarly expanding urban, especially middle-class, clientele. For example, among the 1,500 doctors licensed to practice in predominantly agrarian Ontario in 1877, the majority (55%) were located close to their patients in rural villages and townships. Just 20 per cent worked in urban communities that boasted a hospital. Thirty years later, not only had the number of licensed physicians in the province doubled, but two-thirds of them were located in cities and towns, and half of them in communities with hospital facilities.[23] Bernier has demonstrated that medical practice in Quebec experienced an equally remarkable expansion at the end of the nineteenth century as rural depopulation on the one hand, and urban development on the other, attracted large numbers of young francophones into the liberal professions and focused their aspirations on the needs of the growing bourgeoisie of Hull, Montreal, Quebec, Sherbrooke, Verdun, and Trois-Rivières where hospitals and dispensaries also offered employment.[24]

This proliferation of practitioners, and the increased competition they represented, worried established physicians; they blamed the phenomenon on popular misconceptions of medicine as a lucrative occupation, and on inappropriately low educational standards that permitted "men ... who a few years ago would have taken up telegraphing or bookkeeping" to become doctors. The editor of the *Canada Lancet* surmised that their best hope was a "wealthy wife."[25] As the president of the Canadian Medical Association (CMA) warned in 1903, "The old adage 'There is room at the top' has been overdone." There was too much competition, and the lives of too many general practitioners were being prematurely shortened by the combined strains of hard work and too little financial reward.[26] Estimated average gross annual incomes of $2,000 for established practitioners had to be cobbled together from hospital practice, attending municipal indigents, assessing applicants for life insurance, corporate and lodge contracts, and treating private patients. Some of these activities were professionally questionable others, according to the CMA, downright reprehensible if not unethical. Lodge and corporate practices, in which the physician contracted to provide medical services to the fraternal membership or to all company employees for a flat annual fee, were held in particular disrepute because they disrupted the free market for physician's services based on patient preferences. The only worst practices were contracting for services with "the girls of some cheap bazaar," or advertising free consultations as a come-on to prospective private patients. But in an oversupplied marketplace, the standard of living of the ordinary physician depended on negotiable fee schedules, aggressive recruitment of patients, a broadly based mixed practice, and a tolerance for unpredictable cash flows, not on nice distinctions about the social and professional appropriateness of a doctor's sources of income or about the putative value of physicians' services relative to the benefits they conferred on the patient.[27] Abraham Willinsky's experience was typical of that of young graduates (although he suffered discrimination in his search for a hospital appointment and for admission to post-graduate specialization also because he was a Jew). He first earned a living through rural *locums*, and through contracts with lodges whose members each contributed one dollar annually toward his salary in return for unlimited care. He finally saved enough money to fund post-graduate studies in Dublin (urology) and Vienna (roentgenology), returning to Toronto to rebuild a practice that included "ghost" surgery – performing operations in private hospitals as a substitute for well-established but surgically out-of-date practitioners, without patients' knowledge.[28]

Some observers attributed the surfeit of general practitioners, and the resulting ruinous competition, to the dilettantism of Arts students who stumbled into medicine in the hope of becoming "famous physicians" and who should be weeded out by a premedical curriculum heavily weighted on the side of the laboratory sciences.[29] (Subsequent investigations discovered that among the best Canadian universities, Arts faculties had higher admissions and graduation standards than medical faculties).[30] There is ample evidence that many general practitioners wandered into the profession by chance and naïvely, and that they were ill-prepared by medical school curricula to practise medicine. Most of them graduated with no meaningful clinical experience, and relied on textbooks as their tutors. Hence the initiative, begun before World War One and culminating in the hospital standardization movement, to improve medical education in Canada and the United States by eliminating marginal proprietary medical schools, associating medical education with university-based faculties of medicine, modernizing curricula, replacing didactic teaching with direct clinical experience, and designating selected hospitals as accredited facilities for undergraduate instruction and internships.[31] In any event, whatever their academic backgrounds, at the end of the nineteenth century newly graduated, inexperienced physicians soon encountered the other two principal obstacles to the development of their reputations as practitioners and their material well-being – specialists and hospitals. A "delightful relationship to the family ... was once the glory and the beauty of professional life," lamented one general practitioner in 1894. "Specialism has destroyed all this."[32] So, it was claimed after 1890, had the rapid "multiplication of hospitals" that encouraged large numbers "of sick and injured persons [to] betake themselves to some hospital where they select a bed in a public ward so as to secure free medical and surgical treatment. Even if they do not go into a public ward ... the local doctor loses his ... case and someone on the hospital staff secures the case." The results were "serious reductions ... in the general practitioners' incomes" and the need of doctors to find alternative sources of revenue. Together, hospitals and the specialists who controlled access to them appeared to be siphoning off every patient "who thinks his or her trouble the slightest out of the common."[33] The editor of the *Canada Lancet* thought he saw the handwriting of inevitable redundancy on the wall. "The time may not be so far away [when] the duties of the general practitioner will mainly consist of

presiding at the birth of the child, the injuries occurring in his locali-
ty, and waiting upon those who die ... of old age." It was scarcely a
living or a reason to become a physician.[34]

In comparison to the struggling generalist's tenuous circumstances, the lot of the hospital-based specialist in the new era of surgical efficacy must have seemed gold-plated. As one hospital surgeon
explained in 1912, he saw fifty patients a day, only two of whom ultimately would pay his fees. He therefore maintained a flexible fee
schedule which he adjusted to the patient's financial circumstances
and social status, maximizing his income by charging his richest
patients all that the traffic would bear (as much as $5,000 for a proce-
dure he frequently performed *gratis*), playing on their belief that the
"best" surgical skills available were, by definition, the most expensive. Besides, he argued, the "tension" of operating on a captain of
industry was unimaginable. It was "bad enough ... performing an
operation on an unknown patient from the 'free' wards, but to go
through the same work on a [public] man ... when a slip of the knife
may cause death ... then is the time one's nerves suffer." Surgeons'
incomes, and their professional status, this surgeon contended, simply reflected the "mental agony" associated with this new social
responsibility.[35]

The remedy that general practitioners proposed for their professional crisis was to create a level playing field of medical practice for
specialists and generalists alike by opening the public hospitals to all
physicians so that they would enjoy the privilege of treating their paying patients in the public and private wards, and of collecting fees for
the service. The case for general practitioners' hospital rights and
privileges was explained to the Canadian Hospital Association at
length by Dr J.S. Hart, a Toronto physician. Describing himself as a
mere "camp follower of the army of science" represented by "the pro-
fessors, specialists and members of the hospital staff," Hart envisaged
the hospital as a group practice in which "the average medical man"
and the hospital's specialized "aristocracy of effectiveness" joined
forces to create a "scientific centre" whose success "in getting patients,
in treating patients, and in promoting the best medical ethics" would
flow from the "friendly inter-relation" of specialist and general practitioner. The relationship could not be sustained, however, merely
through "the forbearance of the average medical man" in the face of
the specialist's "too great ... sense of ownership in the ... patient." In
fact, Hart argued, until the family physician's services were no longer
required for treatment, the patient and his fee belonged to the general practitioner. That relationship did not end at the hospital door. The
private physician should follow the patient into the hospital and

remain the primary medical attendant with access to all hospital resources. Even when he was no longer actively treating his patient, the family physician continued to be involved as an indispensable intermediary between patient and specialist. Who knew the patient's medical history, family situation, social and economic circumstances, and heredity better than the family doctor, whose exclusion from the hospital and his patient's course of treatment, said Hart, was tantamount to inscribing over the hospital door "abandon hope all ye who enter here"? If the hospital was the new deity of medical science, patients and their family physicians expected it to be a benign "demigod" that would do no harm either to the patient or to the average physician.[36]

To honorary consultants and attending physicians and surgeons the arguments on the other side seemed equally compelling. Since the unremunerated labour of these doctors was the source of hospital philanthropy to the sick poor, the right to treat all patients admitted to the hospital, to use wards as teaching clinics and sources of research material, to enjoy admitting priority for their own or referred patients (whose fees they sometimes split with the referring family doctor), and to capitalize on the prestige associated with their hospital affiliation as a business advantage seemed to be appropriate, indeed essential, compensation. At the Winnipeg General Hospital, where attending staff were appointed annually on a competitive basis, several physicians who had failed to secure reappointment in 1908 successfully appealed the decision on the grounds that they had "suffered loss of prestige" and in some cases income and related employment as a result.[37] In a city where fewer than 20 per cent of the resident physicians and surgeons enjoyed professional privileges in the largest public general hospital, the opportunities for "professional education and attainment" were jealously guarded.[38] But no more so than in the much smaller community of Brandon, where the hospital's appointed medical staff persuaded the board to deny privileges not only to some of their town colleagues but to all of the area's rural practitioners.[39] Among major urban hospitals, Vancouver General's open door was exceptional. As the board chair explained, "Here in this western country where things are wider open altogether than they are in [the] east or in other lands" an "absolutely open" hospital was simply expected.[40] But at the "closed" Toronto General, even a physician or surgeon fortunate enough to secure an inferior junior attending staff appointment in the outpatient department had to contribute five years' labour in order to win the right to admit and treat just one of his private patients annually as an inpatient.[41]

The consultants' defence of their entrenched privileges was not merely an appeal to historical tradition or to rights accrued through professional selflessness. It was also rooted in the perception that hospital practice was a new career path for clinical specialists whose education, diagnostic skills, and superior – that is, objective – science set them apart from the folksy general practitioner who was out of his depth in the sophisticated scientific and technological environment of the modern hospital.[42] Surgery, according to the editor of the *Canadian Medical Association Journal*, was a case in point.

[A] general practitioner who has been in practice for some years, who has won the confidence of the public as a successful practitioner and the esteem of his colleagues as a scientific and broad-minded man, should be competent to undertake the duties of a hospital physician. It is equally certain that the longer a man has been engaged in general practice without any special opportunities of doing surgical work, the less fitted he is to undertake the onerous duties of a hospital surgeon ... The mere fact that a general practitioner may have achieved success in surgery does not, in itself, qualify him as a competent hospital surgeon, whatever public opinion may say ... The hospital is primarily for the sick, and it is both just and humane that they should have the best that experience and training can give.

In the editor's view, even an experienced general practitioner required a five- or ten-year apprenticeship with hospital staff surgeons before being allowed to perform alone even such routine procedures as appendectomies, using hospital facilities.[43] To ordinary physicians who were accustomed to kitchen-table surgery, who were concerned about their livelihoods, and who were convinced that public hospitals and their specialists were simply stealing their patients, the appeal to scientific and technical rigour was arrant nonsense. At best it was an attempt to create an oligarchy of specialists;[44] at worst, evidence that for nothing more than "a little questionable fame" hospital physicians would "deny the right ... of their regularly licensed confreres" to treat their own patients inside or outside of the hospital.[45] If their privileged colleagues would not be moved, perhaps hospital boards could be persuaded that no patient capable of paying for medical care should be admitted for free treatment by attending staff, and that all paying patients could be treated in hospital by their family doctors.

In the end, what motivated hospital boards to change their policies was the need to attract paying patients whose fees would offset the mounting hospital costs incurred through the care of indigents, and simultaneously fund hospitals' insatiable appetite for expansion and modernization. General practitioners were the most obvious source of a steady clientele who could afford semi-public, semi-private, or private ward care that generated, as doctors soon deduced, "the margin of profit" required to advance hospitals' new mission.[46] Still, some boards moved with greater alacrity than others. When control of the Hamilton City Hospital passed from a committee of the city council to a board of lay trustees in 1894, one of the new board's first acts was to accept the advice of the majority of the city's physicians and permit all paying patients to choose their own doctors. This action peremptorily ended a decade of control by the appointed medical board, whose members promptly resigned. Undeterred, the board then went on to vastly expand the hospital's stock of private and semi-private beds to accommodate the anticipated flow of paying patients.[47] At the Toronto General Hospital the general practitioners' crusade for access took much longer. Other new and established Toronto hospitals routinely opened their wards to private physicians and their patients after 1900, but only in 1911 were general practitioners granted privileges in all but the public wards of the Toronto General Hospital.[48] By 1914 the trend everywhere was toward open hospitals as the proliferation of voluntary community public hospitals, and a reduction in the number of general practitioners, created more opportunities for hospital practice, less competition, and improving incomes. In the end, the realization of the general practitioners' goal, the "joint possession [of the hospital by] all members of the profession,"[49] was essential for professional unity, to the future development of the hospital, and to the welfare of patients.[50] That the discussion of the proposition often generated more heat than light was a measure of the stakes involved for all parties.

Similar emotions characterized the equally divisive, and related, debate over hospital admission policies and the apparent incidence of so-called hospital abuse that further muddied the evolving relationship among boards, specialists, and general practitioners. As hospitalization grew in popularity at the end of the nineteenth century, public hospitals throughout North America confronted the phenomenon of people from every social stratum, including a growing population of *bona fide* indigents, seeking admission either as paying patients or as free patients.[51] As we have noted, it soon became clear to administrations that their budgets could not support indiscriminate indigent admissions, that meeting the needs of the deserving sick poor would require greater expenditures and new sources of income, that hospitals must therefore increasingly cater to patients who would pay for their services, and, consequently, that every patient who could pay must pay. "Hospital abuse," from hospitals' point of view, was the deliberate obfuscation by some patients of their actual financial circumstances, claiming to be able to pay for preferential care and treatment in the private wards, which they in fact could not afford, in order to avoid the social stigma associated with the public wards and their indigent population. This abuse not only provided the abusers with benefits to which they were not entitled, but deprived the hospital of essential income from its preferred clientele. The medical profession, general practitioners in particular, held the opposite view. Almost from the advent of the open hospital, they insisted that "hospital abuse" was widespread among citizens who were demonstrably capable of paying both doctors' and hospital bills but who falsely claimed indigent status in order to receive free hospitalization and treatment, thereby depriving doctors of potential private patients and of their legitimate fees.

In the era of the "closed" hospital whose unpaid appointed medical staffs provided free treatment for indigents in return for the exclusive right to attend all paying patients referred to the hospital, general practitioners blamed specialists and their mentors, hospital boards, for engendering "the abominable evil of indiscriminate medical charity" that threatened medicine's "actual existence as a profession."[52] Ignoring hospitals' legal obligation to accept all indigent patients, private practitioners chose to believe that in the major urban hospitals, especially those associated with medical schools, admissions were simply geared to specialists' need for "bedside material": they would cheerfully "rob some poor, starving, young physician of a few dearly needed dollars" earned from an office or home consultation merely to provide fodder for the instruction of medical students and for research by admitting to the free wards patients who could otherwise afford to pay for hospitalization and for the services of a personal physician.[53] Similarly, private physicians also condemned the boards of closed hospitals for offering paying patients the choice of public, semi-private, or private accommodation that included the free medical attendance of staff doctors in the basic ward fee. This, too, was a form of medical charity that not only excluded general practitioners from the hospital but stole their fees as well.[54] But the worst abuse, according to general practitioners whether they worked in Brandon or Montreal, was allowing "medical communists," "Jews [who] drive away ... grinning at the bargain they had made at the hospital," "well-to-do mechanics, salaried officials and fair wage earners," and "men perfectly able to pay their physician," to use outpatient clinics, or to be admitted as inpatients to the charity wards, in effect getting free medical care for the price of a cab-ride to the nearest hospital.[55] The

unhappy, predictable, results, it was claimed, were voluntary pauperization of patients and "professional suicide" for doctors.[56] Like the
effects of a deep scratch on a vinyl record, the threat apparently posed
by undeserving and dissembling medical indigents to the material
well-being of the medical profession became a refrain endlessly
repeated over the next half century.

As it happened, attending physicians and surgeons became just as
dissatisfied with this situation as were the general practitioners.
Their privileges and prestige notwithstanding, the unremunerated
hospital duties of medical staff rapidly expanded to accommodate
the growing number of public ward patients, including patients
clearly able to pay for physicians' and surgeons' services. The popular attitude, complained one specialist, was that as long as an attending physician's income from private practice provided a diet of
"wind pudding served up with imagination sauce," his hospital
work should be entirely charitable. This misconception, he said, was
responsible for turning the hospital into a "dumping-ground" for
charity cases who did not require hospitalization.[57] But fraudulent
indigents were the worst offenders. The surgeon's "four hundred
dollar [fee lost because] patients who are well able to pay ... take all
they can get for nothing" was "a positive injustice" to specialists
whose charity was meant only for the deserving poor.[58] The blame,
they said, rested squarely with trustees, "whose lust for large [admis-
sions] figures in the annual report seems to overcome their sense of
justice."[59] The *Western Canadian Medical Journal* thought this situation
was proof that the new socially structured public hospital could not
work: better a one-class hospital in which all patients were treated
equally and as economically as possible, preferably at public
expense.[60] But the consensus that ultimately emerged among
appointed medical staff and private practitioners was that all patients
who could pay must pay, that there should be a rigorous process to
distinguish deserving from fraudulent medical indigents, and that
the medical profession should, if necessary, take "some concerted
action" including "refusing [as they would do in the 1930s] their services to any institution that will countenance such abuses."[61]

On the eve of the Great War these tensions among hospital boards,
specialists, and private physicians seemed to have been largely
resolved. The trend toward open hospitals, or at least open private,
semi-private, and semi-public wards whose paying clientele could
choose their own medical attendants fulfilled general practitioners'
aspirations to be at least junior partners in the new factory of scientifically mitigated health care to which they increasingly directed
their patients and their practices.[62] Their hard-won privileges extend-

ed beyond admission and consultation to include access to the operating suites, delivery rooms, and technical services of the hospital which had become indispensable components of a comprehensive, modern, medical practice. As Dr Hart explained, the new model hospital of 1912 benefited the patient by bringing together in one place all that was essential for modern medical practice and for the "mutual instruction" of specialist and generalist – x-ray technology, electrocardiographs, pathology laboratories, diet kitchens, hydro-therapy facilities, and well-trained professional nurses.[63] His list was not exhaustive, but it illustrates the rapidity with which new technologies and untested therapeutic modalities were embraced by a profession long on "supportive and symptomatic" treatment but short of miracles.[64] Dietetics might still be "in its infancy," but doctors could nevertheless "cordially welcome this new advance as one that [would] greatly further the possibilities for exact work."[65] Requests for tissue examinations, urinalysis, serological analysis, and radiographic diagnoses overwhelmed hospital laboratories wherever they were initiated, but no more than did patient referrals for hydro-, physio-, electro-, and massage therapy, which hospitals claimed to have "rescued" from the "onus of quackery"[66] and elevated to the level of scientific practice. As for x-ray therapy, "hospitals attempting to carry on their work without its assistance" were chided for their "audacity."[67] The appeal of novelty must have been, at least in part, a response to popular perceptions and expectations of modern medicine. Looking back from the vantage point of thirty years' experience in a rural practice begun at the turn of the century, one physician thought that he had been just as effective with his medical case, emergency grip, optical refractor set, $10 worth of medicine, and "no hospital within forty miles of me" as he was with access to "x-ray, chemical, or bacteriological examination." His patients, however, "who never dreamed of being sick anywhere but at home, now demand[ed] a hospital bed ... with the attention of numerous experts" and their advanced technologies. Who, then, he asked, was to blame for the soaring cost of health care?[68] But to his urban colleagues a hospital-centred practice represented more than just the gratification of consumer preferences, the institutional legitimation of the individual physician's science, or access to the latest therapeutic fad.

Newly graduated doctors who lacked practical experience had "two principal means of adding to [their] meagre [knowledge], hospitals and books ... Hospitals ... certainly [teach] more of immediate practical value than do books."[69] The idea of the hospital as a continuing medical education centre for general practitioners was a common theme not only in medical and hospital journals but in meetings of local medical societies. It was expected that hospitals would at a minimum maintain medical libraries and reading rooms, sponsor regular open clinics led by their ablest specialists and consultants, and build laboratories for the use of physicians, whose knowledge of anatomy vastly outstripped their familiarity with chemistry and bacteriology. Sir William Osler, the internationally recognized Canadian physician-in-chief of the Johns Hopkins Hospital in Baltimore whose opinions were universally respected, argued that all hospitals should retain a qualified research scientist whose sole responsibility would be to keep general practitioners abreast of the latest developments in biomedical science. The Owen Sound General and Marine Hospital and the local medical society achieved the same goal by co-sponsoring regular seminars conducted by clinicians and researchers from the University of Toronto.[70] There was, of course, a material consideration in all of this activity. The more facilities and services available to physicians in the hospital, the less initial and continuing outlay the practitioner needed to operate his own surgery and stay current with the latest practices in the diagnosis and management of disease. Malcolm MacEachern, the reigning North American expert on physician-hospital interaction in the 1920s and 1930s, urged general practitioners to use hospital space and equipment shamelessly to "cut down overhead tremendously."[71] Even the convenience of having several of their bed-ridden patients hospitalized in one institution instead of scattered across the city in their homes, or in farmsteads around the countryside, saved practitioners time, travel, energy, and expense.[72] In the idiom of the Taylorites, medical libraries, consultation rooms, and "comfortably-furnished" lounges where doctors "may smoke while dictating their ... findings" were essential investments to ensure that "the highest efficiency of the medical staff may be stimulated to the highest order."[73] For all of these reasons, most general practitioners could agree, "hospital appointments, affording, as they do, the highest degree of professional competency, are the places of vantage, the most valuable prizes for which we practitioners compete."[74] The first step in securing such an appointment was lengthy exposure to hospital-based medicine through the privileges now accessible to most practitioners.

The modern hospital's new centrality to the well-being of the medical profession and patients alike was effectively summarized by Manitoba's Public Welfare Commission in 1919. Hospitals, the commissioners, observed, "have been, since their inception, and must always be, instruments for the care of the sick and injured. [The hospital's] chief end is public welfare and its beneficent influence in this regard must not be supposed to begin with the entrance of the patient to the ward and end with his recovery and discharge. It must no longer be a 'boarding house for the sick.' Its responsibility extends outward to ascertain why the patient became sick and having recovered, what his chances of staying well are ... Medical men ... if they are to be of any use, must be informed in all branches of the science, and hospitals are the only place where such knowledge can be gained and nailed fast by the application of known facts."[75]

The era of the hospital as a social institution had passed. The hospital was now the "house of science" supporting the diverse professional interests of theorists and practitioners alike.[76] If the *forte* of late-Victorian medicine at its best had been diagnostic and prognostic accuracy,[77] the modern hospital, with its specialists and its technological apparatus, would become the agency for the perfection and application of those skills as the determinants of effective therapy. The hospital's most urgent task, the commission advised, was to educate "the lay mind ... to understand that the treatment of disease is a secondary consideration to diagnosis. Unless the exact condition from which a patient is suffering can be unerringly determined, it is obvious that *any* treatment is only guess work."[78] In the modern hospital, it was confidently assumed, guess work had been replaced by scientific certainty.

The hospital standardization initiative of the 1920s represented the apogee, before 1945, of a united medical profession's campaign to establish hospital-based medicine as the very model of modern medical practice by defining the minimal clinical environment considered necessary for diagnostic efficacy, standards of professionalism compatible with therapeutic efficiency, and structures of collegial governance and peer group accountability consistent with "medical democracy." The health factory's production "team" thereby assumed collective responsibility for the quality of its output and, more generally, for the institution's reputation, which sustained public confidence in its mission. Thus, in the mid-1920s, the Winnipeg General Hospital's annual reports highlighted the diverse evidence of co-operative group medical practice as the prime example of the hospital's commitment to innovation and excellence.[79] But it seemed to many doctors that their continued investment in this process and hospitals' dependence on it argued for an even greater degree of professional control and authority over institutional priorities and policies. This was not a new theme. While the profession was still struggling to open hospitals that had been closed to the rank and file of practitioners, seats for physicians on hospital boards and the appointment of doctors, rather than graduate nurses or accountants, as senior hospital administrators, had appeared to be the best way to influence, if not direct, institutional policy-making in the interests of the doctors' agenda.[80] But as hospitals' financial, medical, and physical resources were sequentially tested by the immediate postwar social and economic crisis, by inflationary costs, by an accessibility crisis as the 'twenties briefly roared, and finally by the circumstances of the Great Depression, doctors bridled at the unrestricted authority and interventionist managerial practices of lay governing boards who, even a president of the Ontario Hospital Association suggested, "too often consider[ed] themselves divinely appointed."[81]

Particularly at issue were the effects on doctors of hospital financial and admissions policies. As hospitals came under stringent economic and spatial constraints in the 1920s, tensions between doctors and hospital authorities – boards and superintendents – became palpable. Faced with the need to accommodate more patients and enhance revenues, boards aggressively expanded or renovated their institutions especially to accommodate more paying patients, just as persistently raised the tariffs charged to these patients, pursued institutional economies that would contribute to balanced budgets, and increasingly micromanaged all aspects of hospital operations. Doctors felt estranged from the decision-making processes that determined hospital policies and priorities apparently without due regard for their medical implications. At a time when "80 per cent [of the profession] use hospitals and the scientific practice of medicine is impossible without them," the "absolute authority of boards of directors" was not merely intimidating to practitioners; it appeared to demand "obsequious subservancy" to the judgments of laypersons on the part of "the group with the highest degree of scientific training for combating disease," whose "group practice" was synonymous with a hospital's medical importance, and whose philanthropy was essential to a hospital's social responsibilities and financial well-being.[82] Practitioners lashed out in all directions. On one hand, they railed against the hospitals' and the profession's unwelcome burden of medical charity for indigent patients who could not or would not pay for, or did not require, hospitalization as the source of the hospitals' financial woes and its threatened medical inefficiency (see chapter 3). Increased government subsidization of the medically indigent, or better still, weeding out undeserving indigents to reduce hospital costs, were the doctors' preferred solutions. On the other hand, doctors accused boards of "profiteering" at the expense of hospitals' paying patients in order to sustain unworthy indigents and aggrandize their institutions.[83] One of the earliest Canadian references to the "patient of moderate means" as the litmus test of the affordability of modern medicine was made by the medical staff of the Winnipeg General Hospital in 1914 when staff members, outraged at recent increases in maintenance fees and the imposition of "extra" charges for semi-private and private ward patients, recommended partially dismantling the hospital's growing infrastructure of support personnel – nurses and laboratory workers in particular – as a way to control costs and arrest the anticipated loss of paying patients from the hospital.[84] Within a decade, pondering the fate of their "patients of moderate means," that is, their paying patients, had become one of the Canadian medical profession's most persistent preoccupations. The inevitable result of the new admission and financial policies, doctors feared, would be that their private patients, unable to afford hospitalization, soon would be squeezed out of the hospital or, worse, would be medically pauperized, forced to accept indigent hospitalization and free treatment by residents, interns, and appointed medical staff rather than by their family physician. Once again, doctors would lose both patients and fees to hospital medical philanthropy over which they exercised no control. Their solution was cooperative administration of the hospital, to temper "corporate force" with the power of a "united profession" and promote and protect the rights of individual practitioners.[85] As the crisis deepened, hospital boards and administrators for their part become increasingly chary of the "vigorous advocates who talk loudly of Medical Democracy"[86] and of doctors' motives in insisting, in particular, that the individual practitioner's professional judgment should be the sole legitimate criterion for all decisions pertaining to the admission, treatment, and discharge of any hospitalized patient.

All of these complex issues surfaced in an illustrative dispute involving Vancouver General Hospital's board of directors and its attending physicians between 1928 and 1931. For most of the 1920s, the hospital was overcrowded. The numbers of indigents seeking free admission was a particular problem. By 1928 the situation had become so critical that the board declared a moratorium on all admissions except for emergency cases until the problem could be solved. In the superintendent's opinion, too many aged, chronically ill, convalescent, and invalid long-stay patients had been inappropriately admitted to the hospital. This, however, was the source of "a difference of opinion among medical men as to the cases which should be admitted and the length of hospitalization necessary."[87] Some thought that certain family physicians were guilty of abusing their hospital privileges by "dumping" their charity patients in the hospital without adequate medical cause; others that the overcrowding was evidence of a low discharge rate among indigent patients. General practitioners, they claimed, were ignoring or ineffectively treating the indigents they attended, voluntarily, as the price of their hospital privileges because they were too preoccupied with their paying patients.[88] As the problem worsened through 1929, the Vancouver Medical Association (vma), ostensibly to relieve its members of their growing burden of medical charity inside and outside the hospital, recommended to the hospital board that all indigent patients should now be the exclusive responsibility of the hospital's resident interns and appointed attending staff, who would evaluate all such cases for both admission and discharge and in the meantime treat them at hospital expense. The directors quickly agreed because staff control of the admission, treatment, and discharge of these patients was seen as one key to solving the hospital's mounting fiscal and accessibility problems. Then it was revealed that many patients admitted to the public self-pay wards as private patients of general practitioners were in fact indigents who could not pay their hospital bills, but were paying their physicians' fees. In effect, doctors and patients had conspired to protect some indigent patients' preference for a personal physician – and the physician's fees – at the hospital's expense and in violation of the agreement between the hospital and the vma.[89] In the eyes of the board, the "medical men" were, in effect, the authors of a new variant of hospital "abuse."

Blaming the city's general practitioners for duplicity, for unnecessarily hospitalizing patients in any event, for laxity in monitoring the progress of chronically ill and convalescent patients, and, consequently, for adding to the hospital's mounting financial troubles, the board took drastic action in 1929. The hospital's medical staff, who constituted the collegially organized Medical Board, consisted of honorary consultants and attending physicians nominated by the Vancouver Medical Association. The medical board in turn recommended general practitioners for annual hospital privileges. In December 1929 the directors announced that, starting in 1930, they would appoint a medical board whose members' qualifications were acceptable to the board of directors, not to the vma, in order to ensure that the dispensation of hospital privileges promoted the more rigorous admissions and treatment standards that the hospital's medical and financial objectives required. At the same time, the board also decreed that any patient admitted to the hospital who was known to be paying for the admitting physician's or surgeon's services and who claimed to be unable to pay the minimum daily public ward rate in advance would be declared indigent and be required to accept treatment by the resident staff in the free wards. The admitting physician would lose the patient and the fee, and a staff physician would determine whether hospitalization was required, what course of treatment would be followed, and when the patient would be discharged. The message was clear. "The admission of patients at the Vancouver General Hospital [was] the exclusive function of the hospital."[90] The board, not the practitioners, would decide who could receive free treatment and care and on what terms, who was competent to practise medicine in the hospital, and the conditions of that privilege, above all, for general practitioners who would no longer abuse their privileges at great cost to the hospital.[91]

The new regulations came into effect 1 January 1930, setting off eighteen months of bitter feuding among the medical association, the board of directors, the hospital staff, and vgh's senior administrators. In the meantime, a team of external consultants hired to survey the adequacy of Vancouver's hospital services and recommend a future course for the Vancouver General Hospital provided documentation that lent credence to the board's decision. The consultants reported that too much of the hospital's work was left in the hands of unsupervised general practitioners who consistently failed to get the results normally expected from the treatment of typical cases of illness. The consultants calculated that 75 percent of the patients who lingered in hospital long after they should have been discharged, especially large numbers of indigent patients who had undergone surgery, were admitted "with a prognosis of rapid recovery under skilful treatment." Their prolonged hospitalization, and the associated financial losses to the hospital, the consultants continued, represented the hospital's failure to enforce rigorous standards of medical competence among general practitioners, too many of whom "consider that the hospital exists for their personal convenience ... without any corresponding obligation to conform to any standards of professional performance."[92] Noting that, by law, the hospital's board of directors exercised "complete legal and moral responsibility ... for the calibre of medical officers admitted to the privileges of the hospital," the consultants backed the directors' reforms and urged even more sweeping measures, in particular barring general practitioners from the hospital's operating suites entirely, and restricting their freedom to do work, midwifery for example, better left, the consultants insisted and the board agreed, to specialists.[93]

After eighteen months of negotiations with the vma, the hospital's board of directors still refused to rescind its decisions, but agreed to let its newly appointed general superintendent mediate specific cases in which, on sympathetic grounds, a physician might be allowed to follow his fee-paying patient into an indigent ward. The

VMA's Hospital Committee reluctantly recommended that the association accept this process because of the superintendent's reputation for fair-minded diplomacy and because the board was simply adamant in its determination to exercise its authority in these matters.[94] But it was clear that the scales had been tipped in the direction of a less open regime, toward specialists' claims to diagnostic and therapeutic superiority, and on the side of lay control of the rights and privileges of hospital-based medical practice.

These problems were not limited to the Vancouver General Hospital. Amid the growing social and economic strains and tensions of medical practice and hospital service in the 1920s, the Canadian Medical Association in 1928 created a new Department of Hospital Services to address, and mediate, these issues. Its secretary, Harvey Agnew, who anticipated, researched, monitored, and documented problems of mutual concern and served as a liaison between the CMA and national and provincial hospital associations, warned his constituents early in his tenure that just as hospital practice had become more and more essential to physicians' medical and material success, their hospital privileges would be scrutinized in the light of their ability to contribute to hospitals' therapeutic, social, and financial objectives. Less, not more, professional freedom, might be the result. "The problem is to provide that degree of freedom ... which will permit a licensed doctor to give his patient the best of modern care without permitting the unscrupulous, the careless, or the over-ambitious ... to attempt treatment not in the best interests of his patient and at the same time jeopardize the reputation of the hospital ... [The] hospital ... should never fail to protect its patients against inferior medical care ... [No] hospital can rise above its medical staff ... [whose seniority] ... is backed up by [scientific] achievement ... [not merely] ... long years of faithful service."[95] Not surprisingly, general practitioners experienced a sense of *déjà vu* in this veiled resurrection of the old argument that patients' interests were best served by appointed staff specialists on the cutting edge of medical science. The advent of the open hospital had promised a golden age of general medicine. Instead, in just one generation, "the horde of specialists which we have brought into the world," the "vast number of new technical methods in diagnosis," and the confused association of "great medical institutions" with great medicine[96] were again threatening to marginalize the family doctor. All of these fears were exacerbated and magnified, of course, by doctors' experience during the Great Depression.

Physicians, whose rising incomes had encouraged them to attempt to limit, or shift, their responsibilities for medical charity inside and out of the hospital in the 1920s, found themselves significantly poorer and overwhelmed by the demand for medical relief in the 1930s. Surveys conducted by the Canadian Medical Association's Committee on Economics discovered that before the depression doctors' incomes had averaged $6,000–$7,000 annually, higher for specialists ($13,500), lower for rural family doctors ($5,000). In Hamilton, Ontario, between 1929 and 1932 the annual volume of an average medical practice was reduced by 36 per cent, while remunerated work, and income, declined by 30 per cent, accompanied by a corresponding rise in charitable work. Half of the Hamilton doctors surveyed in 1933 were unable to meet their ordinary living and operating expenses from gross income.[97] Among Vancouver doctors, between 1929 and 1933 average incomes of general practitioners and specialists alike fell by 36 per cent.[98] The common perception of the profession was that "the general practitioner ... has felt the hard times almost beyond words. Whether in the country or in the city, many have seen their practices dwindle financially almost to the vanishing point. Plenty of work there has been, but scant remuneration."[99] Doctors understood the social and financial plight of their patients and did not blame them directly for avoiding medical attendance or for seeking charitable medical relief either from their personal physicians or, especially, from hospitals. But given their own financial burdens, doctors chafed at providing unremunerated medical services in hospital indigent wards and outpatient clinics to former paying patients "who [were] within hailing distance of what the Social worker considers to be poverty" while the hospitals collected municipal and provincial grants for their treatment of these same patients.[100] The result seemed to be unnecessary hospitalization for general medical services that could have been provided by any physician in his or her surgery in return for a minimum direct payment or for payment on the patient's behalf. Similarly, doctors resented being asked for free medical care by indigent families receiving direct relief payments from one or another level of government that would not allow welfare or unemployment relief payments to be used for medical attendance. If relief income could be used to purchase food, why not health care? The short-term solution was to end the competition from the hospitals and to change unemployment relief regulations to mitigate the pauperization of both patient and doctor by reviving the private patient-physician relationship. This would be accomplished by reimbursing doctors directly, from public funds, for treating sick welfare recipients at home or in the surgery, rather than in the hospital.[101]

The Ontario Medical Association was the first to negotiate at least a partial solution to the doctors' plight. By an order-in-council, the provincial government agreed late in 1932 to a scheme whereby individuals and families eligible for unemployment relief would also be entitled to medical relief provided by a physician of their choice. Doctors were required to treat these cases for half of their approved fee, but no practitioner could collect more than $100 a month from the scheme. The half-fee payment was to be split, 2:1, between the provincial and local municipal governments; but municipalities were under no compulsion to participate, and pressure from local medical associations was sometimes required to bring local politicians on side (see chapter 3). The major limitation of the plan, restricting it to persons already eligible for direct municipal, provincial, or federal relief payments, meant that it embraced only about 50,000 Ontarians, leaving transients, pensioners, and employed persons with marginal incomes still dependent on medical or hospital charity; and it was of little help to physicians and surgeons whose practices were primarily hospital-centred. But insofar as it targeted the most distressed general practitioners, the "hundreds of doctors whose practices are made up almost entirely of relief cases," this scheme became the model that physicians elsewhere in Canada hoped to emulate.[102] None were more insistent than Winnipeg doctors, who watched their practices evaporate while the number of patients seeking free hospital care soared – up by 66 percent in just two years at the Winnipeg General's Outpatient Department alone.[103] Citing the "unnecessary increase" in the number of patients making use of free hospital services as an "unjust burden" on both the hospitals and the medical profession,[104] Winnipeg doctors in 1932 demanded nothing less than what their colleagues in Ontario had already won. To back up their demands they first threatened the closure of all of the city's outpatient clinics and then the withdrawal of physicians' services in the home, hospital, or doctor's surgery – except in dire emergencies – from all persons receiving direct relief payments from any source.[105] After nine months of unsuccessful negotiations with provincial and municipal authorities, the doctors finally acted on their threat and withdrew their services from all hospital outpatient departments and clinics in July 1933, effectively closing them until civic authorities finally agreed, in February 1934, to the implementation of a Greater Winnipeg Medical Relief Plan, roughly similar to the Ontario scheme. That the Winnipeg Medical Society celebrated its victory with an extravagant party at the Fort Garry Hotel did not go unnoticed by its critics.[106]

What the profession regarded as the decimation of the economics of medical practice during the depression taught its members that a new "generation of physicians [must] concentrate on [the economic] factor with the same intensity with which previous generations have concentrated on [the] scientific and altruistic factors" that contributed to the success or failure of the medical practitioner. As an independent small-business entrepreneur, the general practitioner was a "costly machine" who had been "undersold on the cost of [education] and oversold on the selling price of [the product]."[107] Declining incomes, increased competition from specialists, more stringent conditions for hospital privileges, and an increasing demand for medical charity all threatened a reversion to the dark age of medical practice at the end of the nineteenth century. In 1934, for many physicians the most advantageous way out of this slough of despond seemed to be a national health insurance plan that guaranteed at least minimum professional incomes tied to realistic fees and doctors' actual costs, solved the problem of indigent patient services in home, hospital, or doctor's office, saved the "patient of moderate means" from bankruptcy or the ignominy of medical charity, left physicians ample latitude to charge premium fees to well-to-do patients, and gave the medical profession a significant voice in the governance and administration of the plan. These were the main features of a proposed national health insurance plan devised by the Canadian Medical Association's Committee on Economics and presented to the association's annual meeting in 1934.[108]

In the light of the profession's recent history, the rationale offered for the plan, and the objectives that such a plan was intended to support, are more interesting than the actual details of the scheme. At the heart of the matter lay the traditional doctor-patient relationship "built upon respect and confidence."[109] It had been challenged, said the committee, by governments who "exploited" the medical profession to avoid their responsibilities for indigents, by hospitals that failed to make beds available for practitioners' convalescent and chronically ill patients, and by the ubiquitous and unregulated specialists who, with the support of the hospitals, dealt directly with patients instead of through the family doctor, "the most important unit in medical care."[110] Any scheme of national health insurance, consequently, had to achieve three goals: encourage the growth of general practice, limit the spread of specialism, and make adequate hospitalization available for any and all patients recommended for admission by general practitioners who, the report claimed, could treat effectively 80 per cent of the sick in, or out, of hospital.[111] The report was referred to the CMA membership for reflection and comment, then lay dormant for nearly a decade until the federal government initiated discussion of a national health insurance plan in 1942.

But whereas in 1934 the doctors' plan had been presented as an "antidote for the economic ills of the profession," in 1942 it was transformed into a statement of principles designed to ensure that, in the federal government's blueprint, equity would prevail between the service providers and the insured, and that the more fearful implications of "state" medicine would be minimized.[112]

Meanwhile, in British Columbia, the profession's actual enthusiasm for public, compulsory, comprehensive prepaid health insurance was put to the acid test when the provincial government devised, and proposed to implement in 1935, a provincial health insurance plan. Anticipating this initiative in the fall of 1933, the *Vancouver Medical Association Bulletin* advised its readers that it was time to "abandon our individualism ... to socialize our service largely, to pool our resources for the common good, and to become, to a degree, servants of ... the state."[113] When the draft legislation was made available for public discussion in 1935, however, opposition to it was led by doctors, who were incensed by what they regarded as blatant economic exploitation of the profession by the government. Specifically, doctors objected, first, to the bill's provision for physicians' treatment of indigents at just 50 per cent of the approved fee schedule of the British Columbia Medical Association (BCMA). In effect, physicians would be subsidizing half the cost of indigent health care. Second, the government proposed to require all families with incomes less than $200 per month to participate in the plan, leaving those with higher incomes to subscribe voluntarily in the scheme or to deal individually with their physicians. Doctors, however, wanted the income bar set much lower, at $1,500–$1,800 annually, to maximize their freedom to charge a larger proportion of their paying patients whatever the traffic would bear based on a flexible fee schedule. In short, professional hostility was rooted in the issue of doctors' incomes, hostility that the government attributed to the power, within the BCMA, of the specialists concentrated in the Lower Mainland.[114]

The doctors were not alone in their opposition to the plan. Employers, especially the members of the Canadian Manufacturers' Association, were also instrumental in persuading the provincial government to table the legislation in 1937 on the grounds that it was too costly given the state of business revenues, while employees generally were suspicious of the plan's costs, which would have required a 2 per cent tax on their wages. But it was the doctors' animosity, verging on hysteria, that attracted public attention. As one observer remarked, the government might have erred in putting forward a necessarily "cheap and nasty" proposal; but the profession's "obstinacy in rearguard actions ... would do credit to the highest military tradition" were it not for the symptoms of a "neurosis ill-becoming those who hold our lives in their hands, and who can certify the insane."[115] As it happened, the BCMA also had a long memory. When the provincial government a decade later successfully introduced a new health insurance plan, British Columbia Health Insurance Services, the BCMA's Committee on Economics rang the alarm bells against the "trend toward socialization" and warned that no plan could succeed that was not controlled by, and in the interests of, doctors.[116]

With the failure of provincial health insurance schemes in both Alberta and British Columbia in the waning years of the depression, doctors' attention next became focused on Ottawa where Prime Minister Mackenzie King's thesis about social justice, that "what society fails effectively to prevent, society is in some measure under obligation to mend,"[117] was being put to the test of social and fiscal practicality by the Common's Select Committee on Social Security, and in particular by the Advisory Committee on Health Insurance. In *Industry and Humanity,* first published in 1918, Mackenzie King had thrown his lot in with the progressive movement of social reform, identifying health insurance, which "places the emphasis on personality rather than on property, and on life rather than on wealth," as social legislation that "rejects, as unworthy, the thought that men and women voluntarily incur accident, sickness, disease, enfeebled health, or dependence in distress, any more than they willingly seek enslavement of any kind." Health insurance, he said, was an instance of the state safeguarding "its own assets."[118] To safeguard its members' assets, the Canadian Medical Association in 1941 created a Committee of Seven to serve as its liaison with the federal government in the matter of a national health insurance plan, and the CMA drew up a manifesto of twenty principles representing the profession's minimum conditions for supporting such a scheme. These included provision for both general and specialized medical service, the freedom of patients to choose their own doctors, standard hospitalization and diagnostic services, and insistence that the plan be contributory. The relationship of the Heagerty Committee (see chapter 3) with the Committee of Seven was amicable and productive, and the CMA approved the draft federal proposal in principle. Indeed, the doctors would have supported the legislation if Mackenzie King had succeeded in persuading the provinces to implement it in 1945. But the delay occasioned by the failure to achieve a cooperative federal-provincial agreement permitted the CMA to review its commitment. Members soon decided that there might be "more to this than meets the eye"[119] – state medicine.

By the late 1940s the Canadian medical profession was largely out of sympathy once again with public hospital and medical insurance schemes. The explanation was doubtless in part that, in the era of the Cold War, public health insurance smacked of the "state socialism" abjured by conservative businessmen.[120] But doctors were also pre-occupied with two other historical issues that wartime conditions had either left unresolved or significantly altered. Both were related to the place of the general practitioner in the scheme of things. As Donald Swartz has pointed out, since the late nineteenth century the "social availability" of medicine in Canada was the function of physicians in their capacity as self-employed entrepreneurs selling their unique skills in the marketplace on a fee-for-service basis. General practitioners' independence was the essence of their professional identity, an independence structured around their economic and medical relationship with their paying patients.[121] For half a century that relationship had been nourished and defended in good times and bad, even through the depths of the depression. It could not be surrendered cavalierly either to the untested promises of social, though not state, medicine, or to the resurgence of specialism, which again threatened to minimize the contribution of general practitioners to medical science, particularly in an era of enhanced public funding for medical innovation.

With the growing availability of sulphonamides, penicillin, and streptomycin, with wartime advances in thoracic surgery, and with the identification of cancer, heart disease, and neurological disorders as the new focus of preventive and curative medical intervention, postwar medical science initiated a new model of therapeutic investigation and effectiveness. The new paradigm was structured around intensive pharmacological and biochemical research, the diverse skills of an even wider spectrum of specialists, and capital-intensive, technology-based, hospital treatment centres and research institutes.[122] These trends were sufficiently perceptible by war's end to alarm the general practitioners who had survived the economic and professional depredation of the depression and who now, in better times, saw their hegemony threatened once again by hospitals eager to build reputations as centres of the new medicine, and by medical students, disdainful of the lowly arts of the generalist, anxious to seek fame and fortune as specialists. General practitioners ascribed this threat not only to the better working conditions, higher salaries, and lifestyles that specialists apparently enjoyed but also to the influential example set by heroic military surgeons during the war, and to the determination of teaching hospitals to build graduate schools where they would educate and recruit the next generation of specialists, not family physicians. Worse, these young doctors seemed indifferent to the professional issues surrounding the practice of medicine, especially the question of socialized medicine. There was no way to hold back the tide, except by making general practice as attractive an alternative as possible, and by repossessing the hospital as a centre for the lifelong professional development of the family physician on whose continued professional and economic health depended "the survival of a free medical service."[123] The leading spokesman for Canada's general practitioners in 1950, Dr W.V. Johnston, alluded to one explanation for doctors' hostility to national health insurance when he observed that the "slowness of the medical profession in this country in meeting some of its ... economic and social [responsibilities] ... may be due partly to incomplete cooperation between all its groups. Doctors who are to lead must be more than technically competent professional men. They must have insight into the social and economic problems of medical services. Family physicians are making a contribution that is unmatched; but one that will continue only if they are permitted to share fully in all the latest medical advances." The key was "control of the medical work in [the] hospital ... by its medical staff," among whom the general practitioner was *primus inter pares*,[124] not merely a "camp follower of the army of science." State medicine might promote equity among patients, and between users and providers of medical services. But it threatened the return of the inequity among medical professionals that had engendered the struggle for "joint possession" of the hospital half a century earlier.

The sixty-year quest of the average general practitioner for legitimacy and authority was finally rewarded in 1954 with the creation of the College of General Practice, five years after the Royal College of Physicians and Surgeons had begun certifying specialists' credentials. S.E.D. Shortt characterizes this progression as the "rise, fall, and rebirth" of general practice in Canada. He argues that the years from 1900 to 1930 were a golden age of general practice when the family physician competently served as a respected "Jack of all medical trades" until his or her skills were superseded by the narrower science of the specialist, whose threatened domination of the profession was again arrested by the reinvigoration of general practice in the 1950s.[125] At the very outset of their modern odyssey, family physicians recognized that the new model general hospital was essential to their medical and economic success. The appeal of the hospital as a location preferable to home for treatment and convalescence, its concentrated, superior diagnostic resources, its evolving technology, its trained medical assistants, its batteries of expert consultants, and the absence of restrictions on the physician/surgeon's medical activities – not to mention the convenience of treating many patients in a single location – all made the hospital and its medical privileges an essential adjunct to a successful medical practice. First, however, it was necessary to establish "joint possession" of the hospital with the appointed staff, to end the abuse of hospitals' and physicians' good will by patients seeking to avoid paying for treatment they could evidently afford, and to transform the hospital not only into a doctors' workshop but into a centre for the continuing theoretical and empirical education for the underpractised practitioner. All this had been largely achieved by 1920.

What remained to be addressed was the issue of physician control of the hospital, in particular the increasingly worrisome problem of indigent hospitalization and responsibility for medical charity in the context of public policy and professional self-determination. Doctors, who had come to believe that they were being financially exploited by the system of medical relief for the poor even before the depression, seemed to have all of their worst fears confirmed between 1929 and 1937. General practitioners' incomes plummeted while the demand for doctors' charitable services in and out of hospital skyrocketed. Hospitals, whose privileges were once much prized, became identified with the economic exploitation of the medical profession, and were even the victims of physicians' work stoppages. In the light of their depression experience, doctors' failure to assert control over hospital admissions and treatment policies, or at least to retain the confidence of trustees, in the 1920s was critical because thereafter the profession's agenda was identified as part of the problem of, not as a possible solution to, accessibility to affordable hospital-based community health care. By the time the opportunity arose to use provincial and national health insurance schemes to resurrect their agenda, the "camp followers of the army of science" had been overtaken, in the hospitals, by the shock troops of specialism and a corps of professionally trained hospital administrators determined to forge new alliances for the progress of modern medicine.

5 "Better, Brighter and Kinder Nurses"

Modern hospital care is synonymous with the presence of the professional nurse as principal caregiver and as the intermediary between physician and patient. Since the 1880s nursing science has been inseparable from the purpose and the promise of hospital-centred medical science. Yet, hospitals were not always essential to nursing as a career except for their monopoly over recruitment into and training for the profession, a monopoly that they constantly exploited to their own advantage. Before World War One, private nursing in the home or the hospital, not hospital ward duty, was by choice or necessity the business of approximately two-thirds of Canada's graduate nurses.[1] As late as 1930, just 25 per cent of nursing graduates were employed by hospitals.[2] In most Canadian public general hospitals basic patient care was provided by underpaid, undertrained, overworked student nurses. By 1920 more than 200 Canadian hospitals had introduced nurse training programs that assured them of a steady supply of nursing personnel at, they argued, the most economical cost.[3] With their emphasis on obedience, routine, and a practical understanding of the scientific basis of recuperative care in a sanitized institutional environment, these training schools redefined the content and the standards of nursing science after 1880, and built up the reputation of the hospital as a less hazardous place than the home for the treatment of disease. And under the guidance of the first generation of female nursing and hospital superintendents the social environment of Canadian hospitals was transformed to reflect the expectations, preferences, and tastes of their new clientele of middle-class patients.[4] For the rank and file of three generations of student nurses, however, the dual – and often conflicting – regimen of hospital economy and nursing efficiency would prove to be a barrier to the fullest development of the potential of nursing to contribute to the refinement of the hospital's scientific agenda, and to the advancement of nursing as a self-regulating profession.

The lingering impression of the mid-nineteenth-century public hospital as a Dickenisan horror owes much to the retrospective descriptions of nursing in the pre training-school era penned by garrulous retired physicians and proponents of hospital reform who caricatured the historical deficiencies of hospital staff as anachronisms separating the hospital's modern efficiency from its dubious past. Looking back from a vantage point of fifty years or so, these observers, Sir William Osler for example, attributed nineteenth-century nurses' moral defects and desultory work habits to their lowly origins as "ward servants who had evolved from the kitchen or from the backstairs into the wards."[5] It is unquestionably true that, before the advent of formalized nursing education, inexperienced and ill-trained women often provided essentially domestic care in inadequate hospital facilities with little supervision.[6] There were no minimum standards of nursing care; hospital attendants, both male and female, could be crude, authoritarian, and unfeeling with dependent inmates; and turnover was high, often the result of dismissal for intoxication or alleged sexual impropriety.[7] It is impossible to know, however, the extent to which this behaviour simply reflected the toll of unrecognized, poorly rewarded, unwholesome labour in an abysmally unhealthy, medically and socially dangerous, environment.

From the beginning, hospitals anticipated the shortcomings and prejudices of attending staff by regulating their interactions with patients, physicians, and administrators. In 1863, a year after its founding, New Westminster's Royal Columbian Hospital drafted rules for nurses and patients, defining their interlocking obligations on the principles of deference and obedience. The nurses' foremost duty was to be "most kind and attentive to the Patients, and [to] see in a general way to their comforts." They were also directed to dispense medicine and food at specific times, "obey the orders of the Physicians in the management of the Patients ... see that the latter do likewise," "keep themselves and the Patients neat and clean," and, when the physician was not available (a frequent situation), "be ... responsible for the preservation of order, the maintenance of comfort and cleanliness, and the strict observance of the Hospital Rules."

Failure to comply invited disciplinary action by the board, possibly dismissal. For their part, patients were expected to obey the nurses and, in the absence of any other surveillance, they were urged "to report immediately to their physician any inattention, or unkindness, or want of regularity in the administration of their food or medicine, on the part of the Nurses or attendants, and unhesitatingly to lay before him any complaint they have to make."[8] If a nursing attendant proved trustworthy and capable and did not surrender to the temptation of alcohol or to her sexuality, in time she might advance to become a matron in charge of housekeeping, a superintendent of nursing, or even a lady superintendent responsible for the general management of a hospital.[9]

Contemporary and more recent historical opinion has assumed that these early female hospital workers, whose origins are admittedly impossible to trace, shared much in common with the outcasts they tended. Dr F.J. Shepherd's portrayal of the nurses at the Montreal General Hospital in the late 1860s and after emphasized "age and frowsiness [as] the chief attributes of the nurse, who was ill-educated and was often made more unattractive by the vinous odour of her breath. Cleanliness was not a feature, either of the nurse, the ward or the patient; each one did as best pleased her, and the 'langwidge' was frequently painful and free."[10] But at a time when, with the exception of domestic labour, opportunities for female employment outside the home were limited and most women entered the workforce only in response to extreme economic necessity,[11] few but widows, uneducated, excluded, and otherwise disgraced women at the margins of society would take a job in an institution where "armies of rats frequently disported themselves about the wards, and picked up stray scraps left behind by patients, and sometimes attacked the patients themselves."[12] In this sordid environment, "drunkenness and dissolution were often the way to survive the hospital's horrors and demands."[13] Matrons and nurses in the Victorian hospital worked long hours at considerable risk to their own health for low wages. When it opened in 1864, the Royal Female Infirmary in Victoria employed just one woman to fill the multiple roles of matron, nurse, and housekeeper at $25 per month and $5 for board. If there were no patients in the infirmary, she relinquished her salary but retained the allowances for board, lights, and heat.[14] Whether the disreputable nurse – equated with the self-serving monthly nurse and midwife Sairey Gamp depicted in Dicken's *Martin Chuzzlewit* – was a myth created, as Katherine Williams has argued, "to support philanthropic claims for change"[15] or a reality as perceived by patients and medical staff, Canadian nursing struggled well into the

1890s, more than a decade after the introduction of training schools, to overcome its unsavoury reputation as work "so repulsive and hopeless that there was little to attract a different class," and a refuge for "fat, drunken, old dames."[16]

Even before the advent of nursing and hospital reforms imported from Great Britain in the 1880s, Canadian hospital boards, physicians, and patients had acknowledged the deficiencies of hospital care. In 1866, for example, the Montreal General Hospital (whose patients routinely fled its ministrations), attempted to raise the standards of nursing by hiring a "better class of nurses" responsible only for patient care, not for "cleaning of the windows [and] washing of dishes," duties now to be assigned to charwomen.[17] Hiring better trained nursing personnel became especially urgent in the 1870s and 1880s as "Listerism" gained support in Canada, albeit amid considerable controversy and resistance from within the medical community.[18] The successful implementation of antiseptic surgery required, as Monica Baly has put it, "a more intelligent and conscientious type of nurse" while the accompanying wider use of anaesthetics "called for a more observant one."[19] With higher survival rates, the number of surgical cases rose, generating a need for more closely monitored postoperative care. In this way, nursing became associated with the developing science of medicine, and the parameters of nursing care expanded to encompass concepts and techniques beyond the ability, experience, and judgment of the old domestic servant *cum* nurse. It was no longer enough for nurses merely to attend to patients' basic physical needs and to maintain hospital order.

In the last three decades of the nineteenth century, Canadian hospital boards began to respond to an international movement for nursing reform. The first priority was to recruit better-educated, middle-class women able to understand and execute physicians' instructions, but who would also bring to the hospital's culture "the domestic order created by a good wife, the altruistic caring expressed by a good mother, and the self-discipline of a good soldier,"[20] attributes at the core of idealized, virtuous, Victorian womanhood. It was more than a decade after Florence Nightingale's campaign to establish London's St Thomas' Hospital training school, and thereby legitimize nursing as a middle-class occupation with high standards of care, that Canadian hospitals began to consider similar initiatives. There had been a noticeable exodus, by 1880, of Canadian women to nurse-training schools principally in Boston, where 27 per cent of the applicants to nursing schools from 1878 to 1899 were Canadian-born,[21] in Philadelphia where the Hospital Training School reported in the 1890s that 8 per cent of its students were from Ontario, and in many of New York's largest institutions.[22] As a first step to reform, even before its nursing school was established, the Toronto General Hospital hired Harriet Goldie, not a trained nurse but a woman experienced in British and European hospitals who had recently cared for troops during the Franco-Prussian War, to reorganize its nursing services. To distinguish nurses from other female staff and patients who sometimes wore their street clothes in the hospital, and to reinforce nurses' authority in the wards, Goldie introduced the European rule of "uniform dresses while on duty." Her ultimate goal was a reputable training school.[23]

The first permanent nurses' training school in Canada was opened in 1874 at St Catharines General and Marine Hospital, by then ten years old and "one of the best and most convenient ... in the Province."[24] Two Nightingale-trained women were hired by its superintendent, Dr Theophilus Mack,[25] in an effort to overcome public resistance to hospitalization.[26] Over the next fifteen years, seven other schools were organized in conjunction with general hospitals in Montreal, Toronto, London, Guelph, Winnipeg, Fredericton, and St John.[27] By 1900 twenty-five nursing schools were open across Canada.[28] The incorporation of these nursing schools as part of the infrastructure of the modernizing hospital met varying degrees of acceptance and resistance among existing nursing staffs. As Mary Agnes Snively, longtime superintendent of nurses at the Toronto General Hospital and herself a 1884 graduate of New York's Bellevue Hospital, explained, when the TGH created a nursing school in 1881, "much tact and consideration was required in dealing with those who had heretofore considered that nursing was their own special province and would doubtless be disposed to regard any radical change in this department with disfavour." The nurses already on staff were given the opportunity to enrol at the school if they would pledge two more years to the TGH and could pass an oral qualifying exam. Five of seventeen completed the course.[29] The fate of the others is not known. Judi Coburn has observed that "no mention can be found in writings of the time to elucidate [their] plight ... One would suspect that some were kept on as maids and the rest 'let go.'"[30] In 1875 the first nursing school venture at the Montreal General Hospital failed, even with some advice from Nightingale herself, who recommended Maria Machin, a Canadian formerly employed at St Thomas', to head the project. Machin arrived in Montreal, accompanied by a trained nurse and two students, but her stay was brief because of the hospital's unsanitary conditions, inadequate nurses' housing, financial conflicts with the board, and the untimely death of her fiancé.[31] When the idea of a training school was revived ten years later, the director, Nora

Livingston, a Canadian graduate of the New York Hospital Training School,[32] was able to learn from the experience of other schools and to capitalize on their success; in its first year, the Montreal school accepted 80 probationers from 160 applicants.

Canadian schools endeavoured to reproduce Nightingale's emphasis on character building, obedience, deference to superiors, and practical training in a hospital setting. The physical environment and the limited budgets of the still small Canadian hospitals, however, prevented the wholesale adoption of Nightingale's model, in particular the home-like atmosphere of a nurses' residence, free uniforms, and generous pocket-money. Nor did nursing in Canada carry with it the same anticipation of social status and public admiration that Nightingale deliberately promoted in order to woo British middle-class women away from their domestic comforts in the name of professional altruism.[33] Without the small, but important, compensating inducements of basic creature comforts, Canadian hospitals at first struggled to attract suitable candidates to care for the sick poor, whose living conditions they were forced to share. Nurses at the Montreal General in the 1880s slept in "cubicles built into an old ward, and after a stormy night their beds were festooned with snow."[34] The friends and family of Henrietta Dunlop, an early graduate of the Montreal General Nursing School, actively discouraged her from registering because "the place was [dirty] and overrun by rats, and ... no place for a young girl ...Other people told me what horrid things I would have to do – one was that I would have to wash a dead nigger! Fancy all the niggers waiting to die to accommodate probationers!"[35] The racism of the remark speaks for itself; but the comment succinctly conveys the strong emotions – the uncertainty, doubt, loathing, and the fear of the unknown – that the idea of the hospital evoked in members of the public and in potential nursing students alike.

Until the stigma attached to nursing and to public hospitals began to fade in the final decade of the nineteenth century, nursing was not among the obvious choices for women seeking a vocation as a means of self-support, personal fulfilment, or diversion. The 1901 census recorded just 280 student and graduate nurses in all of Canada. In ten years, however, their numbers would climb to 5,600.[36] As the result of urbanization, industrialization, and immigration, the number of single women joining the labour force out of necessity or choice increased significantly between 1890 and 1914.[37] At the same time, under the aegis of the social reform movement there was an intense public debate over the appropriate role for women beyond the confines of their familial and domestic spheres. Insofar as late-Victorian social convention could accommodate the idea of working women, especially respectable middle-class girls, it identified certain occupations, nursing among them, as being consistent with women's traditional nurturing roles and their responsibility for the social and moral welfare of the family and the wider community.[38] Frederica Wilson, writing in the *Canadian Nurse* in 1906, advised her colleagues to "look on nursing, especially nursing the poor, as the most Christ-like work a woman can undertake ... whatever reason you had for taking up nursing the only motive power is love for your fellowmen and forgetfulness of self in the earnest desire to help others."[39] The spiritual character of the work was reinforced by Nightingale's steadfast perception of nursing as a "calling," not as a profession that would compete with male-dominated medicine and risk alienating public goodwill by situating nursing in the emerging feminist camp.

The National Council of Women of Canada endorsed nursing as a profession in 1900 by virtue of its formalized training requirements "in connection with the great hospitals."[40] But whether nursing should be categorized as a profession is an issue that continues to perplex nursing historians seeking, among other things, an explanation for nursing's failure to surmount such obstacles as the patriarchal hospital structures, implied servitude to the male-dominated medical profession, the lack of solidarity that has characterized nursing associations, and its weak relationship with the organized labour movement.[41] Equality of the sexes was not high on Nightingale's own agenda for nursing reform: as a member of the social elite, she was able, without resorting to feminist rhetoric, to persuade politicians to further her causes. No self-proclaimed radical (even though she apparently did sign at least one petition that included female suffrage), Nightingale emphasized "the importance of educating women and affirmed an educated female approach to health matters."[42] For many Canadian women, especially those raised in small towns and rural areas, wanting to work, to leave home, but not yet, or possibly ever, ready to reject society's conventional views of women's roles, nursing, as perceived and promoted by Nightingale and her followers, seemed an ideal career whose public representation conformed, on the surface, "to a stereotype of a nurturing woman who traditionally cared for the sick and the young."[43] Nurses were set somewhere above the "new women" – lawyers, doctors, journalists – who sought gender equality in the workforce and in public life and threatened late-Victorian social stability by crossing the boundaries into male-dominated territory.

In fact, nurses had more in common with the "new" women than their spokeswomen were willing to acknowledge publicly. A case in point is the preponderance of single women among graduate nurses. Many professional women deliberately chose not to marry. Nightingale believed that, in her own case, self-fulfilment and marriage were incompatible: "she did not wish to deny her own destiny for the sake of a husband's."[44] She did not demand vows of celibacy from her recruits but invoking spinsterhood during training, became, like the uniform, a way to distance nurses from their physically and morally soiled patients. Until the 1970s, being and remaining single was an almost universal requirement for nurse training. This perception of nurses as sexually pure, physically and morally clean, hygienic, and wholesome was sustained by the white or blue – the Virgin Mary's colour – uniforms, which enclosed the trainees like a protective cocoon.[45] There is evidence that some nursing superintendents favoured rural girls as candidates not only because of their capacity for hard work, but because they might be more "morally pure" than their urban sisters.[46] No less than religious orders, nurse training schools were communities of unmarried women where discipline, rules, and a heavy workload were intended to restrict outside social interaction and focus students' energy and their intent on the content of their trade: cleaning bedpans and patients, disinfecting instruments and wounds, assisting during surgery, and preparing the dead, while always practising the "humanity in a hospital [that] is accomplished by a gesture, a look ... which transmits itself to the sufferer and soothes their pain."[47] How to strike a balance among the various aspects of the nursing experience, especially between the ethos of sympathetic care inherent in the ideal of nursing and the materiality of the exhausting nurse training course, would confound students and administrators alike throughout the last decades of the nineteenth and the first half of the twentieth centuries.

Florence Nightingale's legacy of nursing reform has now been re-examined by "a generation of scholars ... sensitized ... to the implications of gender, class, and race,"[48] seeking to explain the subsequent history of nurses' exploitation at the hands of the hospital leviathan, their lack of professional solidarity, and their timidity in confronting their alleged oppressors. This revisionism has shifted the focus from Nightingale and her successors, the elite lady superintendents determined to remake nursing recruits in their own image, to the rank-and-file nurses who struggled to find their place in the workforce through a process of accommodation and resistance and to define the meaning of "profession."[49] Incisive as it may be, this recent perspective does not invalidate Nightingale's impact on the Canadian training schools that adapted her model of nursing education to their needs. Nightingale's philosophy, based on "an uneasy alliance among concepts drawn from the sexual division of labor in the family, the authority structure of the military and religious sisterhoods, and the link between her moral beliefs and medical theories,"[50] served well the modernizing hospital's need for a disciplined, competent, altruistic labour force appropriate to a hierarchical and patriarchal workplace in which, as in the Victorian household, the fundamental division of responsibility and authority was gendered. But whereas Nightingale and her acolytes had envisaged the graduate nurse as the embodiment of this ideal, North American hospital administrators, largely for reasons of economy (false economy in Nightingalian theory), partly to boost the image of their institutions, identified the nursing school itself and its minimally qualified, poorly remunerated students, as the preferred source of "a strictly disciplined labour force [to] do the work ... both uncomplainingly and cheaply."[51] In Ontario, hospital inspectors were quick to endorse this arrangement, which they interpreted as "evidence of good management."[52] By 1900 most Canadian hospitals had adopted a three-year program that took maximum advantage of low-cost student labour. Students seem to have accepted this imbalanced curriculum, perhaps because it was the standard throughout Canadian and American nursing schools. But, as Celia Davies surmises, trainees' submissiveness and compliance with the hospital's self-serving system were also rooted in a society with few employment opportunities for females where, as a result, "women were prepared to be so self-denying, so hard-working and so amenable to discipline."[53] Once dependent on a regular supply of cheap labour, hospitals sacrificed quality and experience in their nurses for economy, a choice that after a short time denied graduate nurses work in the very hospitals where they had been trained.

Deference and self-denial were crucial to the student nurse's survival and ultimate success within a highly structured hospital. A bad grade on an anatomy test might be improved and erased from the record, but failure to follow regulations was anathema to a nursing career. Kathryn McPherson reports that two-thirds of the women in training at the Winnipeg General between 1903 and 1906 graduated; one in seven was dismissed or resigned because of some infraction or a conflict with hospital authorities.[54] Twenty years later, candidates still had difficulty coming to terms with the restrictive routine of the Winnipeg General. Probationers dropped out because "they just couldn't take it, they didn't like the rules and regulations and they wanted to carry on with their social lives, the same as they'd always done and they weren't going to give it up for any training." Those who stayed on were "more or less dedicated ... We certainly weren't going to make any money at it, much."[55] Whether there was a correlation between candidates' backgrounds and work experiences and their persistence and success as nursing students is not clear. Most probationers seem to have had no work-related skills. A small sample of students from the Toronto General between 1882 and 1897 had tried various occupations – teacher, dressmaker, bookkeeper, governess, companion, and telephone operator – while others simply cited domestic duties as preparation for a nursing career.[56]

For at least the first half-century of Canadian nursing, the assumption that domestic skills and household experience, rather than academic ability, would serve the prospective nurse best in her career was probably accurate. The Nightingale model of the highly skilled nurse, "trained in the scientific basis of medicine and the personal needs of the ill,"[57] was hard enough to achieve under the best of circumstances; in late-nineteenth-century Canadian hospitals hampered by inadequate facilities and financing and a shortage of trained staff to provide nursing instruction, the task became almost unworkable. All too aware of the limitations of their nurses even as they graduated, hospital boards nevertheless rejected a more academically rigorous nursing program as too costly to implement. These attitudes began to change only in the 1930s when the Weir Report painfully directed public attention to nursing's faltering reputation, and as hospitals reaped the harvest of their historical dependence on the cheap labour of large numbers of poorly prepared and inadequately educated student nurses.[58]

Admission standards were loose. Formal classroom time was a luxury that Canadian nursing students were not allowed. To facilitate its students' almost immediate entry to the wards, the Toronto General's training school during its first years pursued a program of practical instruction. Lectures on current nursing and health issues were offered by Miss Goldie, though just twice weekly, to the predominantly working-class students whose limited literacy skills made her job all the more difficult.[59] Some hospitals, the Vancouver General among them,[60] had no fixed academic admission requirements for many years, relying instead on a two- to six-month probationary period to identify and weed out unsuitable recruits.[61] "The 'born nurse' theory was a popular argument, supporting the contention that nurses are better off with little education, and by implication, little intelligence."[62] Soon after her arrival at the Toronto General, Mary Agnes Snively introduced a screening process to enable the hospital "to sift our material, and retain only those who seem to give promise of success in the nursing profession."[63] Probationers were required to pass examinations in practical work and in the writing and comprehension of "ordinary English," which she considered essential for instruction in anatomy, physiology, and basic nursing, and for understanding physicians' lectures on diseases of the eye, ear, nose, and throat, lungs, brain, fevers, contagious disease, obstetrics, gynaecology, surgery, and other medically relevant topics.[64] By 1892 dietetics, "the art of cooking for invalids,"[65] had been added to the curriculum under the supervision of a YWCA instructor.[66] All these innovations were directed toward the threefold goals of the TGH training school: "the improvement of the nursing service in the hospital, so that the *poor* of our community who would otherwise find it beyond their means, may have every advantage which skilled nursing can provide ... to be a School of instruction, where women who are fitted by nature and education, can obtain a thorough, theoretical and practical knowledge of the art of nursing, with a view to making this their calling or profession [and] to give the medical profession intelligent and skilful cooperation, in the noble work of alleviating human suffering."[67] The mandate was broadened a few years later to embrace the development of "self-control, self-reliance, executive and administrative qualities in our pupils."[68] Above all, fundamental adherence to firm discipline was inherent in the words "trained nurse."

It was the nurse's primary duty to obey orders and follow the procedures laid down by the superintendents, matrons, physicians, and head nurses in authority above her in the hospital hierarchy. Responsibility for indoctrinating recruits into this highly regulated regime fell to the nursing superintendent or matron, and, if the hospital was large enough to include them on staff, the head nurses in charge of the wards, who served as liaison between nurses and superintendent. These women together constituted a nursing elite that ultimately might control every aspect of a student's personal and working experience in the hospital. In "Notes on Nursing as Given to my Class," published in the *Canadian Nurse* in 1906, Frederica Wilson of the Winnipeg General Hospital clearly defined the head nurse's position in relationship to the hospital organization and her role as the enforcer of its often unspoken disciplinary code based on deeply ingrained Victorian concepts of gender, class, and race. As Wilson saw it, the head nurse, whose foremost attributes were tact, patience, "womanly sweetness combined with strength," and "gentleness backed by force of will," had multiple obligations: to the hospital and its administration, who were owed her "respect and allegiance"; to the attending physicians, who as "superior officers" merited her "respectful adherence to their orders, and, as far as may be, to their wishes and preferences;" to private practitioners, apparently a lesser breed, about whose "professional demerits or blunders" the head nurse was to maintain "absolute silence;" and, lastly, as a role model and teacher, to set an example for the student and graduate nurses under her supervision. Success in her job depended on "the lesson of implicit obedience to authority ... practised ... till it has become a habit of life ... In a hospital, perhaps more than most institutions, it is necessary for military discipline, military precision, military obedience to prevail." [69]

Admission standards, uniforms, whether students should be paid and how much, the quality of accommodations and leisure facilities, and the training school curriculum were all matters of debate during the first three decades or so of Canadian nursing. That discipline was the foundation stone of order within the hospital and harmony among its staff was never questioned in a similarly open way. From the perspective of students and administrators, the meticulous rules and regulations governing individual and collective behaviour in the residence, the classroom, the wards, and the community beyond the hospital represented the essence of the training school experience. Even the architecture of the nurses' residence created an "arena in which the private lives of nursing professionals could be closely supervised and controlled by the hospital administration."[70] For some students, the restrictions were more than compensated for by the sociability among their colleagues in the residence and hospital, and by their intimate understanding of the institution and its processes;[71] but others, whose conduct had perhaps not been as closely monitored before they entered training struggled with the realization that "to be a nurse you had to do as you were told. You don't try to avoid rules and regulations, you make up your mind that as soon as you know about it, you are going to do that."[72] In its early years of publication before the First World War, the *Canadian Nurse* continually reminded head nurses of the need for students' absolute compliance and offered advice on how to enforce it. As C.A. Aikens, a frequent contributor, pointed out in a series of articles about hospital discipline and ethics, "[to] have a girl who will do exactly what she is told, in the manner in which she has been taught, without questioning or arguing ... is to possess a treasure whose value to the institution cannot be measured."[73]

Much of this emphasis on obedience was levelled at the nurses, "simply hand-maidens of the medical profession,"[74] to ensure that they understood how completely subordinate they were to the physicians and surgeons in charge of the hospital's medical services. "What the physician wants," Aikens contended, "is a nurse who has learned to obey, who can be trusted with the patient, and who will refrain from adverse criticism of him or his methods."[75] This conspiracy of silence in the hospital bound nurses to be discreet, and to avoid gossip and discussing "their own or their patient's affairs without conscious effort."[76] But even more vital to a well-run hospital was the trainee's recognition that her opinion about hospital business counted for nothing and that her value to the institution and to society was measured largely by her ability to suppress any sense of curiosity about her working and learning environment in the interests of fulfilling her hospital's mandate to care for as many patients as possible as cheaply as possible. Aiken, whose articles would have been widely read in the nursing community, explicitly warned nurses: "It is no part of a pupil nurse's duty to plan or produce reforms in an institution. If they are wise they will soon recognize that to readjust themselves, to do faithfully, quietly and efficiently, the duties assigned to them, is the best way to improve a situation."[77] For student nurses in most Canadian hospitals, it was the only way to improve a situation. Constantly besieged by the message of duty and obedience, nurses seem simply to have acquiesced, opting for compliance and non-resistance as the easiest defence against the possibility of personal disgrace, loss of privileges, or dismissal.

By the 1920s, more than 200 Canadian hospitals, some with fewer than 25 patients, were taking full advantage of their nursing schools as "the cheapest and most efficient working force available for their purposes" and, as the Manitoba Public Welfare Commission noted, "exacting too much from it."[78] First-year students were sent into the wards with little preliminary preparation. The night shift, when many patients died, was especially stressful for newcomers, who frequently worked unattended and were unable to lean on and learn from more experienced nurses.[79] After just a year of training, the Vancouver General's students, some not yet twenty years old, did night duty alone on a thirty-five or forty-bed ward.[80] Ethel Johns, who became a hospital administrator and editor of the *Canadian Nurse*, recalled that during her first week at the Winnipeg General in 1899, she learned to make a bed, bathe a patient, read a thermometer accurately, take a pulse and "to disinfect the bedpans in the bath tub and to scour them in the unspeakable little sink in the utility room." She worked from 7:00 a.m. to 7:00 p.m. (reversed on the night shift) with one hour off and twenty minutes for meals. Wearing her uniform, a blue gingham dress with a tight fitting bodice and a skirt that "swept the floor," and a "little muslin cap, with its pleated border, all ... made at home ... in accordance with instructions," Johns was assigned to the medical ward where she was immediately expected to respond "with alacrity whenever any one of the thirty patients rapped loudly on her bedside table."[81] Looking back on her introduction to nursing, Johns pragmatically concluded that the board could "hardly be blamed for regarding the school as a heaven-sent and perfectly justifiable source of cheap labour. Patients had to be nursed and nurses had to be trained – it was just as simple as that."[82] But it was more complicated too, because the supply of student nurses was seldom sufficient for the growing case loads, and frugal boards were reluctant to authorize the hiring of higher-priced graduates to make up the staffing deficit.[83]

By the early twentieth century, nurses themselves had begun to realize that "better care would be taken of the sick, fewer mistakes would be made and more intelligent economy would be practiced in all departments" and "the nursing profession would draw nearer to perfection" if most hospital care was provided by experienced graduates.[84] Toward this end, nurse registration legislation was enacted across Canada between 1913 and 1922 in an effort to implement some uniform provincial standards for nursing education leading to the RN accreditation. But, as Judi Coburn points out, "the acts were full of loopholes. The minimum beds a hospital had to have ranged from 'no mention,' to fifteen, to fifty. The curricula outlines were not stringent ... Educational requirements for training school admittance ranged from grade eight (in Alberta), to one or two years of high school."[85] In British Columbia, where registration came into effect in 1918, the minimum educational level was set at one year of high school, the minimum entrance age at nineteen, and "schools were urged not to accept younger women in the interests of the student as well as the profession."[86] During the 1920s, some standards were raised; in Manitoba, for instance, a hospital had to have at least twenty beds before it could qualify for a nursing school.[87] Still, the seemingly low academic criteria for nursing remained a contentious issue for the next twenty years.

How much or how little a trainee learned about patient care and the appropriate treatment for specified illnesses and diseases, and the calibre of her preparation for ward duty, depended very much on the size of the hospital and its nursing school, the quality and commitment of its medical staff, lady superintendent, and head nurses, who supervised the students' studies and work, and on a student's own ability and ambition. In their annual reports nursing schools might, for their public benefactors, list the topics students studied as evidence that they were familiar with the most recent medical developments. But in many schools the lecture schedule was irregular, dependent as it was on the workload of students and supervisors and the availability of physicians willing, like those at the Vancouver

General, to spend an unremunerated evening in the superintendent's living room introducing students to the fundamentals of medical treatment and care in their own specialities.[88] As late as the 1930s, "there was not a full-time nursing instructor in the Maritime Provinces."[89] Most training schools in Canada relied on graduate nurses to lecture on the many topics spread over the course of study apparently according to their difficulty. First year students at the Cornwall General Hospital in 1908 were instructed about hereditary and congenital diseases, the digestive, nervous, and circulatory systems, and some basics of pharmacology. Third year students advanced to the more complicated areas of obstetrics and gynaecological surgery.[90] In most training schools, students rotated through the various wards "sometimes under the supervision of graduate nurses if they had time and sometimes under the direction of other, more 'senior' pupil nurses."[91] The breadth of their knowledge was determined by the nature of the hospital and the age, sex, illness, and number of its patients.[92] Some hospitals, the Vancouver General, for example, which had no maternity ward until after the Great War, sent their students elsewhere for the requisite instruction.

The Winnipeg General's training program in 1909 seems representative of prewar, large, urban hospital nursing schools. There, during Ethel Johns's tenure, students spent two months on probation, six on night duty, two in isolation, maternity, and the operating room, two months at the Margaret Scott Nursing Mission to acquire the fundamentals of public health nursing, and six weeks in the diet kitchen. The balance of their three years, about 18 months, was allocated simply to ward duty as needed.[93] With exponential increases in surgical cases, nurses' responsibilities and workloads grew as well: they "readied equipment and supplies and set up the operating room, prepared patients for surgery, assisted the doctors during operations, and sometimes administered anaesthetic. Postoperative care took place back in the ward, requiring continuous observation by one nurse until patients were fully conscious."[94] As one 1925 WGH graduate put it, "you learned fast in those days. I don't think I killed anyone."[95] Given the potentially lethal combination of inexperienced nurses, minimal supervision, and gruelling schedules, the potential for mishap was high.

The opportunity for error was somewhat diminished by the students' awareness of their ignorance and inexperience during crises and by their scrupulous attention to executing doctors' orders. Student and graduate nurses alike were anxious to please physicians, if only to avoid being reprimanded or shamed by the hospital's medical elite. But this compliance was also deeply embedded in the hospital's complex network of gender relationships. While life in the nurses' residence and most of the training took place within the parameters of an exclusively female environment, in the broader world of hospital routine nurses confronted problems common to many women working in male-dominated institutions. Though they may have constituted a majority of hospital employees, nurses' superior numbers did not translate into influence over hospital business or medical policies, which were the exclusive domain of predominantly male boards of trustees and medical boards.

For nurses and administrators alike, the most troublesome gender relationships involved female nurses and male doctors, although the conduct appropriate for nurses caring for male patients was also an issue of extensive discussion. Few hospitals had either female interns or doctors on staff. After a decade of petitioning by the Local Council of Women, the Vancouver General took on its first female intern, Dr Margaret Burridge, in 1924 and Dr Florence Perry a year later, a quarter century after Toronto General Hospital appointed its first female staff physician, Dr Helen MacMurchy.[96] Even in 1939, the VGH still permitted only one female intern.[97] Nurse/physician relations were doubly complicated by the disparities in their medical education and skills, and by class distinctions between working and lower-middle-class nurses and middle- to upper-class doctors.[98] Many doctors endorsed the perpetuation of nurses' role as their handmaidens. As one physician argued in 1916, doctors needed to exercise discretion about how much medicine nurses should be taught: "Training schools are not intended for medical colleges, nor nurses to be quasi-doctors." The difference, he thought, was nurses' unsuitability for academic learning. His preference was "to lay well the foundation of principles, leaving much of the detail to ward instruction, [rather] than to burden the mind with minutiae, which is unnecessary."[99] Ten years later, the *Canadian Nurse* published a speech on the role of nurses, given by a physician who reaffirmed nurses' subordinate role in patient care and management, and who raised the spectre of nurses' undermining the authority and control of the medical profession in the standardized hospital which required nurses' unconditional allegiance to hospital and doctor alike. "Never by act or word should anything be done that might shake the confidence of the patient in the hospital where he has come to be cared for and ... nothing should be said that might weaken the faith or create doubts as to the methods of the physicians he has selected to care for him."[100] There is no better evidence that this advice was the rule in Canadian hospitals than the observation of 1928 WGH grad Josephine Mann that doctors "came first, last and all the time."[101]

The deference that nurses were expected to show toward the medical profession was no doubt based on a recognition of doctors' professional education and experience; but because, until the 1970s, men were in the majority as doctors, and women as nursing staff, establishing rules and delivering rhetoric for the conduct of doctor/nurse relationships offered a way for hospitals to regulate potentially dangerous sexuality in their growing communities. The *Canadian Nurse* argued that the "delicate" subject of nurses' relations with physicians, male patients, orderlies, interns, and even a patient's male friends should be discussed openly. From her first day, the nurse had to understand that her behaviour, especially in male company, should be above reproach and that while "the whole world [was] not desperately wicked ... a considerable portion [was] desperately weak."[102] As students, at least, nurses self-consciously distanced themselves from physicians. At the Winnipeg General where "if you were entering a room or entering an elevator [nurses] always stood back and let the doctor enter first,"[103] the distance was both physical and intellectual. Many WGH nurses were afraid of doctors; for Grace Parker, a trainee in the early 1920s, her "strange feeling about doctors [who] thought they were on a pedestal" haunted her throughout her life. More than fifty years after graduation, she still had "that fear of them and I know it's my background that makes me like that. Because I'd rather do anything than go to a doctor."[104]

Once beyond the student stage of their careers, when doctors by and large ignored them, however, nurses reported better professional rapport with physicians, who often relied on head nurses to "know how their treatment was progressing."[105] Some doctors continued to undervalue nurses' expertise, fearing their medical reputation with their patients would be jeopardized when, as in the 1920s for example, owing to fiscal restraints nurses were delegated to carry out such procedures as taking blood pressure, administering intramuscular drugs, and giving transfusions – traditionally doctors' exclusive preserve.[106] On the other hand, it is clear that especially in smaller hospitals the experienced graduate nurse's capabilities as a "Jill-of-all-trades," with a knowledge of laboratory analysis, x-ray technology, anaesthesia, and even accounting, were appreciated by doctors and trustees alike.[107] Eventually, with advances in medical technology geared to the treatment of critical care patients, physicians surrendered some of their individual responsibility for prolonging life. As Barbara Melosh has observed, "[the] pace and character of intensive care left no room for the old formulas of nursing deference to medical judgment."[108] In the long run, when working relationships between doctors and nurses were more or less "companionable," most of the credit was due to the nurses, the majority of whom were students in the process of learning to be good women as well as good nurses.[109] Painfully aware of who was "in charge," they "never over-stepped" and "obeyed, even though [they] might have a different opinion."[110]

If nurses' interactions with male doctors were prescribed by the gendered division of professional authority, relationships with their male patients, medical students, and orderlies, were at least the sub-ject of popular speculation. The *Busy Man's Magazine* wondered, in 1906, whether nursing or stenography offered the greatest advantage for young women to pursue their matrimonial interests among suit-able populations of eligible men, and concluded that the number of "vulgar, coarse, and obnoxious" male patients far outweighed desir-able wealthy ones; husbands were more likely to be found in busi-ness establishments.[111] A nurse's "sense of superior social position" afforded little protection in sexual encounters;[112] her penalty for being caught – instigator or not – was summary dismissal.[113] In a few very large hospitals, orderlies tended to the personal needs of male patients, but in most institutions female nurses routinely bathed, catheterized, and gave enemas to male patients with little evidence of outward embarrassment or sexual innuendo in keeping with their mandate to maintain patients' respect and confidence.[114] Isabel Cameron succinctly summarized the attitude of Winnipeg nurses to patient care: "We were there for the patient and not the patient for us and that was our function, to keep the patients happy."[115] The patients – male, female, child, injured, frightened, fatally ill – were all to be considered with respect and treated as more than "just a case."[116] The head nurse was singled out "to interpret in the truest manner possible, the real spirit of the institution. To neglect it is to show clearly that she has a very imperfect understanding of the patients and their human needs."[117]

From the moment patients left the admitting office, nurses attended to their medical requirements, but in hospitals with the capacity to segregate paying and indigent patients, care was strictly differentiat-ed according to the patient's financial status. In addition to choosing accommodation in a one- or two-bed private room rather than a pub-lic ward where ten or twenty-five beds might be crowded together making privacy impossible, patients who could afford it often employed private nurses to take charge of their hospital stay. Because hospitals relied on student labour, in some cases to the almost com-plete exclusion of graduate nurses from their staffs until the 1940s, the majority of Canadian nurses expected to find employment on graduation as private nurses in the home or in the hospital. The ratio of graduate nurses on hospital staffs to those engaged in private care is difficult to estimate. Judi Coburn notes that before 1909 up to 85 per cent of working graduates provided private care.[118] George Weir's *Survey of Nursing Education in Canada* (1932) reported that private duty nursing in its many forms was the choice, or sometimes the only option, for nearly 70 per cent of working nursing graduates.[119] Nurses seeking private assignments might register with employment agencies that coordinated nurses and cases, or they could advertise their services in pharmacies and doctors' offices.[120] Hospitals organized their own agencies, most often to send student nurses into the community, and to collect the fees for service (see chapter 2). Despite its unreliability as a source of regular employment and earnings during downturns in the economy, when many patients reluctantly acknowledged their financial difficulties and took their chances with public ward care, private duty offered some advantages over hospital employment. Wages and personal freedom were the most obvious consideration for women on their own. McPherson estimates that after the First World War, a private duty nurse who worked forty weeks of the year might earn up to $1,000,[121] approximately the wage of a floor duty nurse at a large hospital who put in a minimum of fifty hours a week with three weeks' holiday time.[122]

The comments of a Winnipeg General Hospital nurse suggest that attending to private patients in the hospital was no less demanding than an assignment to the understaffed wards. Exposing her awareness and resentment of the social divide between nurses and private patients, Myrtle Crawford deplored the devaluation of her professional training in a situation where "you were catering to their whims. They were used to servants at home and when they came into the hospital, they looked upon the nurses as servants as well."[123] By inference, being put in this subordinate position by patients affected nurses' ability to take command of the situation. Crawford liked private duty, but preferred the semi-private or semi-public wards and their middle-class patients: "You were professional, looking after a sick person and at the same time establishing a rapport with that patient. [You became] someone that they could unburden themselves to, and ... you could give comfort mentally and emotionally, as well as physically."[124] The public ward was the student nurses' domain. Working twelve-hour shifts until the 1940s, students initially were assigned tasks and responsibilities appropriate to their limited experience, beginning with administrative recording, that is, keeping written accounts of details ranging from patients' possessions to their medical treatments, food intake, and urinary output, test results, and the ward's drug and supply inventory.[125] They soon moved on to the labour-intensive patient care that retained its familiar association with domestic housekeeping and drudgery even as the hospital's medical work became increasingly technologized. The labour of ward nurses was organized around a core of urgent repetitive chores, carrying trays and serving meals, then feeding and bathing patients in readiness for doctors' morning rounds, and cleaning the ward and its equipment. To ensure that nurses were prepared to carry out these responsibilities, training schools routinely included more or less standardized instruction in bed-making, removing stains from linen, maintenance of the utility room, disinfecting bedpans and urinals, and facilitating basic patient comfort.[126] When their costs and admissions soared after the First World War, hospitals tried, some more successfully than others, to apply Taylorism's doctrine of efficiency and uniformity to appropriate ward tasks, forty-two steps to bed-making for example, but this only re-inforced the structural inequities rooted in cheap student labour.[127] As Susan Reverby suggests, in the first half of the twentieth century scientific management of hospital nursing practice was "more rhetoric than reality"[128] except as an excuse, under the rubric of routinization, to reorganize wards so that it took even fewer nurses to "produce" health for still more patients.[129]

In spite of the inherent subordination of nurses to physicians in the hospital, there is ample evidence that time and circumstances often conspired to compel nurses to stand in for physicians, sometimes with alarming consequences. In one incident at the Vancouver General in 1921, the head obstetrics nurse was pressed into substituting for an anaesthetist who failed to appear for an emergency operation in the middle of the night. None of the eight babies born during her absence had been bathed by 10:00 the next morning, and had been left by the student nurse "crowded together in three cots." After investigating the incident, the superintendent of nursing concluded that her staff was "being called upon to perform duties which are properly those of a medical man and at the same time to accept blame because the nursing service is unsatisfactory."[130] Under better circumstances, nursing supervisors sometimes encouraged their charges to take on work delegated by doctors as a professional challenge. Despite the potential for conflict with Toronto General's medical superintendent, who objected to "nurses removing surgical stitches or clips, or ... giving intravenous solutions," Jean Gunn, TGH's superintendent of nursing in the 1920s, deliberately relieved her graduate nurses "of duties which did not require [their] nursing skill or experience" as a way for them to expand their medical proficiency.[131] Eventually, in some larger hospitals the employment of nurses' aides who carried out many of the menial tasks associated with ward routine freed nurses to devote more time to the professional aspects of their work. But hiring nurses' aides was also a cost-saving measure that reduced hospitals' reliance on the labour of nurses, especially after nurses gradually succeeded, beginning in the 1930s, in achieving the eight-hour day.[132]

If the limited opportunities for hospital employment gradually provided graduate nurses with opportunities to hone their medical skills and diversify their qualifications through laboratory work, physiotherapy, and x-ray technology, student nurses' labour remained rigidly focused on institutional housekeeping, especially for the purpose of sustaining the universal principle of modern institutionalized medicine: ensuring cleanliness to prevent the spread of infections in the wards and operating rooms that could ruin the hospital's reputation as a safer place than home during illness and childbirth.[133] In his *Survey of Nursing Education in Canada* (1932) George Weir calculated that one-third of student nurses' time was spent doing "housemaids' work," labour that caused "considerable fatigue" and seriously interfered with their studies.[134] Not surprisingly, these quasi-domestic duties increased in inverse ratio to hospital size.[135] Within the context of the evolution of therapeutic medicine, however, as McPherson suggests, very basic tasks took on crucial significance as part of the "larger system of asepsis for which nurses were responsible."[136] Nurses ignored these practices at their own and their patients' peril. Frequent warnings from their superintendents kept hospital nurses aware that as their workload expanded to keep up with medical advances so did their liability for mistakes and neglect that would slow patients' recovery or, worse, prove fatal. Ironically, perhaps, the nurse's responsibility for the hospital's fundamental appeal as a medical environment made safe from iatrocentric infection contributed to the public's persistent perception of the nurse as a "high grade domestic servant."

That image also belied nurses' responsibility for assessing and managing not only their patients' physical but their psychological needs arising from the impersonal professional relationships, invasive procedures, lack of privacy, and coercive regimentation associated with hospital routine that the patient invariably "negotiated" from "a position of weakness and disadvantage." [137] Writing in the *Canadian Nurse* in 1941, S.R. Laycock underscored the nurse's value in providing security and self-confidence and generally empowering the patient "to master his disability ... to have a real sense of achievement as [he takes] drastic treatments and actively makes an effort to progress towards recovery."[138] But meeting this challenge was almost impossible for young nurses, themselves fearful and inexperienced in the face of death, with little time on night duty in a fifty-bed unit to do more than "just [walk] around all night long looking to see who was alive and who wasn't" and offer a cup of hot milk to their sometimes very distraught patients.[139]

Nurses often admitted to craving the same comfort and compassion that they were expected to dispense to their patients. Apart from close proximity to their work, one of the benefits of the nurses' residence was the camaraderie of communal life among their peers. Although conceived by Nightingale as a respectable and convenient surrogate for her Victorian students' middle-class homes, Canadian nurses' residences rarely realized Nightingale's lofty expectations.[140] Nonetheless, what they lacked in modernity, privacy, and convenience they apparently did compensate for as refuges where women could count on their colleagues' support during emotionally exhausting patient-related situations, conflicts with supervisors, personal crises, or the serious illnesses that debilitated nurses all too often contracted.[141]

A physically and emotionally healthy nursing staff was indispensable to the reputed efficiency of the modern hospital. Time lost to physical or stress-related illness or injury inconvenienced supervisors in large hospitals who had to find replacements for indisposed staff among the pool of private duty nurses. Absenteeism and discontent had even more serious economic and staffing consequences for smaller hospitals. In one of the first critical studies of the problems surrounding nurses' hospital-based training and employment, Vancouver General's superintendent, Malcolm MacEachern, in 1919, identified nurses' physical health, their long working hours, the need for higher educational standards, and the nursing shortage as matters pertinent to producing "a more efficient nursing service."[142] Pointing out how, during the war just ended, the army had recognized, through routine medical examinations, "conditions which would have been a serious consideration to the person if passed over and sent into service," MacEachern contended that, likewise, "nurses must have a well-organized medical service which adequately discovers any disease or physical unfitness, as well as treating such conditions as arise during the training." MacEachern ascribed some of the blame for the ill health of the VGH's nursing students to the training school's failure to assess its recruits' health until after their two-month probationary period. Family doctors were also censured for failing to diagnose pre-existing medical conditions. At the VGH, 10 per cent of the probationers were rejected for health problems, which included heart murmurs (now usually categorized as innocent), malnutrition, spinal curvature, varicose veins, and even tuberculosis.[143] There is no question that nurses' health was, as the Toronto General reported in 1909 when 2,270 nurse working days were lost from illness, a constant "source of anxiety;"[144] but the concern about students' general well-being was invariably compromised by administrators' concurrent worry about its financial toll on the hospitals' inadequate funds. As it was, few hospitals provided the health care required by sick nurses who, allegedly, were often left unattended in their rooms for hours without food or medicine. When the Toronto General built an additional residence in 1932 so that all its nurses could be housed in hospital buildings, it was finally able to open a nurses' infirmary.[145]

Training as a nurse brought with it no guarantee of access to the best medical care. The *Canadian Nurse* in 1915 condemned head nurses' habit of diagnosing and treating their student charges without consulting a physician, citing an instance where neglect had contributed to a trainee's death.[146] MacEachern's suggestion to ensure nurses' health was a daily sick parade carried out by "a competent hospital official" and "the best medical advice and consultation at the disposal of the hospital for diagnosis and treatment." Closer attention to preventive measures might have reduced the number of days lost but, as the 1919 influenza epidemic confirmed, nurses had no special immunity against contagious diseases. They were also susceptible to occupational ailments: fallen arches from working long hours in ill-fitting shoes, dermatitis when bare hands were immersed in irritating solutions, and, most seriously, infections, usually of fingers, from sharp medical instruments. Under the wrong circumstances, a puncture from a safety pin could prove fatal.[147] Until the introduction of effective antibiotics, septicaemia (which claimed at least one VGH nurse)[148] presented a life-threatening risk to patient and nurse alike. Still, of the several areas of hospital nursing that were targeted for MacEachern's constructive criticism, nurses' physical health was perhaps the most amenable to intervention and improvement.

In the 1920s and 1930s, as an examination of The *Canadian Nurse* confirms, dissatisfaction with just about everything associated with student and graduate nursing was widespread within and outside the profession. Nursing superintendents accused other hospital administrators of creating, in their attempts to balance hospital budgets, an environment where individualized patient care was compromised, and in which the burden of work made academic study almost impossible. Faced with severe financial constraints throughout the 1920s, hospitals gave low priority to resolving the problems of their overworked students and underemployed graduates. In mid-depression, Ethel Johns, then editor of the *Canadian Nurse,* stopped short of endorsing a national health insurance plan, but concluded that the solution to the nursing crisis lay not with hospitals or nursing schools but with the whole community, which had to accept greater responsibility for hospital funding.[149] In the meantime, in his 1932 *Survey of Nursing Education in Canada,* a volume that far transcended its terse title, amid meticulous documentary detail on the condition of nursing in Canada, George Weir concluded that nursing was indeed "a profession, however immature in the attainment of professional standards."[150]

The survey, a joint project of the Canadian Medical Association and the Canadian Nurses' Association, was conducted by George Weir, Chair of the University of British Columbia's Department of Education; as a committee of the two organizations stipulated, he belonged to "neither of the professions directly interested."[151] Weir used a variety of sources and methodologies – census data, questionnaires, conferences, and interviews – to address the troublesome question underlying the survey: "How shall the economic gap between the patient of moderate means and the qualified nurse be bridged to their mutual advantage?"[152] Put this way, Weir's mandate clearly linked the unemployment crisis among graduate nurses, and the CMA's growing obsession with the health-care crisis facing doctors' middle-class paying patients, to systemic problems that he proceeded to investigate under three broad categories – economic, educational, and sociological. Weir's mission was also prompted "by the desire of nurses to shift their perspective from one of social reform to that of educational reform." By contrast, the medical association was just as determined to restrain the nurses from unilaterally redefining the components of their professionalism – their knowledge base, entrance requirements, the nature of their work, and the content of hospital-centred nursing education.[153] Weir scrutinized a wide range of issues pertaining to the state of nursing in Canada and the working conditions of its practitioners. Much of the published survey is a compendium of detail, provided by nurses themselves, about age, education, ethnicity, parental occupation, and hometowns, social statistics that Weir believed would help him understand the attraction of the profession and the qualities of nurses. He also administered intelligence tests to 2,280 student nurses: 20 per cent scored below the 90th percentile regarded as normal and were summarily classified as slow.[154] Admitting that intelligence testing was "designed to measure 'ability to learn' rather than willingness to learn or the capacity to be good,"[155] Weir nevertheless concluded that while many nurses were very bright, specifically the women enrolled in the University of

British Columbia's degree nursing course,[156] "unless competently supervised there should be no place in the nursing profession for members of such low mentality,"[157] who were unable to master a rigorous curriculum.[158] "The relatively large numbers of low grade student nurses should," Weir contended, "give the profession and the public food for thought,"[159] perhaps because, as he noted elsewhere, during a convalescence patients found the "uncultured nurse" difficult to tolerate.[160] Clearly, one of nursing's problems was its choice of nurses.

Weir also concluded, on the basis of his evidence, physicians' and hospital administrators' views, and his assessment of the calibre of nursing students and graduates,[161] just as MacEachern and other administrators anxious about the decline in numbers and quality of nursing candidates had done, that most hospital nursing education was at best inadequate, at worst a form of slavery. Hospital nursing programs, Weir argued, urgently required extensive upgrading to keep pace with the changing role of the hospital. In particular, the mainstay of hospital training, the twelve-hour shift on the ward and in the classroom, was "too physically and mentally exacting for the average student nurse,"[162] let alone the less intelligent and poorly educated women accepted at the many small nursing schools across Canada which earned much of Weir's opprobrium.[163]

In the long run, though revelatory in its examination of nurses' backgrounds, career patterns, and job satisfaction or lack thereof, Weir's report simply reinforced, albeit with more authority, what hospital administrators and nursing staff already knew about the shortcomings of the nursing profession. His recommendations restated the demands that nurses had articulated for two decades or more through their professional associations. In the case of hospital training, Weir argued that approved training schools should be compelled to have at least one qualified instructor for every 50 to 75 students,[164] 75 active-care beds, and, at a minimum, departments of surgery, maternity, paediatrics, and contagious and infectious disease.[165] In a recommendation that Florence Nightingale would have appreciated, Weir also advocated junior matriculation as a minimum admission standard to ensure a nurse's competency "to carry out in the sickroom the instructions of the modern specialist in the spirit and with the humanitarian touch of the erstwhile general practitioner."[166] To facilitate students' training, their duty shifts should be reduced to eight hours and less time allocated to housework and more to medical theory;[167] and "hygienic and sanitary [housing] conditions, in residences separate from the hospital ... [not] in the same building as the patients"[168] were essential. Far more significant for the status of nursing was Weir's concept of training schools as educational facilities rather than the agent of nurses' continuing exploitation as a renewable source of cheap labour that perpetuated their "membership in a cult of intellectual serfdom ... as hewers of wood and drawers of water."[169]

Weir's report generated both support and criticism from professional nurses. A few commentators like Ethel Johns took the high road, endorsing the improved material benefits and professional standards that Weir's proposed reforms would promote, but insisting that the value of the nurse's uncommon task of tending "the flame of life at its beginning, in its full blaze, as it wavers, and as it dies out forever ... cannot be governed entirely by inflexible scientific or professional standards."[170] For most nurses the central issues were Weir's recommendation for raising the standards of nursing education through more stringent academic requirements including university nursing degree programs, and his proposal to limit the work responsibilities of student nurses. Their services would be replaced by graduate nurses (thereby solving their employment problems while their experience benefited both doctors and patients). Nursing superintendents in small hospitals feared for the future of their training programs and the costs of employing graduate nurses.[171] Doubts were raised about the feasibility for many women of the university nursing degree programs that Weir favoured. First introduced at the University of British Columbia in 1919 and by 1950 at nine other universities, the degree programs, though deemed essential for an administrative position, were never a popular choice because of the cost and time they involved.[172] Nurses recognized that replacing hospital instruction with university training would eliminate the exploitation of student labour, but, at the same time, they argued that the metamorphosis would then force hospitals to hire "women to work on their wards as practical nurses without making any pretense at training them as professional nurses." The bottom line was, quite simply, job security, and the protection of nursing, which "unlike any other profession [would be] open to unqualified competition on every hand."[173] During the 1930s, however, when public hospitals were in desperate financial straits and graduate nurses struggled to find employment, the debate over the suitable balance between student and graduate nurses remained largely unresolved.

After 1940, as depression conditions eased, hospitals began to adopt some of Weir's suggestions. At the Cornwall General Hospital, where Junior Matriculation (Grade 10) was the minimum entrance requirement, the five new students admitted in 1935 all had at least three years of high school.[174] Incoming students now received a physical during their first month but still had no subsequent checkups. They lost on average twelve sick days per year, likely not preventable in any case, to appendicitis, infections, and contagious disease. The hospital inspector noted that Cornwall's hours of duty "compared favourably" to those of other schools, but the average daytime duty of 57 hours per week and night duty of 67 hours confirms that most hospitals continued to exploit their students.[175] Subsequent inspections suggest that well into the 1940s, although recruits' educational levels rose and students seemed adequately housed in a two-storey home near the hospital, "from a nursing point of view," the CGH's overcrowded wards and congested operating rooms and nurseries mirrored the perpetuation of nurses' unfavourable working conditions throughout the Canadian hospital system.[176]

The local, provincial, and national nurses' organizations, including the Canadian Nurses' Association (CNA), which became more active on nurses' behalf from the early 1920s, were never the staunchest supporters of attempts to improve hospital working conditions for nurses, as the Canadian Nurses Association's disinterested attitude toward a 1928 student nurses' protest at the Guelph General Hospital and their lack of support for the ten-hour day suggest. The agendas of nursing organizations and nursing administrators were singularly focused after 1920 on pursuing issues pertaining to the professional recognition of graduate nurses and creating more hospital employment for them.[177] Hospital boards may have realized that in order to provide a level of care consistent with the expectations of their middle-class patients they would have to acknowledge nursing's priorities; but in the 1930s they had no incentive to move in that direction.

As it happened, the Second World War ushered in a nursing shortage that guaranteed full employment to all qualified graduate nurses, including married women, as hospitals scrambled to replace the almost 4,000 nurses serving in the armed forces.[178] Considering hospitals' previous resistance, the substitution of graduate for student labour was accomplished remarkably quickly, although at significant expense. In some hospitals, Halifax's Victoria General, the Calgary General, and Victoria's Royal Jubilee, for example, students still outnumbered graduates in 1942 by ratios as high as eight to one; but at most other large urban hospitals ratios fell to two to one. Montreal's Royal Victoria with 195 students and 214 graduates on staff, and the Vancouver General, whose 1,029 patients were under the supervision of 175 students and 313 graduate nurses, completely reversed the old pattern.[179] By 1952 the Montreal General's 641 beds were serviced by 181 students, 235 graduates, and 15 ward assistants.[180]

More remarkably, perhaps, Weir's objection to smaller training schools and the CNA's subsequent recommendation that some financially and academically marginal nursing schools might be shut down led to the closure of twelve of British Columbia's nineteen nursing schools alone.[181] By 1945 the transition from hospitals' dependence on students and private duty nurses to the almost exclusive deployment of graduates as their primary caregivers was well underway. Hospital nurses' changed circumstances, however, engendered new, and did little to alleviate old, problems. Doubts still surfaced from time to time as to whether nursing should be categorized as a profession or a trade given the persistence of nurses' inferior role in the health-care field.[182]

Nursing's almost exclusively white English-speaking visage began to disappear, ever so slowly, as First Nations and Afro- and Asian-Canadian women were admitted to nursing schools. Their numbers remained small: "In 1951, 15 'Indians and Eskimos' and 87 Asiatic women were listed as students in the Census."[183] The racist attitudes that assumed, for example, that Asians should only look after other Asians, and had prompted the Vancouver General in 1932 to accept Japanese and Chinese students survived, however, to complicate nurses' working experiences.[184] In a more positive vein, nurses and their work benefited from the numerous medical and surgical advances that materialized in the hospital following the war; salaries, though not high, had become more adequate; living conditions in hospital residences were an improvement on the overcrowded homes of earlier decades; and more regular hours allowed time for recreational and social activities. All this was enough to satisfy many women. Some, like Rita Curley, for example, acclaimed general duty nursing in addition for the opportunity it offered the nurse "to grow through practice, by the daily application of the principles and techniques learned as a student." [185] Others, Annie Laurie, for one, were less trusting of the hospital as a beneficent employer. As she saw it, "eight-hour duty would help to dispense with the too-long hours of work and would be fine, provided enough nurses were employed. I really believe this would make for better, brighter and kinder nurses, and give us a chance to really live instead of just to work and sleep."[186]

In 1950, as in 1890, nurses' relationships with hospitals were conditioned by the status of nursing as an occupation widely acknowledged to be the source of the hospital's medical efficiency, but unable or unwilling to translate its indispensability and its unique skills into a convincing definition and assertion of professional influence within the hospital. There, judged by their industrial workloads, by their

environment, by their susceptibilities to the exigencies of institutional financial priorities, and by their powerlessness to mitigate the circumstances of their apprenticeships and subsequent employment,
nurses shared the essential attributes of workers, not health-care professionals. This historically unequal and exploitative relationship
between nurse and hospital was succinctly summarized by one hospital administrator in 1943:

The hospital is [the nurse's] employer and as such should have her loyalty,
her support and her interest. The hospital is judged by the nurse – her work,
her appearance, and her attitude ... She can be friendly and sympathetic but
not familiar and, with her experience, she will have a better understanding
of her patient's problems. She must be prepared to accept the rules of the
hospital. The first and most important condition is that she be satisfied with
the work she has voluntarily undertaken to do. She has accepted the terms,
and it is her duty to adapt to these arrangements until something is proved
to be drastically wrong.[187]

For the most part, the thousands of nurses who worked in Canada's
voluntary public hospitals from 1880 to 1950 "accepted the terms" by
which others, inside and outside the hospital, defined the theory, the
substance, the quality, and the status of their science.

6 Mrs Jones and Mr Grant

The purpose of the hospital is to heal the sick. How well hospitals succeed in producing health is the ultimate test of their efficiency. But there are no reliable measurements of hospitals' success in the early twentieth century. Hospital boards filled annual reports with detailed tables on income, expenditures, admissions and discharges, surgical procedures performed, hospital morbidity and mortality, the duration of patient stays, the demographic characteristics of patient populations, and the numbers of student nurses trained. These same data were then retailed in annual provincial government reports that comparatively assessed hospital productivity relative to capacity, income, and operating costs per patient day. Hospitals' success became associated with increased volume – patient throughput – inversely related to the costs of production. Failure was measured by long patient stays, rising patient maintenance expenditures, and inaccessibility. Efficiency became associated with medical economics, not therapeutics, quantity rather than quality.

If we cannot ask how successful the hospital was in improving health, we can at least inquire about the nature of patients' experience in the hospital. What were their expectations of, and attitudes toward the hospital? Did people look upon the hospital as a "safe, scientific, and friendly place,"[1] as "a human institution [whose] first interest must be to give good care to the patient at any cost,"[2] as a place where "a special effort is ... made to see the patient from the humanitarian viewpoint, and to treat himself as well as the disease from which he is suffering"?[3] Or, in the expectation of the briefest possible sojourn in hospital, did patients simply tolerate the fear, the insecurity, and the embarrassment of institutional care as objectified diagnoses? How much of the patient's hospital experience was determined by factors such as social class, gender, age, ethnicity, and wealth? What role did hospital staff play in determining the relative quality of life in the wards? And how did hospitals respond to evidence of consumer unhappiness? There are no easy answers to these questions, not least of all because hospital patients and their families, like so many of history's bit players, tended not to have speaking parts. They became articulate only when their expectations, medical and social, were not met. So we must infer patients' institutional experience, and the hospitals' success or failure in shaping it appropriately, either directly from patients' infrequent formal complaints, or indirectly from the words and actions of doctors, nurses, trustees, and administrators responding to patient issues and problems. At one extreme, patients could be regarded as inveterate whiners who, out of ignorance, wasted nurses' and administrators' "too valuable" time with trivial complaints.[4] At the other, any matter relating to patient welfare invoked the rule that "if efficiency is silver, sympathy is golden."[5] As it happened, much depended on whether the patient was Mr Grant or Mrs Jones.[6]

Because the modern general hospital was a work in progress between 1890 and 1950, and given the great diversity of communities and their hospitals, the nature of patients' experiences very much reflected when and where they were hospitalized. A patient admitted to hospital in 1925 encountered an environment noticeably different from the one he or she might have faced in 1900 or 1945. Patients in the Cornwall General Hospital, or the Owen Sound General and Marine in 1900, 1925, or 1945 entered institutions quite dissimilar from their counterparts in Toronto, Winnipeg, Vancouver, or Birtle, Manitoba. Differences in size, in the range of diagnostic and treatment services available, in the complexity of institutional administrative and medical structures, in the qualifications and privileges of the medical staff, in the ratio of staff to patients, even disparities in the quality of food and the physical accoutrements that relative institutional wealth made possible, together defined the unique characteristics of each local hospital as it evolved. Still, all hospitals, large and small, rich and poor, for better or for worse, were the products of common developmental, business, and scientific cultures between 1890 and 1950. Even the physical and material environments of the hospital became standardized as hospital architecture, fittings, furnishings, equipment, and supplies were purposely designed – and priced accordingly – to meet the specialized needs of the new medicine. Over time, hospitals built to resemble the best private homes in the community – maids and nurses in the attic, kitchen and laundry in the basement, patients in between – were replaced by multi-storied, fully articulated medical complexes where form and function coalesced around, and served, the primary activities of the hospital – diagnostic services, surgery, obstetrics, and the patient's successful convalescence.[7] Rapidly expanding workloads, the quest for efficiency, technological innova-tion, and new medical approaches to patient care continuously raised the standards expected of (not least of all by patients) and practised in even the most modest institution. Individual hospital's facilities reflected the ability and willingness of boards to raise (usually bor-row) capital funding adequate to meet at least the minimum standard demanded by current wisdom and practice as defined by the recently specialized world of hospital professionalism. Elevators, communica-tions systems, laundries, central heating, refrigeration, and plumbing and lighting systems had to be constantly upgraded. Diet kitchens to accommodate special meals, the latest improvements in ward furni-ture so that patients "may forget that they are in a hospital," solaria, decorating hospitals in "cheering" and harmonious colour schemes to achieve a soothing "psychological effect" on patients and visitors, and a diverse range of patient services from libraries to occupational ther-apy workshops all became associated, to a greater or lesser degree, with the changing quality of patient life, and contributed to the rising costs of hospitals and of hospitalization. In particular, the costs of hos-pital construction multiplied at least tenfold between 1900 and 1930. Hospitals that had been built for less than $200 per bed had to be expanded or replaced at $1,800–$3,000 per bed ($1,300 per room for nurses' residences).[8] Medical technology marched to its own drum-beat: the cost of an x-ray unit was $300 in 1900, $3,000 in 1920, $7,500 in 1930, and at least $10,000 in 1940.[9] The link between institutional wealth and institutional progress simply became inexorable as time passed.[10] It is hardly remarkable that the aspirations of hospitals, large and small, always outdistanced their resources, and that the rationale for hospitals' inevitable fee increases and for their unapologetic solic-itation of the public for voluntary charitable financial support rou-tinely juxtaposed the miracle of modern medicine against the threat of debt-driven medical ineffectiveness or redundancy. As a spokesman for the Canadian Medical Association bluntly informed a *Chatelaine* reporter, "modern medicine, if properly practised, is expensive and cannot be otherwise."[11]

Each local hospital's physical environment and standard of service represented income-dependent variations on this larger theme. In the same way, while every patient's hospital experience was unique in time and place, throughout the period elements of a common patient culture emerged from the interaction between the modernizing hospital and the diverse, dependent, but nevertheless voluntary, clientele that it served. Whether, and how, this interaction translated into patient satisfaction, or disaffection, was a matter of some importance to hospitals. Now it would fall under the heading of "accountability," the evaluation of institutional success in achieving defined goals with a prescribed resource base. In this earlier era, patients' responses to hospitalization belonged in the realm of public relations. Complaints in particular were interpreted as the hospital's failure "to educate the public [about] the changes that [were] taking place from day to day in hospital service" so that an "intelligently informed" – that is, tractable – population of patrons and patients would acquiesce in the scientific merit of hospitalization, in the conditions of patient care and treatment, and in the costs of service as defined by hospitals in order to sustain their appetite for the extremely expensive tools of medical progress.[12]

The public, for its part, developed ambivalent, sometimes conflicting, expectations of and feelings toward hospitals as a result of their growing insistence on the necessary interdependence of business-like efficiency, medical efficacy, and corporate humanitarianism. Hospitals' visible, extraordinary medical resources, acquired under the banner of community philanthropy, offered treatment and recuperative care demonstrably superior to home care during a brief residency in the equivalent of a good hotel in return for payment according to the paying patient's means, or free, to indigent patients, in the name of medical charity. What hospitals delivered with their medical services, however, were social and medical judgments, rules, regimentation, routine, and, in the matter of finances, a reputation for ruthlessness, all based on recognizable contemporary assumptions about class, gender, ethnicity, race, and the social determinants of sickness and health. Consequently, patients' perceptions of and responses to hospitalization came to have as much to do with non-medical issues as with the unknown terrors of their illnesses and treatment. As one mother explained, at a time when the hospitalization of her sick child filled her with "fear and insecurity" for the child's welfare, "where the money shall come from" to pay the hospital bill, and her personal responsibility for the hospital's annual balance sheet, were not only irrelevant, but merely heightened her sense of hopelessness. On both fronts, however, medical and monetary, the hospital had assumed control of her life, the price she paid for the anticipated restoration of her child's health.[13] Not surrendering unconditionally to institutionalism meant, above all, paying for care. Important issues of privacy, individual preferences, deference, comfort, and control hinged on the distinction of self-pay from indigent patients in the newly socially-structured hospital's ladder of preferment. So did many patients' perceptions of their self-worth and personal dignity, at first, perhaps, as a cultural memory from the era of the charity hospital, but in time as the result of their direct experience or indirect knowledge of the modern public ward. Hospitals may have downplayed the link between differentiated care and the quality of patient life, insisting that "a hospital should be judged by its ... free ward ... service," which, if it provided "the poorest patient [with] every possible facility for the maintenance of life" was "fulfilling its obligation to the community ... and in terms of true hospital service [could not] do any more."[14] But the reality was that patients quickly learned all too well the first lesson of medical consumerism: for a paying patient, "any reasonable request [would] be fulfilled";[15] for the rest, hospitalization was synonymous with varying degrees of institutional intractability, discrimination, judgmentalism, dehumanization, and *noblesse oblige*.[16]

Patients' hospital experience began at the admitting office where, ideally, they were to be met by a "neatly dressed" woman with a "million-dollar smile" whose *forte* was "kindness and leniency tempered with firmness, persistence, and sound business methods."[17] The most important formality was the issue of payment. What individual patients, or their guardians, were willing to pay for hospitalization determined the level of accommodation and the services to which the patient was entitled in hospitals where even the public wards held two distinct classes of patients.[18] Although undoubtedly skewed by the effects of the depression, two patient surveys conducted in the 1930s provide some insights about the social status and financial situation of patients admitted to hospital. A census of patients discharged from Ontario hospitals on 31 March 1937 revealed that nearly 48 per cent were indigents, 36 per cent were self-pay private and semi-private ward patients, and 16 per cent were self-pay public ward patients (see Appendix P). One-fifth of the self-pay public ward patients reported that they had borrowed money to pay for their hospitalization, presumably to avoid the stigma of public charity even during the depression.[19] The daily fees collected from the 52 per cent of patients who paid were inflated by an amount roughly equivalent to the total costs of supporting one-third of the charity cases, reflecting hospitals' historical shortfall in maintenance income for indigents. A second survey documented that only about 30 per cent of discharged patients, who spent on average two and a half weeks in hospital at an average cost of about $120 a week, had no difficulty paying their hospital bills. The rest encountered varying degrees of stress. For about 15 per cent, hospitalization represented extreme financial duress. The longer the stay, the greater the hardship. Patients requiring in excess of sixty days' care were "so deeply in debt that they could not hope to extricate themselves." Yet several reported that they had accepted personal bankruptcy as an alternative to hospitalization as indigents; and very few of these "patients of moderate means" thought that hospital charges were unjustified. What they resented was "the system" that made those charges necessary, in turn threatening the economic and social security of their families.[20]

On admission, municipal and other non-paying indigents requiring hospitalization were assigned to a segregated free public ward if one existed, otherwise to a public ward. Public ward self-pay patients might or might not be housed with indigents depending on the size and complexity of the hospital; but unlike the charity cases who were attended by the appointed medical staff, paying public ward patients in "open" hospitals could be treated by their personal physicians. In some hospitals, semi-public wards offered modest improvements on the crowded conditions in the public wards and were designed to appeal to the social sensitivities of patients determined to avoid the public wards, but unable to afford semi-private or private ward care. For the well-to-do and even (the hospitals hoped) for the "patient of moderate means," semi-private and, especially, private accommodation promised, at the very least, privacy, quiet, comfort, a relaxation of hospital regulations and regimentation, the particular attentiveness of the staff, and special privileges, for example, the employment of private nurses. Variations on the grandeur of private accommodations depended on the size of the hospital. At the Toronto General and the Vancouver General private patients were housed in segregated pavilions, in smaller hospitals on separate floors or wings. But the purpose was the same – to enhance the hospital's income and reputation by providing differentiated services to attract those patients who could afford them and desired them. As one administrator explained, "we preach the value of hospital services to all. But ... we realize that ... we are often talking to Mrs Jones ... who has been brought up in comparative luxury ... [It] is very unfair to all the Mrs Joneses to expect them to come to us under [the] conditions" of the public wards. If the Mrs Joneses were accustomed to "foodstuffs that would be the envy of any ordinary dietitian," smoking, having friends around for afternoon tea, flowers in their rooms, ultra-modern furniture and custom-made beds, air-conditioning, and tranquillity, "we should provide a service compatible with their standard of living."[21] Few hospitals would have met this standard of private ward service; but in every hospital the private wards were a magnet equally to patients who could afford them and those who could not. The principal duty of admitting officers was to separate the Mrs Joneses from everyone else.

The Vancouver General was typical of hospitals that, having unsuccessfully pursued through debt collection agencies private ward patients whose accounts went unpaid (see chapter 2), instituted weekly payment in advance for semi-private and private accommodation, or a third-party guarantee that the patient's bill would be paid in full on discharge. The woman who, after being prepped for an emergency radical mastectomy, was followed into the operating room by an admitting clerk still seeking confirmation of her husband's ability to afford private ward post-operative care, was not an exceptional case.[22] Testifying at the public inquiry into the management of the Vancouver General Hospital in 1912, a husband claimed that he and his wife were kept waiting in the admitting office for an hour, she in great pain from appendicitis and in need of immediate surgery, until his financial status was verified. In another instance, a dying clergyman's friends, who had paid for his private ward care in advance, were shocked to learn that when their initial payment was exhausted the hospital, in its haste to give the bed to a paying patient, summarily and without consulting either his family or his benefactors, moved the man into a segregated free ward usually reserved for lunatics.[23] It was from instances such as these that hospitals acquired a reputation for being, at worst, mercenary, at best "efficient" to the point of insensitivity.[24] From the hospitals' perspective, private and semi-private wards were their cash cows, the difference between balanced budgets and crippling deficits. With perpetual waiting lists for differentiated service at least until they felt the full impact of the depression, hospitals assiduously promoted the benefits of, and guarded access to, this resource which they expanded at every opportunity to increase their intake of paying patients. From the public's point of view, the fact that many "a man goes into the hospital and when he comes out forgets that he owes for anything"[25] might have been morally reprehensible, but no more so than hospitals' policy of assuming that patients already traumatized by pain, fear, or insecurity were, first and foremost, potential financial liabilities. In any case, given the alternatives, the attractions of a private room were probably worth some dissembling.

Once past the admitting office, patients (especially patients destined for the free and public wards) surrendered their personal effects, bathed, exchanged their street attire for hospital gowns, and were put to bed, all part of what Guenter Risse describes as a formalized "induction" ritual intended to signal the transfer of control from the now depersonalized individual to the authority of the uniformed hierarchy of hospital staff responsible for the next tier of rituals, the daily routine of patient care.[26] The ward was awakened at seven o'clock in the morning. Patients having surgery were to be prepped, on the operating table, and anaesthetized by eight. Doctors were never to be kept waiting. Breakfast, dinner (at noon), and supper were served at prescribed times by nurses either from ward kitchens or on trolleys wheeled from the main kitchen. Physicians and surgeons attended and wrote their orders in the mornings. Afternoons were reserved for visitors who, in the public wards, were limited to two hours daily, compared with five in the private wards. Lights went out at eight p.m. Between times patients were expected to comport themselves in a manner appropriate to their convalescence, to the business of the ward, and to "the discipline of the hospital." No food from external sources unless approved by the head nurse, no leaving the ward, no smoking (a privilege reserved for male doctors), no alcohol, no swearing or displays of rudeness, strict obedience to attending physicians, "silent and respectful" deference in the presence of hospital authorities and medical staff, and no disruptions of the "regularity of the management" of the hospital were the essential restrictions on patients' behaviour.[27] But of course the discipline of the hospital, and the patient culture it anticipated, was predicated on expectations of normality. For most of its early history, however, the modern general hospital was in a state of constant upheaval as it attempted to cope with too many patients and their doctors chasing too few resources, and too many competing interests attempting to define and prioritize its responsibilities. The realities of life – and death – on the public wards frequently overcame the ideal of tranquillity, order, and efficiency.

Overcrowding in the public wards, the result of both patient demand and hospital policy, was commonplace. Patients endured cramped, poorly ventilated, often barracks-like rooms, or they were housed in corridors, in alcoves, and in elevator foyers. There was no sense of privacy in the best of circumstances, and in the worst patients recuperated from major surgery, or died, without the benefit of segregation from other patients and ward visitors amid a noise level "that would not be tolerated in a factory."[28] "Night noises" that reverberated through ferroconcrete construction were particularly disturbing to ward patients, but no more so than the groans from the next bed, frightening overheard prognoses, and the bedside weeping of a wardmate's relatives and friends.[29] A former patient in the Mission (B.C.) Memorial Hospital remembered wards so cramped that when two patients died during his stay each had to be lifted out over his bed.[30] Before the Great War, hospitals blamed these overcrowded conditions on Canada's flood of recent immigrants and hospitals' unwelcome responsibility for municipal indigents; and they sought to alleviate the problem through outpatient departments and, later, social service bureaus (see chapter 2). After the war, the growing population of incurable and chronically ill indigents was commonly identified as the source of unnecessary hospitalization, overcrowding, and waiting lists. Hospitals laid responsibility for this problem squarely at the feet of governments for failing to build sanatoria for the care of tubercular patients and nursing homes for the elderly, and blamed general practitioners for hospitalizing patients in general, the chronic cases in particular, merely for the doctors' convenience.[31] The result, in any case, was that public ward patients of every age and condition were (with some exceptions) thrown together to endure their illnesses in public. Infectious patients, to whom hospitals could not refuse admission, were isolated from the general patient population; but only the largest metropolitan hospitals could maintain separate buildings for patients suffering, for example, from tuberculosis, scarlet fever, diphtheria, or whooping cough. Consequently, isolation wards for these patients might be in close proximity to the public wards. The spread of infection to other patients was a constant threat to be feared by staff and patients alike, depending on the adequacy of the hospital's sterilizing equipment and procedures – in one case a wet sheet tacked over the door of the isolation ward.[32] Nor was infectious disease the only danger from which the general patient population, it was thought, had to be protected.

As of 1907, Vancouver General Hospital maintained a basement ward (Ward "H") for the reception of Chinese and Japanese patients. Later defended as a "special effort to care for these people," who were considered to be "apathetic" about health care,[33] the "Oriental Ward's" original purpose was racial segregation: Ward H was created in the same year that race riots tore the city apart as armed supporters of the Asiatic Exclusion League descended on Vancouver's Chinese and Japanese enclaves, inflicting severe property damage and personal injury.[34] The hospital became a microcosm of race relations in the city. Subsequently, in an attempt to deal with the problem of overcrowded public wards and to create space for more private wards, the board decided to use Ward H as well to house so-called dirty indigent cases – terminal cases best hidden from the sensibilities of other patients – irrespective of ethnicity; hence the fate of John Grant. Grant, an elderly indigent suffering from senile dementia, was dying from a gangrenous foot. He was strapped in a bed in Ward H, sedated with alcohol from time to time, and left largely unattended in the usually undersupervised and understaffed ward whose Asiatic inmates had to endure Grant's ravings and his stench. When a friend brought Grant's treatment to light *post mortem*, a public hue and cry ensued over the hospital's explanation that Grant could not have been assigned a room "fit for a respectable white man" because he could not pay for it; and in any event as a "dirty" case he had to be segregated from sensitive white public ward patients. The investigator of the complaint concluded that it was perfectly reasonable to assign charity cases whose "conditions are obnoxious to most white patients" to racially segregated wards rather than creating special wards in space better utilized to house paying patients.[35] The line between medical and social judgment in the hospital remained blurred. Twenty years later the VGH, following widely accepted practice, segregated prostitutes with venereal disease, alcoholics, and drug addicts from the general patient population; but it still had no special facilities for the care of "particularly offensive cancer cases" or of women who had developed septic infections following childbirth or abortion except among the social derelicts in Wards W and X, the successors to Ward H.[36]

Amid the hostile and intimidating conditions of the public wards, the principal intermediary between patients and their insecurities and fears was the nurse, more particularly the student nurse. If private ward patients tended to treat nurses as highly qualified domestic servants whose purpose was to "cater to their whims,"[37] public ward patients were more likely to develop a dependent relationship with their nurses which defined the relative quality of their hospital experience. As a professional caregiver, the nurse was trained to protect and promote the "sacredness of impersonal routine" as the essence of nursing science.[38] In practice, "nurturing good relations with patients was central to nurses' daily work" since cooperative patients eased the nurses' burden, forestalled complaints, and reduced conflict, even if the nurse had to bend rules and become more personally involved with patients' concerns than her training or hospital regulations might have dictated.[39] Fraternization did not extend to discussing patients' diagnoses or prognoses with them: it did involve attempting to gain every patient's confidence by conveying an understanding of each patient's humanity, individuality, and perception of the obstacles hindering personal participation in his or her recovery.[40] Running interference for doctors with patients who resented being treated as "a little bit stupid," helping patients, in particular women with families, overcome feelings of guilt for abandoning their domestic responsibilities, acting as an intermediary between patients and their families, or merely persuading shy and embarrassed patients to accept the necessity of having their bodies and bodily functions more or less publicly explored, all fell equally within the circumference of nurse-patient relationships.[41] For this reason, very early in the history of the modern hospital nurses were recognized by medical professionals and patients alike as essential contributors to the "psychic" ambience of the hospital as a healing institution.[42] But by the same token, nurses who subsequently failed to retain the confidence of individual patients amid the competing demands of all their charges bore the brunt of complaints, no matter how trivial, that reflected the patient's perceived loss of individual identity. The 373 patients who participated in a 1932 survey overwhelmingly characterized themselves as "average" persons, neither demanding nor "fussy," and largely satisfied with the nursing care they received. Yet 25 per cent of them reported that they had lodged a complaint against a nurse.[43]

Not surprisingly, the most common grievance of public ward patients against nurses was their inattentiveness and unresponsiveness when they failed to answer call-bells promptly or to respond immediately to table thumping or shouted demands for attention while they were busy with other patients. Nurses were thought to be particularly unresponsive, or at least slow, during the night shift and in segregated wards where difficult patients appeared to be left unattended, sometimes wallowing in their own filth, for prolonged periods of time. One VGH patient complained in 1912 that in desperation he had to play "mother of the ward" fetching tea, coffee, and water for his fellow patients because "the nurse [who] is supposed to look after patients" was not doing her job.[44] No doubt there was a more or less exact correlation between the time available to attend to the prescribed routine care of a student nurse's twenty-four patients during a twelve-hour shift and the residual time available to satisfy the idiosyncratic needs of individual patients. But to patients inclined to judge nursing services as "if it had been [their] own daughter" providing them, the standard of public ward care was an easy target for the disaffected and discontented.[45]

An easier target was hospital food. At the end of the nineteenth century the standard daily menu, week in and week out, in the wards of the Toronto General Hospital consisted of tea, bread and butter, and porridge for breakfast, beef, mutton, or fish, boiled potatoes, and bread or rice pudding for dinner at midday, and at supper bread and tea.[46] This essentially working-class diet, filling but low in nutritional value,[47] was still the staple of hospital food services two decades later. Hospital kitchens could produce full, light, or fluid variations of the basic menu on doctors' orders; but neither the state of nutritional science nor the tight provisions' budget of a two-hundred bed hospital responsible for 150,000 meals a year, nor the larders of small hospitals that, until the Great War, relied on personal donations of foodstuffs to make ends meet, permitted much latitude for gustatory creativity. Patients lamented that hospital food was, variously, too coarse, too heavy, unrefined, unvarying, inedible, and nauseating, depending, no doubt, on the nature and extent of their own illnesses. What recuperating patients seemed particularly to crave were more "dainties" and comfort foods, especially sweet desserts. Knowledgeable doctors and hospital superintendents agreed that an unrelieved diet of large dollops of meat and potatoes was "not the kind of food a sick person wants," particularly when it was "presented in its most indigestible form;" but "chicken salad, strawberries and cream" were beyond the pale of hospital budgets except for patients prepared to pay for premium service.[48] It was not until the 1920s that hospitals began to promote "right living" through "hygienic rectitude" with the aid of "model normal diets" designed by qualified dietitians whose objective was inexpensive, properly cooked, palatable, and nutritionally balanced meals as much for the education, as for the healing, of the patient.[49] But even in the late 1930s the *Canadian Medical Association Journal* reckoned that in all but the largest Canadian hospitals most hospital food was "better adapted ... to the boys' camp than to the sick room."[50]

To this catalogue of complaints about impersonality, insensitivity, inattention, poor service, and bad food patients were quick to add their observations of the unsanitary conditions that prevailed in hospitals from time to time. Patients understood that cleanliness was the modern hospital's ruling imperative. One Vancouver General public ward patient who was issued clean bed linen just once a week, and who had seen patients sharing towels, asserted that everyone knew that in a hospital "everything should be spotlessly clean."[51] Evidence to the contrary – noxious odours, stained linens, unclean patients, shoddy housekeeping, and, above all, vermin – elicited pointed complaints and strenuous rebuttals. And in these matters, patients were not the only source of critical observations. Depending on political jurisdiction and the specific charters of individual hospitals, "visiting governors," grand juries, municipal medical health officers, and provincial hospital inspectors also monitored hospital conditions with greater, or lesser, degrees of perspicacity. The Winnipeg General, the Cornwall General, and the Royal Columbian, for example, had Hospital Visitors whose task was to make monthly inspections and to file written reports on the physical condition of the hospital and the concerns of patients. Of course, the mice appeared at their own, not the visitor's convenience, and the cockroach always surfaced in the patient's, not the inspector's, soup. Vancouver General Hospital had "nice fat shiny fellows" according to several public ward patients whose reports were vigorously denied until a public official found cockroaches in the kitchen, leading to this bit of journalistic doggerel:

Said the doctor to the nurse,
"Oh, what do you have to drink?"
Said she, "Since you're so kind,
Some Cockroach soup, I think."

Oh, the microbe's on the spoon,
And the cockroach in the soup.
If the photo man don't come soon
We'll never get the group.[52]

Hospital authorities tended to interpret these criticisms as trivial, uninformed expressions of ingratitude from people who were restored to health, at someone else's expense, by the combined scientific and financial power of an institution the complexity of which was beyond ordinary understanding.[53] What the public knew was that a "patient is taken to the operating room, given something to put him to sleep, is operated upon, [and] returned to his bed to let nature takes its course." What remained unseen and unappreciated, said the administrators, were the costly infrastructures of "mere" patient maintenance that underpinned this apparently simple medical process, structures whose regrettable but inevitable shortcomings could be attributed to a single factor, money, not to the hospital's failure to use its limited resources more appropriately as defined by patients' overactive sensitivities.[54] The final proof of the hospital's efficiency, in any event, was medical effectiveness, the test, as one doctor put it, of whether "science as young as the aeroplane or the radio [was] craw[ling] out its application ... in [a] stage coach."[55]

Medically, the patient population of a fully articulated public general hospital in the late 1930s consisted of three principal groups: women admitted for ante natal care and childbirth (and, subsequently, their newborns); other acute-care cases (primarily pre- and postoperative surgical cases) of both sexes and all ages but tending toward younger rather than older patients; and chronically ill and incurable male and female patients of all ages but generally elderly. The census of discharged patients conducted for the Department of Health's *Survey of Public General Hospitals in Ontario* in 1937 reported that 22 per cent of patients were mothers and their newborn infants, 24 per cent other acute care (including surgical) patients, and 54 per cent chronically ill and incurable (including surgical) patients. Indigents accounted for 53 per cent of the chronic and incurable cases, and for nearly two-thirds of the total number of days of chronic care provided (see Appendix P).[56] This distribution clearly was badly skewed, but not caused, by the depression. The predominance of maternity cases was a phenomenon of the 1920s when public and professional concern over unacceptable levels of infant and maternal mortality persuaded more women and their doctors that the hospital was a safer birth venue than home. Similarly, postwar social and economic dislocation, as well as demographic change, brought to the hospital a swelling population of indigents and chronically ill social dependants unable to find alternative sources of care.

The presence of so many chronic and incurable cases diluted the hospital's preferred mix of acute and chronic patients to an extent that doctors, hospital boards, and administrators found alarming and wrong-headed, medically, socially, and financially.[57] A 1936 investigation into the medical causes of long stays in Ontario hospitals identified, in descending order, chronic cardiac and arterial disease, cancer, tuberculosis, non-tubercular pulmonary diseases, arthritis, and osteomylitis as the leading causes of extended chronic care.[58] A more comprehensive analysis two years later added venereal disease and certain diseases of the central nervous system as major contributors.[59] Apart from surgical intervention in some cases, medicine had no remedies for these conditions. Patients' symptoms were treated while their money or their entitlements to charity lasted. It is important to note that not all long-stay patients were chronically ill or incurable. Some were the unwilling victims of institutional and medical inefficiency. Others outstayed medical need by choice. On the other hand, most chronic cases, especially among the indigent, were also long-stay patients whose primarily custodial existence was the result of many factors. Homelessness, poverty, the refusal of families and relatives to accept discharged patients, and the limited availability of convalescent or other facilities for the care of incurables, the chronically ill, or the merely elderly all contributed to the re-emergence of the hospitals' archaic and unwelcomed role as a warehouse for the sick poor who once defined the hospital's identity, and after 1920 comprised its swelling resident underclass.[60]

The hospital's modern mission, on the other hand, was exemplified by the growth and importance after the Great War of its newest clientele, birthing women. By 1940 the institutionalization of childbirth across Canada was very nearly complete, led by Vancouver where, in 1940, 92 per cent of all live births took place in a hospital.[61] This development was fuelled by one of Canada' major public health and medical failures, unacceptably high – indeed, some of the highest in the Western world – rates of maternal and infant mortality. Amid growing concern in the 1920s on the part of medical and social service professionals and public health authorities, and demands from female activists for a "national and nonpartisan" crusade to "spread the gospel" of "the dangers of the midwife, the fatality of exhaustion, the necessity of medical care and the realization of its availability from the beginning of pregnancy to term,"[62] doctors and hospitals successfully convinced growing numbers of women (especially middle-class women) that the best interests of mother and newborn lay in routine professional prenatal supervision followed by the safety and the convenience of hospital deliveries, including medical intervention to hasten birth and render it painless (through drugs, most commonly the "twilight sleep" procedure).[63] As the frequency of hospital births grew, however, so did the evidence that hospitalization did not reduce maternal and infant mortality and, for reasons that remain unclear, probably exacerbated both before the 1940s. In Ontario by the mid-1930s the hospital rate of maternal mortality (5.3 deaths per 1,000 live births) was twice as high as the rate for home births, and the death-rate among parturient women who contracted puerperal sepsis in hospital was 27 per cent. Worse, the maternal mortality rate among those (principally middle-class) women whose labour was controlled or intervened in by a doctor was four times higher than for women in the hospitals' public and indigent wards who were left alone to experience natural labour.[64] Hospital authorities and clinical obstetricians were quick to blame general practitioners, or imperfectly trained generalists posing as obstetricians, for this sad record, in particular for succumbing to the temptation of "meddlesome midwifery" either for their own or the patient's convenience, intervening in the birth process when only "watchful waiting" was necessary until nature required modest assistance.[65]

A more serious charge was physician incompetence. The Vancouver Hospital Survey Commission's 1931 report categorically denounced the assumption that "every practitioner … is competent to do forceps applications, versions, genital repairs and other major surgical manipulations" related to childbirth, and demanded that the vgh (which had no obstetrician with post-graduate training in that speciality on staff) enforce rigid rules for obstetrical practice.[66] Hospitals argued that it only appeared to be more dangerous to give birth in their facilities because, by definition, they received a disproportionate share of the most difficult cases.[67] If deaths following abortions are included in obstetric mortality rates, the hospitals' claim has some merit. By the mid-1930s, when maternal mortality rates were showing signs of significant improvement, abortion-related deaths accounted for 46 per cent of all maternal deaths in British Columbia as more and more women turned to abortion as a secondary form of birth control and family limitation.[68] But most evidence suggests that, as patients in Canadian hospitals before 1940 at least, women in childbirth were at best trading off their own and their infant's safety against convenience for their physicians and the dubious benefits of a restful environment and a hazy remembrance of a painful interlude in their lives.

The hospital's other acute-care patients, principally surgical cases, had always been regarded as the defining clientele of the new model hospital, all the more if they were paying, short-stay examples of the therapeutic efficacy of invasive surgery. Their patterns of, and reasons for, admission were established early in the history of the modern hospital. At the small Cornwall General Hospital in 1908, when about 45 per cent of patients treated annually were surgical cases, previously exceptional abdominal and genito-urinary surgery accounted for 60 per cent of all the operations performed.[69] At the much larger Winnipeg General Hospital, abdominal, genito-urinary, and throat (tonsillectomies) surgery constituted nearly 70 per cent of all surgical work at about the same time.[70] This pattern remained largely unchanged for the next thirty years. In Ontario in 1937, the most common causes of hospitalization for acute treatment (after childbirth) were tonsillectomies, appendectomies, accidental injuries, herniotomies, stomach ulcers, cholecystitis, and genito-urinary problems requiring surgery.[71] What had changed in the meantime was the safety and security associated with surgical intervention. As Appendix Q illustrates, between 1900 and 1946 the percentage of surgical patients, as a proportion of all patients treated at the Winnipeg General Hospital, increased from less than a third to nearly 60 per cent. At the same time, surgical mortality per 1,000 operations was reduced by 45 per cent and, notwithstanding this vast increase in the number of operations performed, the contribution of surgical death to total hospital mortality remained fairly constant. These results made surgery the jewel in the crown of medical specialization in

Canadian hospitals, a record of performance assiduously promoted by hospital boards and administrators, and jealously defended by surgeons against the threatened depredations of amateurs. Professor Jasper Halpenny, the senior surgeon in the Winnipeg General Hospital, sounded the alarm at the 1919 meeting of the Canadian Medical Association. "It should be settled beyond a preadventure that the entrance of a patient on the roll of a reputable hospital should carry with it a guarantee [from the hospital board] that any surgical procedures undertaken will be reasonably well done ... It must be candidly admitted that many necessary operations are badly done ... and that sometimes unnecessary operations are done." If patients lost confidence in hospital surgery, Halpenny warned, hospitals could cease to exist. He thought that there were already signs of patient mistrust in his own institution,[72] fears that must have been exacerbated a year later when at least 23 WGH surgical patients in two months developed acute postoperative streptococcal peritonitis attributed to contaminated surgical gauze. Six of them died.[73]

Halpenny's critique came just as the debate over "closed" and "open" hospitals had been largely settled in favour of the general practitioners and at the outset of the standardization movement which was intended to enhance the medical efficiency of hospitals and the medical authority of physicians and surgeons. But Halpenny saw standardization as a conservative movement to entrench medical democracy by making it possible for more doctors to participate in the work of the hospital as long as they paid lip service to the processes defined by the new standards. Standardization, he contended, would discourage innovation and excellence and, in the case of surgery in the open hospital, simply open up surgical opportunities for untrained practitioners who were indifferent to diagnostic accuracy and for whom surgery was a form of "carpentry."[74] Thirty years later, when general practitioners were again on the defensive against elite specialism and seeking to protect, through the articulation of new standards of general practice, their continued access to completely open hospitals, they frankly admitted that the principal criticism levelled at them, serious "errors of commission in ... surgery," was probably warranted.[75] It is difficult to provide historical chapter and verse on the relative frequency of these errors of commission on the busiest service of the country's general hospitals where, to all intents and purposes, the rate of surgical success, at least as measured by mortality rates, was quite acceptable, and appears to have been no worse in small town hospitals than in large metropolitan institutions.

Where intensive investigations were undertaken, they tended to identify a familiar litany of problems some of which put patients at risk, and others that further incapacitated or at least greatly inconvenienced patients and added to the costs of their hospitalization. For example, the consultants who investigated the Vancouver General Hospital in 1929–30 advised that there was too great "a tendency to rush patients to the operating room with the claim that the situation [was] an emergency when, in fact, no emergency exist[ed]." The problem was inaccurate diagnosis which, when followed by unnecessary or inappropriate surgery, led to prolonged convalescences for patients who should never have been hospitalized, or who would have responded to more appropriate treatment much more quickly and with better results. The consultants guessed that 75 per cent of the hospital's long-stay postoperative patients fell into this category.[76] Similarly, a 1936 analysis of long-stay patients in Ontario general hospitals identified unnecessarily lengthy preoperative hospitalization when no useful diagnostic work was done, disagreements among surgeons over appropriate therapy, and unjustifiably prolonged convalescence from herniotomies and appendectomies in particular, as evidence of medical inefficiency and as major sources of inflated hospital costs and inconvenience – not to mention pain, suffering, and expense – to patients.[77] In both of these instances it was indigent patients who were the principal, but not the exclusive, recipients of inappropriate, ineffective, untimely, or unwarranted surgery that tended to prolong even further their typically – due to social factors – extended sojourns in hospitals. But paying patients were not immune from these excesses that, if nothing else, exacerbated the financial and medical plight of "the patient of moderate means."

A 1932 survey of 1,000 Canadian hospital workers – doctors, nurses, and administrators – attempted to assign responsibility for excessive hospitalization that contributed to overcrowded wards, higher operating costs, and increased patient financial liability. Forty per cent of the respondents blamed doctors, 40 per cent patients, and 20 per cent hospital administrators. Patients, it was claimed, were too frequently hospitalized merely for the convenience of doctors, who would also readily agree not to discharge either a paying or an indigent patient who insisted on remaining in hospital. Administrators, on the other hand, appeared to restrain their authority to deal with the problem equally out of concern for the hospital's public relations, and out of fear for the legal liability that might ensue from arbitrary decisions about admission and discharge. Many patients, finally, were not motivated to leave the hospital, either because they could afford, in the case of well-to-do patients, the comparative luxury of private accommodations and service, or, in the case of indigents, because they had nowhere else to go. Whatever the cause, the report concluded, on any given day the well-being of one-fifth of Canada's hospitalized patients would have been better served in some other environment.[78] If this estimate had been inflated by the number of women at risk giving birth in the hospital, it would have been considerably higher. But it is also too easy to question, in hindsight, the motives and actions of doctors, patients, hospital authorities, and governments who, in attempting to cope with the staggering evidence, and the physical, psychological, and social effects, of sickness and disease, used the resources of the public hospital unashamedly, and sometimes inappropriately, given the limited tools at their disposal to address matters of life and death.

As one physician remarked, comparing the success of the public health movement with the vicissitudes of individual health care, the "medical army as it attacks disease in communities is fairly modern and effective. As it attacks disease in individuals it is almost a mob, with little concerted action, little co-ordination, no one plan of campaign. Indeed, it can scarcely be said to attack disease at all. The individual medical soldier has to wait until disease attacks, then engage as best he can, pretty much on the primitive plan of 'When you see a head, hit it.'"[79] This comment neatly captures the essence of the thesis advanced by some medical historians, Charles Hayter for example, that "enthusiastic empiricism" on the part of clinicians eager to enhance the physician's role as healer was at least as important as basic laboratory science in expanding the actual effectiveness, and the promise, of medical science in the early twentieth century. Hayter cites the example of the widespread use of radiation therapy by inexpert generalists, and the subsequent struggle of community hospitals, general practitioners, and patients to promote local control over this dangerous but potentially life-saving technology in the face of attempts to restrict and centralize its employment to a few expert scientists in large metropolitan hospitals.[80] To individual physicians and their patients, the potential of the technology to prolong life not only outweighed its unknown dangers but was also a powerful argument for general accessibility by a society that increasingly equated medical "science" with the ability to postpone death.[81] From this perspective, in spite of its limitations, before the age of miracles the modern hospital was the place where medicine's footsoldiers refined their tactical weaponry through the trial and error processes of actual, not theoretical, combat.

In the final analysis, the "patient etherized upon the table" was the essential symbol of medical progress between 1890 and 1950. For the rest, the principal tasks of doctor and hospital were to assemble all of the evidence on the patient's condition "like ... a court trial, with the diagnosis as the verdict,"[82] then to assist the patient to overcome his or her fears and anxieties about the prognosis, and, finally, to lead the patient, through self-knowledge, to the necessary acceptance and accommodation of biological reality.[83]

Charles Rosenberg has observed that within just two decades of the hospital's modern transformation all of the criticisms commonly levelled at American hospitals today had already been articulated.[84] This was the Canadian experience as well. Patients encountered, and resented, hospital service that was socially judgmental, therapeutically challenged, discriminatory, paternalistic, bureaucratic, impersonal, demeaning, frequently inaccessible, sometimes harmful, and, depending on the patient's ability to pay, downright inhospitable. Governments insisted that hospitals were wasteful, inefficient, and elitist. Among members of the medical profession, the specialists and the general practitioners promoted their respective views that hospital-based medical practice was either too democratic or too restrictive; but both were united in condemning governments and hospital authorities – laymen all – for pursuing policies that restrained the free exercise of medical judgment and authority by sustaining a system in which the responsibilities and costs of social medicine undermined the efficiency of scientific medicine. Caught in the centrifuge of criticism, hospital boards and administrators publicly clung to the voluntarist conception of the hospital as a civic obligation to provide equitable health care for all by taxing the most affluent members of the community in order to provide medical charity to the least of its members; and they defended the efficiency of the model of hospital organization and management that they had invented to meet those obligations. Among themselves, hospital authorities bemoaned the system that required them to divert their hospital's wealth from the creation of temples of medical progress to meet public responsibilities still rooted in Victorian social morality and the image of the defunct charity hospital. Yet, nearly everyone – patients, doctors, trustees, administrators – agreed that the new hospital was an absolute necessity as the community's primary source of progressive acute care and preventive medical science for the whole population.

They also agreed that what had gone seriously wrong with their creation between 1890 and 1940 was precisely that its benefits increasingly accrued, however disproportionately, to the Mr Grants and the Mrs Joneses at the expense of everyone in between. The ability of "patients of moderate means" to access, on middle-class incomes, essential hospital services consonant with their presumed

social status had been compromised to the point where hospitalization threatened to pauperize, socially and financially, the very users
who had spawned the modern hospital and upon whose continued
patronage the future of the model depended. The failure of the hospital, and, more generally, the "system," to insulate the middle class
from the prospect or the reality of public ward – worse, indigent –
hospitalization was a constant theme in hospital and medical journals, in government reports, and of hospital public relations between
the wars. The patient's perspective was succinctly condensed in a
three-part investigative report published by *The Chatelaine* magazine
in 1929. For the average patient, the report claimed, the hospital had
become a "mysterious and exasperating" institution in which the
patient was an uninformed and unwitting participant in a "drama he
does not understand." Hospital boards, administrators, and doctors
had obscured the hospital's purpose in order to promote their respective agendas, creating a "mongrel combination of philanthropic,
professional, and business" objectives that militated against the necessary definition of the hospital as a patient-centred "public utility
for all taxpayers." The result was a secretive, autocratic, paternalistic
institution in which standards of care were determined, at one
extreme, by "the fussy Jones[es]" and at the other by the limits of
public philanthropy to the indigent sick who, provided they were
willing to endure the humility and the regimentation of medical charity, were given more thorough diagnostic evaluations and more comprehensive care than middle-class patients who only received the
care they could actually afford.[85] Affordability, the report concluded,
was simply beyond the average middle-class patient because the
"extortionate and unjustifiable" costs of hospital and medical services were determined by the unregulated interplay of professional
self-interest, institutional inefficiency, and inappropriate public policies that, for example, permitted the cost of a single procedure to
range from $50 to $1,000, depending solely on the patient's ability to
pay. The irony was that the people of moderate means who supported the hospital with their taxes and who shunned medical charity
were the least likely to be able to afford these services at any price.[86]
For them, the author concluded, affordable health care for all had
taken on the urgency of a new national policy.[87]

When the House of Commons Select Committee on Social Security
finally stated the case for national health insurance, it felt compelled
to offer both a general and a "special" defence of its proposed plan.
The general case was based on the concept of the "social minimum"
standard of health care for all Canadians. The special case was the
minimum standard acceptable to, and appropriate for, the "patient of

moderate means."[88] It was an acknowledgment that, fifty years on, and with the best of intentions, the new model of hospital-based community health care that had emerged after 1890 still succeeded best in doing what Victorian medicine had done, treating the rich and warehousing the poor. Socialized medicine was the Canadian solution to the problem of providing continued, equitable accessibility to health care for the middle class, just when an international revolution in medical therapeutics was about to alter permanently the scientific, social, and economic parameters of the people's health.

Health Care Déjà Vu

In the interval between Mackenzie King's first abortive postwar attempt to introduce national health insurance and the promulgation, in 1957, of the federal government's *Hospital Insurance and Diagnostic Services Act*, Canada's inventory of general hospitals grew by 58 per cent. The number of patient days provided annually by these 750 hospitals increased by two-thirds; but the cost of providing them leapt by 185 per cent, while yearly total general hospital expenditures increased by nearly 400 per cent. In the hospital insurance scheme's first year of operation under provincial legislation, hospital expenditures nationally were inflated by 30 per cent.[1] A decade after the passage of the *Medical Care Act* in 1966 and its implementation in 1968, Canadians had the highest rate of hospitalization in the western world, Canadian health-care costs had climbed to $1.5 billion annually, and future demand was estimated to be 'literally unlimited" as chronic and degenerative diseases related to lifestyles and longevity drove health-care costs constantly upward.[2] By the late 1970s, provincial governments were convinced that containment of the demand for, and the cost of, the therapeutic promises of modern hospital-centred medicine was an urgent social and fiscal priority. Their search for a functional model of hospital and medical services consistent with the limitations of the public purse, the needs and expectations of the sick, and the aspirations of medical science is a work still in progress. It has been in progress since the beginning of the twentieth century when the Victorian charity hospital was first transformed into the community general hospital providing scientific, hospital-based medical care to men, women, and children of all class-es. *Who pays?* is the only question that seems to have been more or less settled in the last hundred years. Who requires, and benefits from, hospitalization? What are the legitimate functions of the hospi-tal relative to other modes of health-care delivery? What are the cost/benefit implications of the diminishing returns from expensive diagnostic technologies and therapeutic procedures largely employed to psychologically anaesthetize patients perpetually wor-ried about, but helpless in the face of, their own mortality? Why have we come to regard death as evidence of the failure of the health-care system?[3] All these issues, rooted in the often conflicting priorities of politics, patients, and health professionals, were inherent in the rise of the modern hospital as the temple of scientific medicine.

A century ago, when the advent of safe surgery, modern nursing science, diagnostic technology, and vigorous professional competi-tion first engendered a buyer's market for scientific health care, contemporary observers predicted the exponential growth of hospital-based medical services and the costs for their provision as the bene-fits of scientific progress became more popular. Hospital boards and health professionals optimistically reasoned, however, that costs could be contained and accessibility maintained by hospitals' com-mitment to diagnostic accuracy, the therapeutic potential of surgical intervention, the recuperative effectiveness of professional nursing care, and the efficiency of modern business methods. These strengths would coalesce in an institution dedicated to timely, successful inter-vention in cases of acute, treatable illness. The demise of the general hospital's unsavory Victorian reputation as a medically irrelevant custodial facility for the infectious and the poor would be followed by an era in which the reach of scientifically-mediated and special-ized health care for all was limited, apparently, only by hospitals' ability to accommodate demand. The costs – never cheap – to the new paying consumer were justified in terms of hospitals' demonstrable success in returning patients speedily to health and productivity from the terrors of once-fatal illnesses. Moreover, there was a level of hospital service geared to each patient's ability to pay, from the spar-tan public ward to the most luxurious private suite, so the spectre of "the cost" arguably had less to do with medical necessity than with the physical amenities required to satisfy the dictates of social and economic status, or pretension. Confident that on these terms the public, as paying patients, as municipal taxpayers, and as subscribers to hospitals' charitable obligations, would support the purpose, the priorities, and the financial requirements of the new model public general hospital, the voluntary boards of directors who responded to and nurtured this new opportunity set about making it work. Their own voluntarism was their guarantee of unimpeachable intent, unquestioned control their bible of management, and Taylorite "efficiency" the litmus test of their medical, financial, and social accountability. The factory whose product was health, whose surgeons were its skilled craftsmen, whose nurses kept the line moving with military discipline, and whose managers practised economy to a fault promised a double dividend – not just health, but health affordable to all but the indigent.

From the outset, however, the new public general hospital's medical and scientific priorities, and the economic assumptions that underpinned them, continued to be challenged by the presence of the indigent poor, whom the hospitals were not allowed to abandon in their quest for scientific legitimacy and popular approbation. A creature of the conflicting Victorian impulses of responsibility for, and control of, the improvident, the general hospital began life as the product of a social contract among provincial governments, municipalities, the medical profession, and private philanthropists to provide medical relief to the deserving sick poor. The hospital's modern priorities were superimposed upon this inherited responsibility in the expectation that continued public generosity, medical efficiency, a starkly economical free service – neither more, nor less, than the poor deserved – and the expansion of professional philanthropy as the trade-off for hospital-centred medical practices, would carry the hospital's historical burden of charitable care and treatment without detriment to its new scientific mandate. But events conspired to thwart this optimism. The business cycle's regularly occurring valleys, immigration, demographic shifts, social structural transformation, and changing patterns of disease and population health repetitively inflated the quantity, the scope, and the costs of the public hospitals' charitable obligations to the extent that, especially after the First World War, they sapped the public and private resources available to sustain hospitals' legal responsibilities for medical charity. Boards turned to the only available sources of this required income – fees charged to paying patients in the public, semi-private, and private wards, and institutional debt – in order to generate the resources both to sustain a minimum standard of hospital services for all patients, and to satisfy hospitals' appetite for medical progress. Throughout the 1920s hospitals inflated the fees of paying patients and implemented a catalogue of diagnostic surcharges that further elevated the cost of hospitalization. The potential of this strategy had already been exhausted, at least in terms of consumer tolerance, when the Great Depression finally exposed – to the point of impending total collapse – the historical tenuousness of hospitals' financial structures, social assumptions, and public policies. They required hospital-centred community health care to provide the services of a public utility using a business model better suited to an industrial enterprise and inconsistent with the economic circumstances of half the population who simply could not afford health care.

Of the remaining 50 per cent of the population, the majority fell into the category of "patients of moderate means," middle-class families whose incomes would tolerate brief periods of hospitalization for acute treatment, but not prolonged care. Moreover, they were caught in a conundrum partly of their own making and partly the product of hospital merchandising. From the beginning, middle-class paying patients shunned the cheaper public wards (sometimes with good reason) which they associated with indigence, and demanded differentiated care defined by greater personal privacy, comfort, choice of medical attendants, and the undivided attentions of care-givers. Hospitals responded by creating, and promoting the attractions of, hotels for paying patients constructed on foundations in which the poor – sometimes literally – were accommodated. The socially structured voluntary hospital thus reflected the class distinctions of the community in which "keeping up with the Joneses" and the defense of privacy were the essence of respectability. But the tolerance of middle-class patients for the price of medical respectability was not infinite. By the 1920s, as the costs of hospitalization soared, the potential impact on middle-class standards of living raised serious concern among hospital boards, managers, and members of the medical profession, who began to measure the health of their institutions and their practices in terms of their continuing ability to attract paying patients. There was already ample evidence of consumer resistance to a regime in which the measurable benefits of modern medicine – privacy and aesthetics aside – seemed to accrue inequitably to the very poor and the very rich, while the middle-class paying patient, whose fees largely sustained the hospitalization of the sick poor, was gradually being squeezed out of the hospital under the threat of financial ruin or medical pauperization. The subsequent wholesale retreat of paying patients from the hospital during the 1930s provided the pretext for a re-examination of the problem of health-care accessibility for all Canadians; and the medical plight of the middle class subsequently became the "special" argument for a national health insurance scheme, one that still permitted, for those who could afford it, differentiated care within a socially acceptable universal level of basic care – the centrepiece of postwar social and economic reconstruction. Whatever other benefits it conferred – on the poor, on rural and remote areas historically deprived of health services, on the chronically ill, and on the incurable – national hospital, and later medical, insurance at last relieved the middle class of the direct responsibility for the medical welfare of all Canadians, a burden they had largely acquired since the emergence of the modern hospital.

The least enthusiastic of the partners essential to any public hospital or health insurance scheme was the medical profession, in particular general practitioners. This hardly seems surprising in the light of their most recent experience with governments when, during the depression, municipal, provincial, and federal unemployment relief policies left doctors either unpaid, or only partially remunerated, for continuing to provide full medical services to relief recipients in their surgeries and in public hospitals. This reversal of economic fortune, soon to be compounded by a threatened loss of the general practitioners' professional status, in the mid-1940s, with the re-emergence of hospital-centred specialism as the preferred focus of medical education and practice, seemed to portend the end of a golden age of medicine, the age in which physician's professional and material success had derived from their hard-won hospital privileges, the cornerstone of general practice since the beginning of the century. Then, the rank and file of medical men, in search of professional advantage and scientific credibility, had convinced reluctant boards and proprietary specialists that joint possession of the new model hospital was good for business, better for patients, and best for medical science. Group practice brought the whole medical armamentarium of the hospital to bear on the patient's well-being, the patient, in the first instance, of the ubiquitous family physician who was thus an indispensable source of the hospital's preferred clientele. In this way, the "surgeon's workshop" also became the independent general practitioners' subsidized place of business, centre for continuing education, source of scientific legitimacy, and monument to their claim to professional exclusivity. For the next three decades doctors worked assiduously to end hospital abuse by patients fraudulently seeking medical charity, to define the limits of medical philanthropy in relation to hospitals' social responsibilities, to exclude medical "cults," and to expand the doctors' role in the hospital's medical, managerial, and political processes. For the most part they succeeded. But in the end, the "open" hospital proved to be a "closed" shop in at least one important respect, the limit of physician control.

As it became more and more difficult for hospitals to hold demand, accessibility, income, and costs in equilibrium in the interests of paying and indigent patients alike, doctors moved to ensure that hospitals' only legitimate priorities were medical priorities as determined by the practitioners' vested interest in maintaining the widest possible institutional latitude for professional freedom of action. Boards, on the other hand, became less and less tolerant of the license with which practitioners interpreted their privileges, of the apparent lack of quality control in a self-regulating profession, and of the assumption that medical priorities were the only legitimate driver of hospital policies and processes. When hospital boards consequently sought to restrain professional *laissez-faire* in the interests of institutional probity, the symbiosis between the "camp followers of the army of science" and their institutional partners began to dissolve in disputes. Their culmination was the withdrawal in the 1930s of physicians' services from hospitals, and the denunciation of compulsory public hospital and medical insurance, in British Columbia for example, as a threat to the continued independence of the individual physician in a free market for medical services. By the 1940s, when a national health insurance scheme seemed inevitable, the profession was once again in full defensive mode, insisting, as doctors had at the creation of the modern hospital a half-century earlier, that the essential criteria for any new system of health care must be physician control and the centrality of the hospital, the doctor's workshop, in which the recently tarnished principle of equitable ownership was to be fully restored.

Nurses, hospitals' other skilled medical workers, had pretensions to no similar proprietary claims over their workplace, if only because the master-servant relationship between the predominantly student nurses and their medical, nursing, and lay superiors, reinforced by the gendered division of work, meant that hospital-centred nursing was neither a recognizable occupation nor a profession with an agenda to pursue. It was a novitiate – for a higher calling – characterized by learning through obedience instilled by rigorous regimentation and discipline whose aim was to create a medical assistant who would respond predictably and consistently to the instructions of doctors, the needs of patients, and the routine of the sick room in, or out, of hospital. For the majority, graduation promised independent employment as private duty nurses; for some, professional advancement as a specialized nurse, head nurse, matron, or lady superintendent in a hospital, or perhaps as a public health nurse or social worker; for others, "jill-of-all-trades" employment as laboratory technicians, technologists, physiotherapists, and even anaesthetists in hospitals too small or too poor to support a full complement of paramedical assistants. Meanwhile, the generic hospital nursing student, the institution's essential worker, part domestic servant and part acolyte, served, frequently in return for third-rate training geared to students of often indifferent abilities, at the pleasure of an institution that valued her first because of the economies that flowed from her essentially indentured labour. Hospital nursing in Canada thus fell considerably short of Florence Nightingale's ideal of the physician's handmaiden recruited from the middle classes to improve and elevate the quality of medical care through her unique combination of intelligence, natural nurturing instincts, social values, and specialized training. Nevertheless, the presence, and the nature, of skilled nursing services in Canadian hospitals after 1880 had contributed significantly to the growing attraction of the public general hospital to paying patients by the turn of the century. If this attraction was partly the appeal of having someone akin to a servant – a disappearing breed – as close as the patient's silent call bell to answer every need real or imagined, it must also have come from the reassuring presence of a sympathetic, attentive, knowledgeable, tactful, non-threatening, social equal who acted as intermediary between the individual patient with his or her fears, expectations, apprehensions – and pain, and an institution that, even as it was being reborn, had to ask itself whether patients were "persons" or "cases."[4] For all of these reasons, between 1900 and 1930 the number of hospital nursing schools in Canada grew disproportionately to the number of general hospitals that could fairly offer academically rigorous training programs, because until the 1920s nursing and nursing education were largely unregulated. When provincial regulation and nurse registration were introduced, hospitals successfully resisted changes that would have further exacerbated their already precarious financial arrangements had they redressed the balance of student nurses' academic and ward responsibilities. Only when war, alternative employment opportunities for young women, and the postwar explosion of demand for hospitalization forced hospitals to hire large numbers of graduate nurses, at enormous cost, did the historical false economies of student nursing come home to roost. Meanwhile, three generations of Canadian nursing students served as the public hospitals' first line of deference to the wishes and needs of patients and practitioners alike.

Between 1890 and 1950, hospitalization for patients in an institution large enough to support diagnostic technology, the latest surgical techniques, specialized obstetrical care, a nursing school, and both private and public wards, was an experience that varied markedly with the patient's medical, social, and financial circumstances. In general, any given public hospital population consisted of patients who paid and medical indigents; patients with treatable acute illnesses and those whose diseases were chronic or incurable; and patients who medically required hospitalization and those who required it for social and economic reasons. The correlation among paying patients, treatable diseases, and short stays, on one hand, and, on the other, medical indigents, long stays, and chronic or incurable diseases was manifest from the outset. General hospitals' medical stock-in-trade, their unique contribution to the people's health, was diagnostic skill and surgical dexterity. Consequently, hospitals marshalled their resources to provide the best medical and convalescent services available to people suffering acute illnesses who would benefit most from this limited, but effective, diagnostic and therapeutic regime, irrespective of the patient's ability to pay. But social condition, financial circumstances, race, ethnicity, gender in some cases, and even the nature of their diseases, relegated some patients to the status of regimented inmates in free and special wards where conditions frequently were not much of an improvement on nineteenth-century hospitals. The free wards contrasted starkly with the elegant tranquility of the private and semi-private wards restricted to the hospitals' essential clientele, short-stay paying patients. The general hospital thus developed a reputation for being socially as well as medically judgmental in addition to its legendary financial imperiousness.

Nevertheless, for a quarter-century hospitals successfully defended these institutional biases that they attributed to the dictates of the marketplace, medical necessity, social utility, and institutional efficiency. But for a growing number of middle-class Canadians after the First World War, financial self-reliance when faced with hospitalization threatened to become the path to pauperization as the price of health care soared ominously. Consumer resistance to hospitalization on these terms steadily developed throughout the 1920s, fuelled by paying patients' fears about the preservation of individual choice in hospital services. Those fears materialized as the social reality of the 1930s, when doctors and hospitals were overwhelmed by the demand for free treatment and care. Hospitals ascribed this debacle to the historical failure of public policy to provide adequately for the medical relief of the poor, imperiling in the process the independence of the middle-class consumer and jeopardizing the medical utility of the hospital for all patients. But there was also an accumulating body of evidence that excessive hospitalization and inappropriate medical intervention were also driving hospitals' related problems of costs, prices, and accessibility. Hospitalization frequently was medically inappropriate, unnecessary, unjustifiable, or merely convenient for patients or doctors. Similarly, the treatment available was often unsuitable, incompetently administered, or predictably ineffective, given the state of medical knowledge and practice. Hospitalization was wasted on, or failed to benefit, at least one in four patients. But for the sick, the community hospital simply had become synonymous, between 1890 and 1940, with the promise and the expectation of healing and recovery accessible to all.

By 1945, the fulfilment of the promise was seen to be only a question of political will to guarantee universal accessibility to standardized hospital services everywhere, irrespective of individual circumstances, as an objectively good, historically justified, national social policy. Individual health thus became a public responsibility in Canada just as the postwar therapeutic revolution launched a new stage of modern medicine. It would test the limits of Canadians' political commitment to the new culture of hospital-mediated health for all at any price.

Appendices

I   Distribution of Patients by Hospital Service, Winnipeg General Hospital, 1911–1930

J   Admissions, Length of Stay, Capacity and Usage, Ontario General Hospitals, 1880–1946

K   Hospital Statistics, British Columbia and Royal Columbian Hospital, 1924–1950

L   Hospital Statistics, Manitoba and Winnipeg General Hospital, 1930–1950

M   Hospital Statistics, Ontario and Owen Sound General and Marine Hospital, 1925–1950

N   Index Numbers for Hospital Costs and Income, and Patient Charges, Per Patient Day, 1900–1946 (1913=100)

O   Ward and Method of Payment, Ontario Hospital Patients, 1948

P   Distribution of Acute and Chronic Care by Patient Classification, Ontario 1937

Q   Hospital and Surgical Mortality, Winnipeg General Hospital, 1900–1946

Hospital Costs, Income, and Income Sources, 1878–1930

	RCH 1878	TGH 1885	Ontario 1890	WGH 1900	Ontario 1910	Manitoba 1913	OSG&M 1919	B.C. 1924	WGH 1930	Ontario 1930
% Income patient fees	2.6	10.7	16.2	20.6	51.7	37.1	73.3	52.4	82.3	67.4
% Income govt. grants	97.4	63.8	61.1	24.1	30.7	28.2	18.1	44.3	16.7	22.9
% Other income	0	25.4	22.6	55.3	17.6	34.7	8.6	2.3	1.0	9.7
Cost/Patient day	1.1	0.6	0.7	1.9	1.3	2.6	2.3	4.4	3.6	3.6
Patient contribution to cppd										
$	N/A	0.08	0.1	0.1	0.6	0.7	1.8	1.8	2.5	2.7
%	N/A	12.9	19.4	10	50	29.1	78.2	41.7	70.5	73.9
% Bed capacity used				66.3	50			65	66.5	64

Sources: Province of Ontario, Legislative Assembly, Sessional Papers; PAM, Province of Manitoba,Legislative Assembly, Sessional Papers; PABC, Province of British Columbia, Department of the Provincial Secretary, Hospital Reports, 1924; Owen Sound G&M Hospital, Annual Reports; CVA, Royal Columbian Hospital, Board Minutes; PAM Winnipeg General Hospital, Annual Reports; Toronto General Hospital, Annual Reports; CVA, Royal Columbian Hospital, Board Minutes

RCH = Royal Columbian Hospital, New Westminster, B.C.

TGH = Toronto General Hospital, Toronto, Ontario

WGH = Winnipeg General Hospital, Winnipeg, Manitoba

OSG&M = Owen Sound General and Marine Hospital, Owen Sound, Ontario.

APPENDIX B

Classification by Medical Diagnosis of Patients Admitted to Hospital

	SCG&M % 1877	WGH % 1891	OSG&M % 1901	WGH % 1911	OSG&M % 1926	Ontario % 1983–84
Infectious/Parasitic	24.8	19.1	30.8	23.4	4.5	1.7
Neoplasm			2.9	3.5	3.9	6.7
Endocrine/Metabolic				0.6	1.4	2.1
Diseases of the blood			0.4		0.2	0.6
Mental disorders			4.6	0.2	0.9	4.5
Nervous System/Sensory	4.7	4.1	2.7	8.3	3.2	4.6
Circulatory			3.0	1.1	2.6	11.8
Respiratory	5.5	4.9	5.7	1.9	20.2	9.7
Digestive	7.9	9.9	17.8	18.8	13.1	11.3
Genito-urinary	4.4	7.9	8.1	5.2	6.7	8.1
Pregnancy/Childbirth	6.6	5.6	3.1	6.1	12.1	13.9
Skin diseases	4.7			1.2	0.3	1.4
Musculo-skeletal	7.4		4.6	4.2	1.4	5.4
Congenital anomalies				0.6		0.9
Perinatal					0.1	0.3
Ill-defined	7.4			1.1	0.7	0.6
Injuries/Poisoning	17.9	10.1	8.4	12.3	7.1	7.9
Others	8.5	39.4	11.3	11.4	11.1	3.1

Sources: Province of Ontario, Ministry of Health, *Hospital Statistics 1983–84* (Toronto, 1985)
PAM, Winnipeg General Hospital, Annual Reports, 1891, 1911
St Catharines General and Marine Hospital, Patient Register, 1877
Owen Sound General and Marine Hospital, Patient Register, 1925–26

APPENDIX C

Surgical Cases as Proportion of all Hospital Admissions, 1891–1930

		1891	1895	1900	1904–05	1907	1909–10	1912–13	1914	1915	1920	1925	1927	1930
WGH	#	415		813	1042	1250	2295	2574	3473	4100	7504	6776		7821
	%	36.6		31.6	26.9	24.3	38.6	45.9	41.5	44.4	58.4	50.9		55.1
VGH	#					760		2235		4532		9317		10311
	%					31.6		44.6		63.0		64.5		65.7
OSG&M	#		21				137		455	302				
	%		18.7				34.2		53.6	58.1				
RCH	#				244								1342	
	%				49.0							52.1	41.3	
CGH	#			108			240							
	%			34.0			48.9							
TGH	#	369			946		1791							
	%	10.1			24.1		32.5							

Sources: Annual Reports, Owen Sound General and Marine Hospital, Vancouver General Hospital, Royal Columbian Hospital, Winnipeg General Hospital, Cornwall General Hospital, Toronto General Hospital

WGH = Winnipeg General Hospital
VGH = Vancouver General Hospital
OSG&M = Owen Sound General and Marine Hospital
RCH = Royal Columbian Hospital
CGH = Cornwall General Hospital
TGH = Toronto General Hospital

APPENDIX D

Growth of Attending Medical Staff, Winnipeg General Hospital

	1884	1889	1892	1893	1897	1901	1908	1914
Surgery	1	1	1	1	4	3	4	4
Gynaecology						2	2	2
Ophthalmology								3
Otolaryngology			1	1	2	2	2	2
Paediatrics								1
Orthopaedics							1	2
Obstetrics	2	2	2	2	2	2	2	2
Anaesthesia						1	1	1
Pathology					1	1	2	1
Contagious diseases				2	2	2	3	4
General medicine	6	6	6	6	3	4	7	6
Radiology							1	2
Total	9	10	10	13	14	17	25	30

Source: PAM, Winnipeg General Hospital, Annual Reports

APPENDIX E

Winnipeg General Hospital Annual Patient Data, 1891–1930

	1891	1900	1905	1910	1915	1920	1930
No. in-patients treated	1,133	2,649	4,366	5,935	9,234	12,839	14,273
Avg. stay (days)	24.5	20.5		19.4		15.0	16.1
Cost/patient day ($)	0.86	1.09		1.58		3.77	3.61
% Revenue from pay patients	12.5	27.6		48.8		67.9	82.3
% Revenue from private wards	7.7	22.1		21.9	39.1	68.8	55.5
Patient fees as % of op. costs	15.8	32.9		49.2		73.1	70.5
No. operations	415	813		2,295	4,100	7,504	7,821
Surgical patients % of total	36.6	30.7		38.7	44.4	58.4	54.8
% Patients public ward	88.9						60.1
% Patients private ward	11.1						39.9
No. outpatients treated	1,105	1,435	5,735	7,660	22,583	26,408	50,441
No. x-rays	n/a	n/a	100	2,131	5,578	14,158	29,986
No. pathology exams			2,143	14,146	24,238	29,908	35,742
No. births	56	70		178		835	949
No. deaths	64	156		405		586	532
% Female patients		42.8		38.8	43.9		51.9

Sources: PAM, Province of Manitoba, Sessional Papers, 1885–1930; PAM, Winnipeg General Hospital, Annual Reports

APPENDIX F(1)

Proportional (%) Contributions to Hospital Operating Income, Ontario, 1890–1930

	1890	1895	1900	1905	1910	1915	1920	1925	1930
Governments	56.6	46.8	34.7	31.1	30.7	37.8	23.6	25.9	23.1
Patients	18.1	19.3	35.3	47.6	51.7	50.8	64.7	64.3	68.1
Voluntary	25.2	33.9	29.9	20.3	17.6	11.4	11.6	9.8	8.8

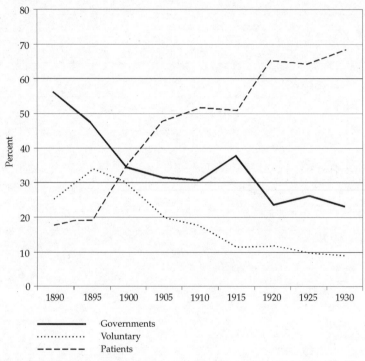

—————   Governments
·············   Voluntary
– – – – –   Patients

Source: Ontario Sessional Papers, 1880–1930

APPENDIX F(2)

Proportional (%) Contributions to Hospital Income, Quebec, 1918–1937

	1918	1922	1925	1928	1932	1937
Governments	7.5	10.1	16.1	25.2	36.5	43.3
Patients	38.7	49.5	33.2	36.9	34.9	34.9
Voluntary	20.8	11.5	9.8	8.2	6.5	4.7
Other	31.7	24.6	44.9	26.5	18.2	15.8

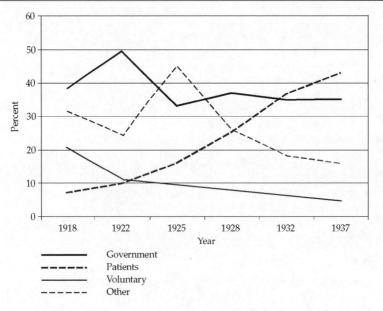

Source: Quebec, Annuaire statistique/Statistical year-book, 1918–1940

APPENDIX F(3)

Distribution of Paying and Indigent Patients,
General, Maternity, and Foundling Hospitals, Quebec, 1918–1937

	Full pay	Part pay	Indigent	% Increase in admissions
1918	36.5	24.2	39.3	
1922	32.3	22.1	45.6	9.6
1925	37.3	22.1	40.6	19.6
1928	36.7	28.1	35.2	32.6
1932	28.8	30.1	41.1	23.2
1937	17.3	38.8	41.1	39.1

Source: Quebec, Annuaire statistique/Statistical year-book, 1918–1940

APPENDIX G

Percentage of All Births Occurring in General Hospitals, Ontario, 1901–1949

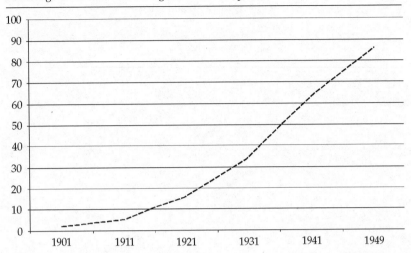

Source: Ontario, Ministry of Health, *Report of the Ontario Health Survey Committee*, Volume 1 (Toronto 1950), Table A35.

APPENDIX H

Average Duration of Patient Stays (Whole Days) by Diagnostic Classification,
Owen Sound General and Marine Hospital, 1901–1941

	1891	1900	1905	1910	1915	1920	1930
All patients	26	19	16	15	14	12	12
Infective and parasitic	30	21	21	31	31	7	18
Neoplasms	16	14	18	15	12	15	30
Allergic, endocrine	n/a	13	23	49	17	9	23
Blood and blood-forming organs	n/a	n/a	n/a	363	n/a	5	30
Mental, psychoneurotic	21	9	11	6	1	n/a	10
Nervous system, sensory organs	11	18	21	35	11	10	16
Circulatory system	22	13	13	15	8	32	16
Respiratory system	36	11	14	6	3	2	4
Digestive system	24	20	18	16	15	15	12
Genito-urinary system	18	20	21	14	10	12	17
Pregnancy, delivery, puerperium	16	14	12	12	12	11	10
Skin and cellular tissue	n/a	49	16	6	26	9	18
Bones and organs of movement	38	21	32	27	10	49	9
Congenital malformations	n/a	n/a	3	n/a	n/a	n/a	6
Neonatal, perinatal	n/a	n/a	7	n/a	14	n/a	3
Senility	n/a	20	27	21	n/a	264	19
Special admissions	27	46	2	61	7	6	4
Accidents/poisoning/ violence	27	31	27	16	17	16	17
Not stated	32	11	11	11	21	14	6
Live births	14	11	12	10	11	11	10

Source: Owen Sound General and Marine Hospital, Patient Registers, 1901–1941

APPENDIX I

Distribution of Patients by Hospital Service,
Winnipeg General Hospital, 1911–1930

	1911	1930
Medicine	22.5	20.5
Surgery	40.9	26.6
Gynaecology	4.3	6.5
Obstetrics	4.5	7.8
Births	1.9	7.1
E.E.N.T.	11.9	22.7
Urology	3.7	1.9
Orthopaedics	4.6	4.9
Other	5.5	2.1

Source: PAM, Winnipeg General Hospital, Annual Reports

APPENDIX J

Admissions, Length of Stay, Capacity and Usage, Ontario General Hospitals, 1880–1946

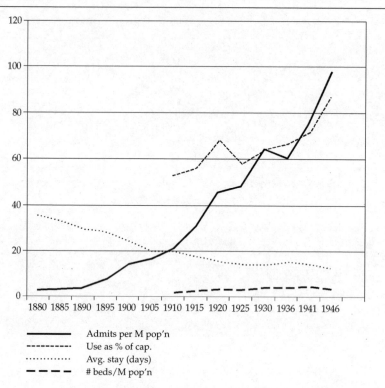

Legend:
- Admits per M pop'n
- Use as % of cap.
- Avg. stay (days)
- # beds/M pop'n

Source: Province of Ontario, Sessional papers, 1880–1946

APPENDIX K

Hospital Statistics, British Columbia and Royal Columbian Hospital, 1924–1950

British Columbia						
	1924	*1933*	*1939*	*1944*	*1950*	*1924–50*
Increase in admissions (%)		19.8	52.4	40.1	53.9	293.9
Increase in patient days (%)		27.7	23.9	16.6	40.7	159.8
Average stay (days)	14.4	14.3	13.2	11.9	9.9	
Payroll as % of expenditures	41.1	50.5	50.3	55.3	59.9	
Staff/100 patients	3.6	4.3	4.0	3.9	3.9	
% Revenue from patients	53.1	51.1	88.1	75.1		
Cost/Patient day ($)	4.44	3.29	3.78	4.85	11.23	
Public ward days as % of total			80.1	72.0		

Royal Columbian Hospital					
	1924	*1933*	*1939*	*1944*	*1950*
Increase in admission (%)		32.0	32.6	49.0	81.8
Increase in patient days (%)		66.6	1.9	37.7	60.4
Increase in total income (%)		6.6	50.0	83.3	320.7
Increase in total expenditures (%)		22.7	52.3	110.6	331.2
Cost/Patient day ($)	2.79	2.06	2.92	4.37	11.83
Average stay (days)	12.9	15.1	15.7	10.9	10.6
Payroll as % of expenditures	41.5	48.5	49.9	55.9	66.3
Staff/100 patients	3.4	4.2	4.4	4.4	5.1

Sources: Province of British Columbia, Department of the Provincial Secretary, Report on Hospital Statistics and the Administration of the "Hospital Act," 1924–1950; Vancouver City Archives, Royal Columbian Hospital, Annual Report Files, 1930–48

APPENDIX L

Hospital Statistics, Manitoba and Winnipeg General Hospital, 1930–1950

Manitoba				
	1930	1935	1940	1947
Increase in admissions (%)		10.2	12.1	44.3
Increase in patient days (%)		13.6	12.1	−10.8
Average stay (days)	14.9	15.4	15.4	10.6
Increase in total income (%)		−7.5	18.9	103.9
Increase in total expenditures (%)		−4.3	24.4	64.8
Cost/Patient day ($)	3.33	2.8	3.11	5.76
Wages as % of expenditures	32.2	39.7		44.7
Occupancy rate (%)	84.1	65.1	65.6	77.4

Winnipeg General Hospital					
	1930	1935	1940	1945	1950
Increase in admissions (%)		0.7	4.7	1.2	27.5
Average stay (days)	16.1	15.1	13.6	13.9	11.9
Cost/Patient day ($)	3.41	3.59	3.39	4.81	8.39
Increase in outpatient visits		−15.1	10.1	−16.4	52.4
Private patient fees as % of revenue	50.1	28.8	31.7	44.4	40.7
Diagnostic services as % of revenue	14.7	20.7	24.1	31.6	37.9
Surgical cases (%)	55	60	57	60	52
Public ward patients as % of total	31.7	44.0	69.7	22.9*	14.4*

*Note: By 1945 these data appear to represent *indigent* hospitalization only.

Sources: PAM, Province of Manitoba, Legislative Assembly, Sessional Papers, Annual Reports of the Department of Public Welfare, 1930–1950; PAM, Winnipeg General Hospital, Anneal Reports, 1930–1950.

APPENDIX M

Hospital Statistics, Ontario and Owen Sound General and Marine Hospital, 1925–1950

	Ontario				
	1925	1930	1935	1941	1946
Increase in admissions (%)		41.6	1.1	16.7	60.4
Increase in patient days (%)		7.6	13.4	64.3	–4.8
Average stay (days)	14	14	15	14	12
% Revenue from patients	64.3	68.0	57.8	69.6	77.5
Cost/Patient day ($)	3.35	3.97	3.46	3.84	5.03
Staff/100 patients	7.7	5.8	5.4		3.4

	Owen Sound G&M Hospital					
	1925	1930	1935	1940	1945	1949
Increase in admissions (%)		51.4	37.2	14.6	79.7	0
Increase in patient days (%)		46.1	7.8	14.6	47.1	0
Average stay (days)		14	11	11	9	9
Increase in total income (%)		62.2	12.1	40.1	118.9	missing
Increase in total costs (%)		84.3	2.7	27.7	123.5	68.8
Cost/Patient day ($)	2.83	3.57	3.48	3.79	5.76	9.80
Surgical cases as % of total (*1927)	*61.8	44.6	51.7	48.8	60.4	64.8

Sources: Province of Ontario, Legislative Assembly, Sessional Papers, Reports on General Hospitals, 1925–1950; Owen Sound General and Marine Hospital, Anneal Reports, 1925–1950.

APPENDIX N

Index Numbers for Hospital Costs and Income, and Patient Fees, Per Patient Day, Ontario, 1900–1946, where 1913=100

	Costs	Income	Fees
1900	53.5	57.1	36.7
1905	77.1	75.7	65.8
1910	91.6	87.9	82.3
1915	109.2	115.7	105.1
1920	199.9	198.4	230.4
1925	239.7	236.1	272.2
1930	257.1	279.4	340.9
1936	215.7	243.3	251.9
1941	244.3	270.6	337.9
1946	354.1	393.2	548.1

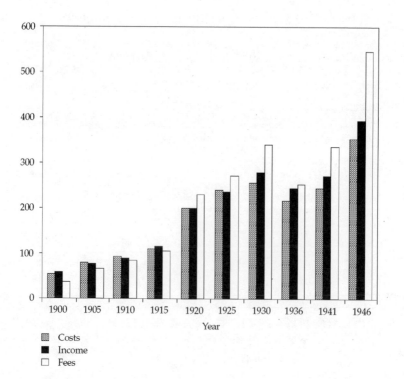

APPENDIX O

Ward and Method of Payment, Ontario Hospital Patients, 1948

	Private/Semi	Public
Total %	50	50
% Self pay	67.4	61.3
% Blue Cross	25.3	17.5
% Other	7.3	22.1

	Self Pay	Blue Cross	Indigent	Other
Total %	64.4	21.5	7.5	6.5
Private/semi	52.8	59.5	n/a	55.4
Public	47.2	40.5	100.0	44.6

	Self Pay Private/Semi	Self Pay Public	Blue Cross Private/Semi	Blue Cross Public	Indigent
Average stay (days)	9.1	8.1	8.7	8.2	25.1

Source: Adapted from Ontario, Minister of Health, *Report of the Health Survey Committee*, Volume I (1948), 23.

Distribution of Acute and Chronic Care by Patient Classification, Ontario, 1937

	% Total Patients	% All Acute Care Patnts	% All Chron. Care Patnts	% All Days of Care	% All Days Acute Care	% All Days Chron. Care
Self-pay public ward	16.5	17.6	15.6	20.3	16.3	21.5
Private/Semi-private	35.8	41.0	31.2	18.2	35.3	13.5
Indigent	47.7	41.4	53.2	61.5	48.4	65.0
All patients		46.3	53.6			
All days of care					21.6	78.4

Source: Province of Ontario, Department of Health, Division of Medical Statistics, Survey of Public General Hospitals in Ontario, 1940, Part V, Table XXII, p. 39.

Hospital and Surgical Mortality, Winnipeg General Hospital, 1900–1946

	1900	1905	1911	1915	1920	1925	1930	1935	1940	1946
Hospital mortality per 1000 patients	58	76	71	36	44	37	39	42	39	39
Surgical mortality per 1000 operations	44		29				22	27	26	24
Surgical patients as % of all patients	30.7	20.1	43.7	44.4	56.9	50.9	58.2	59.6	56.7	59.3
Surgical mortality as % of all hosp. deaths	23.1		18.4				32.7	38.2	37.2	36

Source: PAM, Winnipeg General Hospital, Annual Reports

Notes

ABBREVIATED ENDNOTE REFERENCES

Archives

BCMA British Columbia Medical Association
CVA   City of Vancouver Archives
HCA   Hamilton City Archives
PABC Public Archives of British Columbia
PAM   Public Archives of Manitoba
PAO   Public Archives of Ontario
UMA   University of Manitoba Archives

Government Records

BCSP Province of British Columbia. Legislative Assembly. Sessional
      Papers
MSP   Province of Manitoba. Legislative Assembly. Sessional Papers
OSP   Province of Ontario. Legislative Assembly. Sessional Papers

Institutions

CGH   Cornwall General Hospital
HCH   Hamilton City Hospital
OSGM Owen Sound General and Marine Hospital
RCH   Royal Columbian Hospital

SCGM   St Catharines General and Marine Hospital
TGH   Toronto General Hospital
UMFM   University of Manitoba Faculty of Medicine
VCH   Vancouver City Hospital
VGH   Vancouver General Hospital
WGH   Winnipeg General Hospital

Journals

Note: *Full references for academic journal articles are provided in the bibliography. Full references for articles from historical professional journals and magazines are provided in the notes, which make use of the following abbreviations:*

CL   *Canada Lancet*
CD   *Canadian Doctor*
CH   *Canadian Hospital*
CMAJ   *Canadian Medical Association Journal*
CN   *Canadian Nurse*
CP   *Canadian Practitioner*
DMJ   *Dominion Medical Journal*
HW   *Hospital World*
MMAB   *Manitoba Medical Association Bulletin*
MMAR   *Manitoba Medical Association Review*
MMR   *Manitoba Medical Review*
SW   *Social Welfare*
VMAB   *Vancouver Medical Association Bulletin*
WCMJ   *Western Canada Medical Journal*

INTRODUCTION

1 This historical process is summarized in David Gagan, "For 'Patients of Moderate Means,'" 151–4.
2 See Risse, *Mending Bodies, Saving Souls*, esp. chapters 7–9.
3 Woodward and Richards, "Towards a Social History of Medicine," 44.
4 Rosen, "The Hospital: Historical Sociology of a Community Institution," 2.
5 Haller, *American Medicine In Transition*, 321. The foregoing discussion is based on Starr, *The Social Transformation of American Medicine*; Rosenberg, "Inward Vision and Outward Glance"; Rosenberg, "George Rosen and the Social History of Medicine"; and Stevens, *In Sickness and in Wealth*, esp. ch 1. Vogel, *The Invention of the Modern Hospital* is a useful representative of this historiographical approach.
6 Starr, *The Social Transformation of American Medicine*, 159.

7 See Rosenberg, *The Care of Strangers*, esp. ch 12; Grob, "The Social History of Medicine and Disease in America: Problems and Possibilities," 401; Achenbaum, "American Medical History: Social History and Medical Policy," 344; McKeown, "A Sociological Approach to the History of Medicine," 14.

8 Rosen, "The Efficiency Criterion in Medical Care, 1900–1925;" Howell, *Technology in the Hospital*, 30–9; and see Goebel, "American Medicine and the 'Organizational Synthesis': Chicago Physicians and the Business of Medicine."

9 Stevens, *In Sickness and in Wealth*, esp. ch 6; Stevens, *American Medicine and the Public Interest*, 47; Lawrence, *Medicine in the Making of Modern Britain*, 14–15; Digby, *Making a Medical Living*, 236; Pickstone, *Medicine and Industrial Society*, 251–5; Naylor, *Private Practice, Public Payment*, 98–133.

10 Perron, *Un siècle de vie hospitalière au Québec*; Connor, *Doing Good*; Reaume, *Remembrance of Patients Past*. Examples of commissioned histories include: Gagan, *'A Necessity Among Us'*; Hollobon, *The Lion's Tale*; Lewis, *Royal Victoria Hospital, 1887-1947*; Howell, *A Century of Care*; Robertson, Marcellus, and Dandy, *Mission's Living Memorials*; Sullivan and Ball, *Growing to Serve*; Savage, *To Serve With Honour*; MacDermot, *A History of the Montreal General Hospital*.

11 For the history of the medical profession in Canada see: Gidney and Millar, *Professional Gentlemen*; Bernier, *La médicine au Québec*; Howell, "Medical Professionalizaton and the Social Transformation of the Maritimes, 1850–1950"; Carr and Beamish, *Manitoba Medicine*; Gérard Bouchard, "Naissance d'une élite: les médecins dans la société saguenayenne (1850–1940)"; Hamowy, *Canadian Medicine: A Study in Restricted Entry*; and Naylor, *Private Practice, Public Payment*. The definitive histories of nursing in Canada are McPherson, *Bedside Matters*, and Petitat, *Les infirmières: de la vocation à la profession*; and see Cohen and Bienvenue, "Émergence de l'identité professionnelle chez les infirmières québecoises, 1890–1927." On medical technology, see, for example, Hayter, "The Clinic as Laboratory: The Case of Radiation Therapy, 1896–1920." Paramedical services are discussed in Fahmy-Eid and Piché, "Le savoir négocié: les stratégies des associations de technologie médicale, de physiothérapie et de diététique pour l'accès à une meilleure formation professionnelle (1930–1970)." On hospital record-keeping see Craig, "The Role of Records and of Record-keeping in the Development of the Modern Hospital in London, England, and Ontario, Canada, c. 1890–c. 1940."

12 See Anctil, et al., "La santé et l'assistance publique," generally, and esp. 56–60 for a commentary on these historical tensions; also Petitat, *Les infirmières*, esp. ch 3 for their relevance to the history of the hospital.

13 Risse, *Mending Bodies, Saving Souls,* 4.
14 See Craig, "The Canadian Hospital in History and Archives."
15 Ibid., 52.

1 PAO, RG8, Ontario, Department of the Provincial Secretary, Inspector of Hospitals and Charities, Annual Report, 1894.
2 Ibid., 1905.
3 Ibid., 1904, 8.
4 See Katz, Doucet, and Stern, *The Social Organization of Early Industrial Capitalism.*
5 OSP, 1974, VI, Part 1, No. 2, 128–9.
6 Owen Sound *Times,* 12 June 1893.
7 Gagan and Gagan, "Working-Class Standards of Living in Late-Victorian Urban Ontario."
8 Gagan, *'A Necessity Among Us,'* ch 1.
9 Cortiula, "Social Class and Health Care in a Community Institution: The Case of Hamilton City Hospital."
10 Howell, *A Century of Care,* ch 1.
11 CVA, RCH, A.C. Lawrence to Lord Milton, 27 Nov 1863; "Appeal to Miners and Other Inhabitants of British Columbia," August, 1863; Governor's Secretary to Board, Feb. 13, 1865.
12 See MacDermot, *A History of the Montreal General Hospital,* 1–60; Crosbie, *The Toronto General Hospital, 1819–1965,* 43–71; Sullivan and Ball, *Growing to Serve,* 25.
13 OSP, 1890, No 10, Inspector of Hospitals and Charities.
14 Connor, *Doing Good,* 123.
15 BCSP, 1879, Hospital Returns for 1878; SCGM, Patient Registers, 1877, 1889–90; OSP, 1880–1914; PAM, WGH, Annual Report, 1900.
16 Howell, *A Century of Care,* 14; and see Mitchinson, *The Nature of Their Bodies,* 55–6.
17 Unattributed editorial comment cited in Angus, *Kingston General Hospital,* 33.
18 SCGM, Patient Register, 1889–1890; OSGM, Patient Register, 1900–1901; TGH, ACC 0030, Annual Report, 1891; and see Barber, "The Women Ontario Welcomed: Immigrant Domestics for Ontario Homes, 1870–1930."
19 See R. Gagan, "Mortality Patterns and Public Health in Hamilton, Canada, 1900–14"; Palmer, *A Culture in Conflict,* esp. ch 2; Warsh, "'John Barleycorn Must Die': An Introduction to the Social History of Alcohol." Kealey, ed., *Canada Investigates Industrialism* relays many first-hand accounts of the frequency and nature of accidents in the workplace.

20 Rosenberg, "And Heal the Sick: Hospital and Patient in Nineteenth-Century America," 121 argues for this view of early American hospitals.
21 Woodward, *To Do the Sick No Harm*, 139–42.
22 Sullivan and Ball, *Growing to Serve*, 25.
23 OSP, 1880–1900; Gagan, *'A Necessity Among Us*," 32–4. By 1900 the removal of tubercular patients to sanatoria and the refusal of hospitals to admit tubercular patients, and the inroads made by public health reform on seasonal and infectious diseases may have accounted for much of this change.
24 PAO, RG8, Ontario, Department of the Provincial Secretary, Report on General Hospitals, 1879.
25 Sullivan and Ball, *Growing to Serve*, 47.
26 Cortiula, "The Social Transformation of the Clinic in Hamilton, 1880–1917," 114.
27 MacDermot, *A History of the Montreal General Hospital*, 66.
28 TGH, Annual Report, 1891; Hamilton, *The Spectator*, 12 August 1887.
29 "Home Hospitals," CL, 9 (July, 1877), 343. Woodward, *To Do the Sick No Harm*, 142, notes that Victorian hospital mortality rates below 10 per cent would have represented a "remarkable degree of success." Compare this with the Kingston General Hospital's annual mortality rate of 3.4 per cent by 1914 as noted in Angus, *Kingston General Hospital*, 94.
30 Splane, *Social Welfare in Ontario*, 81, 209.
31 Petitat, *Les infirmières*, 110.
32 "Hospital Investigation," *Manitoba Daily Free Press*, 26 April 1880.
33 Hamilton, *The Spectator*, 6 December 1889, 29 May 1894.
34 HCA, HCH, Board Minutes, 25 July 1893.
35 OSGM, *Rules and Regulations, 1893*.
36 Hamilton, *The Spectator*, 26 November 1889.
37 CVA, RCH, Rules for Patients, 1862.
38 Rosenberg, "Inward Vision and Outward Glance," 20.
39 Gibbon and Mathewson, *Three Centuries of Canadian Nursing*, 124.
40 See Gagan and Gagan, "Working-Class Standards of Living," 176–184.
41 Gibbon and Mathewson, *Three Centuries of Canadian Nursing*, 146–51; PAM, WGH, Visitors' Committee Report Book, e.g., 15 August 1879, 7 December 1880, 23 December 1883, 17 January 1885; Gagan, *'A Necessity Among Us*,' 18; R. Gagan, "Mortality Patterns and Public Health, in Hamilton, Canada, 1900–14."
42 Angus, *Kingston General Hospital*, 54.
43 *Manitoba Daily Free Press*, 20 February 1880, 17 March 1880.
44 Howell, *A Century of Care*, 25–6.
45 PAM, WGH, Visitors' Committee Report Book, 20 September 1891.
46 SCGM, Annual Report, 1870.

47 R.W. Bruce Smith, "The Responsibilities of Hospital Superintendents,"
    CL, 40 (May, 1907), 776.
48 SCGM, Annual Report, 1889–1890, 4.
49 "Hospital Abuses," DMJ, 10 (March, 1898), 125.
50 PAO, RG8, Ontario, Department of Health, General Hospitals, Annual
    Reports, 1904, 8; 1903, 7.
51 Compiled from Urquhart and Buckley, eds., Historical Statistics of
    Canada, Series A20–A24.
52 Artibise, Winnipeg: A Social History of Urban Growth, 1874–1914, 182–242.
53 See Copp, The Anatomy of Poverty; Fingard, The Dark Side of Life in
    Victorian Halifax.
54 See R. Gagan, "Mortality Patterns and Public Health in Hamilton,
    Canada, 1900–14," and McKinnon, "Mortality Reductions in Ontario,
    1900–42."
55 PAO, RG8, Province of Ontario, Department of the Provincial Secretary,
    Report on General Hospitals, 1913, 17; Splane, Social Welfare in Ontario,
    114, quoting Goldwin Smith; and see Bacchi, "Race Regeneration and
    Social Purity: A Study of the Social Attitudes of Canada's English-
    Speaking Suffragists" on the fear of "race suicide."
56 The historiography of social reform in Canada is extensive. See, in par-
    ticular, Cook, The Regenerators; Valverde, The Age of Light, Soap, and
    Water; Allen, The Social Passion.
57 Kinnear, A Female Economy, 72; Bradbury, Working Families, 180, 217–19,
    Table 4.3, Table 5.1; Parr, "Rethinking Work and Kinship in a Canadian
    Hosiery Town, 1919–1950," 221–6; Strange, Toronto's Girl Problem, 50–2,
    Table A.2; Barber, "The Women Ontario Welcomed: Immigrant Domes-
    tics for Ontario Homes, 1870–1930," 120; R. Gagan, "Mortality Patterns
    and Public Health in Hamilton, Canada, 1900–14," 170.
58 C. Howell, "Medical Professionalization and the Social Transformation
    of the Maritimes, 1850–1950," 11.
59 Godfrey, " 'Into the Hands of the Ladies': The Birth of the Moncton
    Hospital," 37.
60 Bernier, La médicine au Québec, 102–4.
61 "Hospital Abuses," 125; "The Pay System At Hospitals," CL, 27
    (December, 1894), 126–7; "The Hospital Facilities for Clinical Teaching
    in the Centres of Medical Education,: CL, 37 (December, 1903), 353
62 TGH, ACC 0030, Series A9, Annual Reports, 1905, 23.
63 Lewis, Royal Victoria Hospital, 40–5.
64 Quebec, Statistical year-book, 1915, 382.
65 Sullivan and Ball, Growing to Serve, 58.
66 "Hospitals and Charity Patients," CL, 39 (January, 1906), 462.
67 Tomes, The Gospel of Germs, 9.
68 See Granshaw, " 'Upon This Principle I Have Based a Practice': The

Development and Reception of Antisepsis in Britain, 1860–90"; Meade, *An Introduction to the History of General Surgery*, esp. 224–324.

69 See Roland, "The Early Years of Antiseptic Surgery in Canada;" Connor, "Listerism Unmasked: Antisepsis and Asepsis in Victorian Anglo-Canada."

70 "Antiseptic Surgery at Bellevue Hospital," CL, 16 (February, 1884), 105–7.

71 "Hospital Troubles in Halifax," CMAJ, I (March, 1911), 256.

72 PAO, RG8, Ontario, Department of the Provincial Secretary, Report on General Hospitals, 1883.

73 "Management of the Sick Room," CL, 19 (September, 1887), 16; and see McPherson, *Bedside Matters*, 27–9.

74 "The Life of a Nurse," (Toronto *Globe*, 8 October 1886) in Tauskey, ed., *Sara Jeanette Duncan*, 29.

75 "Trained Nurses," CL, 17 (December, 1885), 120.

76 "Management of the Sick Room," 15.

77 OSP, 1890, No. 14, Inspector of Prisons and Charities.

78 See McPherson, *Bedside Matters*, 29–39.

79 CVH, VGH, Annual Report, 1907; PABC, GR785, Province of British Columbia, Royal Commissions and Commissions of Inquiry, Commission of Inquiry, Vancouver General Hospital, 1912, *Investigative Proceedings*, 275–82.

80 Ibid., 297; Vancouver *Daily World*, 14 February, 25 February 1911.

81 OSGM, Report of the Committee to Gather Information on the Advisability of Establishing a Training School for Nurses, 12 October 1900.

82 Godfrey, "Into the Hands of the Ladies," 35, quoting the Moncton *Daily Times*, 14 January 1895.

83 Sullivan, "Sanguine Practices: A Historical and Historiographic Reconsideration of Heroic Therapy in the Age of Rush"; Tomes, *Gospel of Germs*, 6; Maulitz, "'Physician *versus* Bacteriologist': The Ideology of Science in Clinical Medicine," 91–3; Bonner, *Becoming a Physician*, 279–90.

84 Hayter, "The Clinic as Laboratory," 671; Gidney and Millar, "The Reorientation of Medical Education in Late Nineteenth-Century Ontario," 77–8.

85 Ibid., 76.

86 These arguments are summarized in Sturdy, "The Political Economy of Scientific Medicine," 125–9.

87 "Canadian Medicine," CMAJ, 1 (February, 1911), 150.

88 Bonner, *Becoming a Physician*, 290.

89 Sullivan and Ball, *Growing to Serve*, 97–8.

90 Rosenberg, *The Care of Strangers*, 152.

91 Hayter, "The Clinic as Laboratory," 681–2.

92 See Connor, "The Adoption and Effects of X-Rays in Ontario."

93 J.D. Howell, *Technology in the Hospital,* 116.
94 Connor, "The Adoption and Effects of X-rays," 98; Petitat, *Les infir-
    mières,* 125; PAO, CGH, Annual Report, 1908; PAM, WGH, Annual Report,
    1906; CVA, VGH, Board of Directors' Minutes, 31 December 1906 and 31
    December 1907; OSGM, Board of Governors' Minutes, 8 April, 28 May
    1914.
95 J.D. Howell, "Machines and Medicine," 116.
96 CVA, VCH/VGH, Medical Board/Medical Staff Minutes, 4 June 1900, 24
    September 1905, 5 November 1907, 7 January 1908, 2 March 1909; OSGM,
    Annual Report, 1917; OSGM, Board of Trustees' Minutes, 12 February
    1919, 14 September 1922; Owen Sound *Sun Times,* 13 December 1918, 17
    February 1923.
97 Owen Sound *Sun Times,* 17 February 1923.
98 PAM, WGH, 1902–1930.
99 In 1934, for example, the Ontario College of Physicians and Surgeons
    disqualified the Owen Sound General and Marine Hospital's former
    radiologist for offering patients a money-back guarantee if his private
    radiology clinic failed to cure goitre, skin and glandular disorders, and
    tonsillitis painlessly, without surgery. See Gagan, *'A Necessity Among
    Us,'* 92–3.
100 See Sturdy, "The Political Economy of Scientific Medicine," 129.
101 Stevens, *American Medicine and the Public Interest,* 40–6; and see Weisz,
    "Medical Directories and Medical Specialization in France, Britain,
    and the United States."
102 This discussion is based on a quantitative analysis of *The Ontario
    Medical Register, 1877.*
103 These data are derived from an analysis of a 20 per cent sample of *The
    Ontario Medical Register, 1907.*
104 Stevens, *American Medicine and the Public Interest,* 44–50.
105 "Professional Courtesy," CL, 27 (November, 1894), 84.
106 Weisz, "Medical Directories and Medical Specialization in France,
    Britain, and the United States," 36.
107 Fahrni, *Prairie Surgeon,* 48.
108 J.S. Hart, "What the Average Medical Man Expects of the Hospital,"
    HW, 1 (January, 1912), 36.
109 Petitat, *Les infirmières,* p. 120.
110 Gagan, *'A Necessity Among Us,'* 34–5, 69–70.
111 PAM, WGH, Annual Report, 1911.
112 "The Future of the Medical Profession," CL, 40 (November, 1906),
    367–8.
113 J.D. Howell, *Technology in the Hospital,* 58–65.
114 PAO, RG8, Department of the Provincial Secretary, Report on General
    Hospitals, 1910, 10.

115 Kelly, *Quest for a Profession*, 2.
116 "Hospitals and City Life," CL, 42 (February, 1909), 404.
117 PAO, RG8, Province of Ontario, Department of Health, General Hospitals, Annual Report, 1906.
118 "Equipment of the New Toronto General Hospital," HW, 1 (April, 1912), 239–42.
119 TGH, Series F, "Private Patients' Building," 1913.
120 OSGM, Annual Report, 1912; Owen Sound *Sun*, 20 June 1911, 1 April 1916.
121 PAM, WGH, Annual Reports, 1890–1908. The quotation is from the 1908 Report, 12.
122 CVA VGH, Annual Report, 1922.
123 "President's Address," HW, 1 (May, 1912), 307.
124 PAM, WGH, Annual Report, 1918.

CHAPTER TWO

1 OSGM, Annual Report, 1920.
2 MacMurchy is of interest in her own right as one of Canada's leading proponents of eugenics and as a child welfare activist in the age of social reform. See Dodd, "Advice to Parents: The Blue Books, Helen MacMurchy, MD, and the Federal Department of Health, 1920–34."
3 PAO, RG8, Department of the Provincial Secretary, Report on General Hospitals, 1916.
4 "The Hospital Field in Canada," CH, 8 (September, 1931), 52–5; "The Progress of Radiology," CMAJ, 15 (October, 1925), 1062.
5 TGH, Annual Report, 1905.
6 "More Publicity Is Needed," CH, 5(September, 1928), 11.
7 PAM, MSP, 1903, Department of Public Works, Annual Report.
8 See Godfrey, "'Into the Hands of the Ladies'"
9 OSGM, Board of Trustees, Minutes, 30 November 1909.
10 "Brief Sketch of the Origin and Progress of Hospital Aids," CH, 7 (February, 1930), 28.
11 PAM, WGH, Annual Reports, 1918, 1919.
12 TGH, ACC 0030, Series F, "Social Services in the Toronto General Hospital, 1911–1949."
13 Goulet et Paradis, *Trois siècles d'histoire médicale au Québec*, I, "Les institutions hospitalières (1639–1939)," esp. 120–71, provides useful comparative summaries of the terms of incorporation of many varieties of hospitals in the province, 1890–1930.
14 PAM, WGH, Annual Reports, 1903, 1913.
15 Starr, *The Social Transformation of American Medicine*, 146.
16 PAO, RG8, Department of the Provincial Secretary, Report on General Hospitals, 1920, 12.

17 PAM, MSP, 1919, Second Interim Report of the Public Welfare Commission of Manitoba, February, 1919, 7, 36.

18 Goulet et Paradis, *Trois siècles d'histoire médicale au Québec*, "La loi d'assistance publique," 40; "Loi établissant le service de l'assistance publique au Québec," 152; Quebec, *Annuaire statistique/Statistical yearbook, 1925*, 249. Municipalities had been required to support indigent hospitalization since 1879, but there was no provincial subvention until 1921, and it remained unadjusted for inflation for the next two decades. See Petitat, *Les infirmières*, 56, 120.

19 PABC, GRO785, Royal Commissions and Commissions of Inquiry, Vancouver General Hospital, Commission of Inquiry, 1912, *Commissioner's Report*, 90; and see RSO 1897, c 320, s 1 (1912).

20 PAO, RG8, Department of the Provincial Secretary, Report on General Hospitals, 1913, 13.

21 PAM, MSP, 1903, Department of Public Works, Annual Report.

22 Gagan, *'A Necessity Among Us,'* 41–3.

23 Risse, *Mending Bodies, Saving Souls*, 471.

24 E.E. Dutton, "A Hospital Problem Survey," *CH*, 3 (February, 1926), 12.

25 Malcolm T. MacEachern, "Some Hospitalization Problems: Hospital Standardization," *CMAJ*, 12 (August, 1922), 522.

26 PAM, WGH, Annual Report, 1921.

27 PAM, MSP, 1919, Second Interim Report of the Public Welfare Commission of Manitoba, February, 1919, 11–12.

28 Ibid., 12.

29 PAM, WGH, Annual Report, 1901; and see J.D. Howell, *Technology in the Hospital*, 30–2.

30 Taylor, *The Principles of Scientific Management*.

31 The foregoing synthesis owes much to the analysis presented by Haber, *Efficiency and Uplift: Scientific Management in the Progressive Era, 1890–1920*, ix, xii, 54, 55, 60–2.

32 Perron, *Un siècle de vie hospitalière au* Québec, 119–20.

33 D.A. Stewart, "The Care of the Sick," *CMAJ*, 16 (December, 1926), 1512.

34 Flexner, *Medical Education in the United States and Canada*, 100.

35 Perkins, "Shaping Institutional-Based Specialism: Early Twentieth-Century Economic Organization of Medicine."

36 D.A. Stewart, "The Care of the Sick," *CMAJ*, 17 (January, 1927), 94.

37 Starr, *The Transformation of American Medicine*, 178–9.

38 See PABC, *Rules and Regulations of the Vancouver General Hospital*, November 8, 1906; OSGM, Board of Trustees, Minutes, 1893–1930.

39 R. Bruce Smith, "The Responsibilities of Hospital Superintendents," *CL*, 40 (May, 1907), 776.

40 HCA, HCH, Board of Governors, Minutes, September 27, 1922.

41 "Medical Representation on Hospital Boards," *WCMJ*, 12 (February, 1912), 50.
42 PAM, MSP, 1919, Second Interim Report of the Public Welfare Commission of Manitoba, February, 1919, 12–14.
43 Rosenberg, *The Care of Strangers*, 254; Stevens, *In Sickness and in Wealth*, 37–9.
44 OSGM, Board of Trustees, Minutes, 4 May 1909.
45 "The Pay System at Hospitals," *CL*, 27 (December, 1894), 126–7.
46 R.M. Richards, "Manitoba Medical Matters," *CL*, 47 (July, 1904), 1030.
47 "Hospitals and Charity Patients," *CL*, 39 (January, 1906), 462.
48 "Toronto General Hospital," *CL*, 39 (September, 1905), 69–70.
49 HCA, HCH, Hospital Committee Minutes, 16 December 1902; CVA, VGH, Annual Report, 1908; PAM, WGH, 1912.
50 PAM, WGH, Annual Report, 1911, 13.
51 PAM, WGH, Medical Staff, Minutes, 17 November 1913, 25 August 1914.
52 See Gagan and Gagan, "Working Class Standards of Living"; Piva, *The Condition of the Working Class in Toronto, 1900–1921*; and Bartlett, "Real Wages and the Standard of Living in Vancouver, 1901–1929."
53 Vancouver *Daily Province*, 16 May 1912; PABC, VGH, Inquiry, 1912, *Report*, 23–4.
54 PAM, WGH, Annual Report, 1907; TGH, Annual Report, 1925.
55 "The Ontario Medical Association," *CL*, 36 (January, 1903), 357; "The Toronto General Hospital," *CL*, 39 (September, 1905), 69–70.
56 "The Need for Private Rooms," *CH*, 5 (June, 1928), 15.
57 CVA, VCH, Board of Directors, Minutes, 11 August 1904; OSGM, Board of Trustees, Minutes, 9 September 1914.
58 HCA, HCH, Hospital Committee Minutes, 18 March 1902, 17 October 1905.
59 PABC, VGH, Inquiry, 1912, *Investigative Proceedings*, 100–19, 625.
60 Vancouver *Daily Province*, 27 May 1912.
61 Stewart, "The Care of the Sick," (1927), 97.
62 TGH, Annual Report, 1916.
63 PAM, WGH, Annual Reports, 1903, 1907, 1915; CVA, VGH, Annual Report, 1908.
64 PABC, VGH, Inquiry, 1912, *Report*, 87.
65 PAO, RG8, Province of Ontario, Department of the Provincial Secretary, Report on General Hospitals, 1911, 1912.
66 See Rosen, "The Efficiency Criterion in Medical Care, 1900–1925."
67 PAM, WGH, Annual Report, 1903, 1904, 1905.
68 Fahrni, *Prairie Surgeon*, 48.
69 CVA, VGH, Annual Reports, 1917, 1932; BCMA, Vancouver Medical Association, Minutes, 17 December 1914, 18 January 1917.

70 See Burke, *Seeking the Highest Good*, esp. ch 2.
71 J.M. Kniseley, "Medical Social Work in the Toronto General Hospital," *SW*, 13 (February, 1931), 93–6.
72 PAM, WGH, Annual Reports, 1916–1925.
73 OSGM, Board of Trustees, Minutes, 14 December 1927.
74 PABC, VGH, Inquiry, 1912, *Report*, 54–5.
75 PABC, VGH, Inquiry, 1912, *Proceedings*, 321.
76 MacDermot, *A History of the Montreal General Hospital*, 89.
77 PAO, CGH, Annual Reports, 1900–1911.
78 See, for example, HCA, HCH, Hospital Committee Minutes, 15 April 1902; PAM, WGH, Medical Staff , Minutes, 25 August 1914; OSGM, Board of Trustees, Minutes, 12 June 1912.
79 "Pupil Nurses," CN, 9 (November, 1913), 736.
80 A.E.B., "Should Nurses in Training Be Paid?" CN, 4 (September, 1908), 412–15.
81 OSP, 1928, No. 14, Division of Nurse Registration, Annual Report, 1928
82 J.D. Howell, *Technology in the Hospital*, 66–7.
83 Ibid., 521; Stevens, *American Medicine and the Public Interest*, 73; Stevens, *In Sickness and in Wealth*, see ch 3.
84 Ibid., 522–5; Agnew, *Canadian Hospitals, 1920–1970*, 32–3.
85 MacEachern, "Some Hospital Problems," 526.
86 Ibid., 522.
87 CVA, RCH, Board of Directors, Minutes, E.A. Wismer to Board, 20 March 1929.
88 Philip Hilkowitz, "The Results of Hospital Standardization and Extent of Their Adoption," CH, 5 (April, 1928), 23–5.
89 CVA, VGH, Series C, v. 9, File 47, M.T. MacEachern, "Progress and Application of Hospital Standardization in the Vancouver General Hospital," nd [typescript]; CVA, VGH, Standardization of Hospital Treatment and Records, W.C. White to M.T. MacEachern, 29 July 1921.
90 See Stevens, *In Sickness and in Wealth*, ch 3.
91 Risse, *Mending Bodies, Saving Souls*, 470.
92 See, Canada, Dominion Bureau of Statistics, *The Small General Hospital in 1957: A Statistical Summary* (Ottawa: Queen's Printer, 1960); and Canada, Dominion Bureau of Statistics, *The Large General Hospital in 1957: A Statistical Summary* (Ottawa: Queen's Printer, 1960).
93 MacEachern, "Some Hospital Problems," 526.
94 Agnew, *Canadian Hospitals, 1920–1970*, 4.
95 See Twohig, "Organizing the Bench," esp. 148–58; and Twohig, " 'Local Girls' and 'Lab Boys,'" 1–41.
96 Lois Stewart, "The Place of the Dietitian in the Hospital," CH, 3 (January,

1926), 20; "The Physiotherapy Department in the Hospital," *CMAJ*, 24 (February, 1931), 298.

97 Fahmy-Eid and Piché, "Le savoir négocié."

98 At the Owen Sound General and Marine, for example, in 1931 employee wages represented about 30 per cent of total annual hospital expenditures, in 1951, 57 per cent, in 1956, 67 per cent. See Gagan, '*A Necessity Among Us,*' 113, Table 11.

99 Flexner, *Medical Education in the United States and Canada.*

100 Goulet, *Histoire de la Faculté de Médicine de l'Université de Montréal,* 130–1.

101 Flexner, *Medical Education in the United States and Canada,* 320–5.

102 McPhedran, *Canadian Medical Schools,* 63, 118, 144; UMA, UMFM, Dean's Office Files, "Location of Internes, Session 1928–29," nd; University of Manitoba, Faculty of Medicine, *Annual Announcement, Session 1920–21,* 13–15.

103 Goulet, *Histoire de la Faculté de Médicine de l'Université de Montréal,* 147.

104 Fahrni, *Prairie Surgeon,* 149; Sullivan and Ball, *Growing to Serve,* 123. At the new Toronto General Hospital in 1912, the University of Toronto's Faculty of Medicine controlled 500 public ward beds.

105 Flexner, *Medical Education in the United States and Canada,* 100.

106 OSGM, Annual Report, 1912.

107 Stevens, *In Sickness and in Wealth,* 107.

108 PAM, WGH, Annual Reports, 1902, 1926, 1930.

109 Strong-Boag and McPherson, "The Confinement of Women: Childbirth and Hospitalization in Vancouver, 1919–1939," 145.

110 Urquhart and Buckley, eds., *Historical Statistics of Canada,* Series B51–58, Series B92–99.

111 See Dodd, "Advice to Parents;" and Oppenheimer, "Childbirth in Ontario: The Transition from Home to Hospital in the Early Twentieth Century."

112 See Strong-Boag and McPherson, "The Confinement of Women."

113 See Comacchio, *Nations Are Built of Babies,* esp. ch 4.

114 A.K. Heywood, Malcolm T. MacEachern, and W.H. Walsh, *Report of the Vancouver Hospital Survey Commission upon the Hospital Situation of Greater Vancouver* (Vancouver, 1930), 89, quoting Dr W.G. Cosbie [hereinafter *Hospital Survey of Greater Vancouver*].

115 PAM, WGH, Annual Report, 1902, 15; Annual Report, 1918, 33.

116 PAM, WGH, Annual Report, 1912, 11.

117 Stevens, *In Sickness and in Wealth,* 107.

118 Starr, *The Transformation of American Medicine,* 159, and Stevens, *In Sickness and in Wealth,* 48–9 describe the same pattern in American hospitals.

CHAPTER THREE

1   R. Fraser Armstrong, "Hospital Service to the Patient of Average Means," CH, 8 (August, 1931), 13.
2   Carr and Beamish, *Manitoba Medicine*, 75.
3   PAM, WGH, Annual Reports, 1917, 1918; OSGM, Annual Reports, 1917, 1918.
4   Gagan, *'A Necessity Among Us,'* 66; *The Story of VGH*, 13.
5   Gagan, *'A Necessity Among Us,'* 67. The history of the epidemic in Canada is summarized in McGinnis, "The Impact of Epidemic Influenza: Canada, 1918–1919."
6   Urquhart and Buckley, eds., *Historical Statistics of Canada*, Series J135, J139, J147.
7   The indexes in Appendix N were calculated from the data compiled in OSP, Reports on General Hospitals, 1890–1946.
8   See Gagan, *'A Necessity Among Us,'* Table 6, 80.
9   PAM, WGH, Annual Reports, 1920–1926; G.F. Stephens, "Problem of Patients," MMAB, 10 (November, 1930), 4–5.
10 *Hospital Survey of Greater Vancouver, 1930*, 41, 60, 85; "Hospital Bed Shortage," VMB, 4 (March, 1928), 142–3.
11 Anctil *et. al.*, "La santé et l'assistance publique," 51.
12 See Struthers, *No Fault of Their Own*, 32–7.
13 Kubat and Thornton, *A Statistical Profile of Canadian Society*, Table P-4.
14 "A National Hospital Day," CMAJ, 11 (May, 1921), 364.
15 "Paying the Hospital Bill," CH, 4 (November, 1927), 9.
16 "Hospitals Handicapped By Meagre Grants," CH, 4 (November, 1927), 11–12.
17 M.T. MacEachern, "The Financing of Public Hospitals," CMAJ, 40 (May, 1921), 313.
18 "Representative Deputation Presses Claim at Parliament Buildings," CH, 5 (February, 1928), 14.
19 PAO, RG63, Series A7, "Profit and Loss Statement, Year Ending September 30, 1928, of 138 General Hospitals."
20 Quebec, *Annuaire statistique/Statistical year-book, 1932*, 170.
21 See Petitat, *Les infirmières*, 122. It should be noted that the data available from the Quebec government's *Annuaire statistique/Statistical year-book* for this period are not reliable with regard to total hospital admissions and the breakdown of patients by admission category (full pay, part pay, indigent). As Petitat demonstrates, the evidence from individual hospitals suggests that their dependence on patient fees escalated much more rapidly than Appendix F(2) indicates.
22 "Is the Public Out of Touch With the Hospital?" CH, 6 (July, 1929), 11.
23 Comacchio, *Nations Are Built of Babies*, 28; Naylor, *Private Practice*, 40–1.

24 MacDermot, *A History of the Montreal General Hospital*, 111–12.
25 D.A. Stewart, "The Care of the Sick," CMAJ, 16 (December, 1926), 94–7.
26 Toronto *Globe and Mail*, 26 August 1929.
27 Stewart, "The Care of the Sick," 97.
28 Naylor, *Private Practice*, 29–37.
29 PABC, Province of British Columbia, Royal Commissions and Commissions of Inquiry, Commission on Health Insurance (1919–1921), Report on Maternity Insurance, 1921, 9.
30 Ibid., Report of the Health Insurance Commission, 1921, 43.
31 Ibid., Report on Maternity Insurance, 10.
32 Ibid., Report of the Health Insurance Commission, 88.
33 Ibid., 41–2.
34 Ibid., 57, 90, 101.
35 Ibid., 101, 104, 107–8.
36 Ibid., 94.
37 Ibid., 73–4.
38 Naylor, *Private Practice*, 40–1.
39 James Govan and B. Evan Parry, "Hospital Problems in Cities and Large Towns," CH, 6 (June, 1929), 15–16.
40 The metaphor is Rosemary Stevens's, in *In Sickness and in Wealth*, 48.
41 Rosenberg, "Inward Vision," 36.
42 See Morton, *Manitoba: A History*, 422–3; Britnell, "Saskatchewan, 1930–35," *Canadian Journal of Economics and Political Science* [CJEPS] 11 (May 1936), 144; Innis, "Economic Conditions in Canada, 1931–32," *Economic Journal*, 42 (March, 1932), 13; Guest, *The Emergence of Social Security in Canada*, 86; Struthers, *No Fault of Their Own*, 94–118, Appendices 1–3.
43 Horn, ed., *The Dirty Thirties*, 12.
44 Thomas, ed., *The Making of a Socialist*, 227.
45 PAM, MSP, Department of Health and Public Welfare, Reports, 1930–1936; "The Medical Health Officer and the 'Hospital Aid Act,'" MMAB, 13 (June, 1933), 505–7; Province of Manitoba, Legislative Assembly, *Statutes of Manitoba*, S.M. 1933, c 15, s 1, "The Hospital Aid Act."
46 PAM, WGH, Annual Reports, 1930–1939.
47 Naylor, "Canada's First Doctors' Strike."
48 Ibid., 1936, 30.
49 CVA, *Proceedings of the Thirteenth Annual Convention of the British Columbia Hospital Association*, 1930, 19.
50 See Ormsby, "T. Dufferin Patullo and the Little New Deal," esp. 44–5; Robin, *Pillars of Profit*, 20–9; Andrews, "The Course of Medical Opinion on State Health Insurance in British Columbia, 1919–1939," esp. 139–42; and Irving, "The Doctors versus the Expert."
51 CVA, RCH, Annual Reports, 1930–1935.
52 CVA, RCH, Board of Directors, Minutes, 28 December 1933.

53 CVA, RCH, "Arrangements for unemployed to pay off their accounts to RCH..." March, 1935.

54 CVA, RCH, Annual Reports, 1930–1936; CVA, VGH, W. Walsh, "Report of a Study of the Vancouver General Hospital With Special Reference to the Efficiency and Adequacy of the Physical Phase of the Institution," 1936, 11.

55 Naylor, "Canada's First Doctors' Strike," 155–6.

56 CVA, City of Vancouver, Social Services, Series S, Director's Files, Statistics, 1937.

57 Province of Ontario, Royal Commission on Public Welfare, *Report to the Lieutenant-Governor in Council* (Toronto: King's Printer, 1930).

58 Ibid., 15.

59 Ibid., 14.

60 J.M. McCutcheon, "The Study of the Public Welfare Commission with Regard to Hospitals," *CH*, 8 (January, 1931), 27, 24.

61 "The Provincial Hospitals Act for Ontario Becomes Effective October 1, 1931," *CH*, 8 (August, 1931), 16.

62 Province of Ontario, Department of Health, *The Hospitals of Ontario: A Short History* (Toronto: King's Printer, 1934), 21–2.

63 Province of Ontario, Department of Health, *A Survey of Public General Hospitals in Ontario* (Toronto, 1939–40).

64 Ibid., Part 3, Tables 4, 5, 6, 30; Part 1, 12.

65 Ibid., Part 1, 20–5.

66 Ibid., Part 3, Table 47.

67 Gagan, '*A Necessity Among Us*,' 87–92.

68 Ibid., 94.

69 Owen Sound *Daily Sun-Times*, 15 October 1938, 3, 11, 23 March 1939.

70 League for Social Reconstruction, Research Committee, *Social Planning for Canada* (Toronto, 1935), reproduced in Horn, 205, 207 (italics ours).

71 PAM, WGH, Annual Report, 1941, 30; OSGM, Superintendent's Report re: Training School, July, 1940; Owen Sound *Daily Sun-Times*, 3 February 1941, 5 February 1943, 11 February 1944.

72 "Hospitals Rated As Essential Service," *CH*, 19 (May, 1942), 15; "Hospitals Seriously Affected by Government Order Fixing Room Charges," *CH*, 19 (February, 1942), 15.

73 Province of Ontario, Minister of Health, *Report of the Ontario Health Survey Committee*, vol. 1(1951), 24.

74 PAM, WGH, Annual Reports, 1941–1951.

75 *Hospitals in Manitoba: Report of a Study*, Manitoba Welfare Supervision Board, 1944, 16.

76 CVA, VGH, Annual Report, 1940, 36–7.

77 Urquhart and Buckley, eds., *Historical Statistics of Canada*, Series B138–141.

78 Anctil et al., "La santé et l'assistance publique," 90.

79 Edna Nicholson, "The Problem of Long-Term Illness," CD, 12 (February, 1946), 92.
80 Hospitals in Manitoba, 38, 42.
81 Report of the Ontario Health Survey Committee, I, 58, 91–2.
82 Ibid., 58.
83 Smith and Nickel, "From Home to Hospital: Parallels in Birthing and Dying in Twentieth-Century Canada," 55.
84 Report of the Ontario Health Survey Committee, I, 91, 92; Survey of Public Hospitals in Ontario, Part IV, 20.
85 "The Shortage of Hospital Beds," CMAJ, 46 (April, 1942), 373.
86 Canada, Department of National Health and Welfare, Hospital Care in Canada: Trends and Development, 1948–1962, Health Care Series, Memorandum no. 19 (Ottawa, 1964), 9.
87 Urquhart and Buckley, eds., Historical Statistics of Canada, Series B225.
88 See "Ontario Plan for Hospital Care to be Launched Shortly," CH, 18 (March, 1941), 40; "British Columbia Institutes Plan for Providing Hospital Care," CH, 20 (December, 1943), 39.
89 George F. Stephens, "Group Hospitalization: the Logical Solution," CH, 18 (February, 1941), 14.
90 Naylor, Private Practice, 163; Report of the Ontario Health Survey Committee, I, 23; Canada, Department of National Health and Welfare, Hospital Care in Canada: Recent Trends and Developments, Health Care Series, Memorandum no 12 (Ottawa, 1960), 77–8; Taylor, Health Insurance and Canadian Public Policy, 113 estimates that among commercial health insurance carriers premium costs were equal to 170 per cent of the benefits paid to subscribers.
91 Urquhart and Buckley, eds., Historical Statistics of Canada, Series B225.
92 Hospital Care in Canada (1960), 16, 77.
93 Ibid., 75. There were, however, significant provincial variations. For example, the Manitoba Health Advisory Survey Committee estimated in 1952 that about 48 per cent of provincial general hospital revenues came from self-pay patients, 30 per cent from hospital insurance plans, and 17 per cent from government This appears to have been the result of the fact that participation in the Manitoba Associated Medical Services' plan was primarily an urban phenomenon. See, Province of Manitoba, Department of Health and Public Welfare, Manitoba Health Advisory Survey Committee, Report on Health Services, Facilities and Personnel, and Recommendations, 1952, 111.
94 Report of the Ontario Health Survey Committee, I, 21.
95 Urquhart and Buckley, eds., Historical Statistics of Canada, Series B173; Taylor, Financial Aspects of Health Services, 14.
96 These data were extrapolated from Dominion Bureau of Statistics and

Department of National Health and Welfare, *Canadian Sickness Survey, 1950–51* (Ottawa, 1953), Tables 1–8.

97 Taylor, *Financial Aspects of Health Services*, 9.

98 Pellagrino, "The Sociocultural Impact of Twentieth-Century Therapeutics," 246.

99 The following discussion is based on *Health in Manitoba: A Presentation to the Canadian Council on Mental Hygiene*, Manitoba Pool Elevators, 1939; *Study of the Distribution of Medical Care and Public Health Services in Canada*, National Committee for Mental Hygiene, 1939; F. S. Moorhead, "Manitoba Hospital Services Association," *Manitoba Medical Review*, 10 (January, 1940), 13; *Public Health in Manitoba: Report of a Study by the American Public Health Association*, 1941; *Submission to the Hospital Survey Committee, Manitoba Federation of Agriculture, 1943; Hospitals in Manitoba: Report of a Study*, Manitoba Welfare Supervision Board, 1944; *Report of the Royal Commission in reference to the Costs of Hospitalization*, 1949; "Hospital Beds," *Manitoba Medical Review*, 19 (July, 1949), 371; *Report on Health Services, Facilities and Personnel, and Recommendations*, Manitoba Health Advisory Survey Committee, 1952. The versions of all of the foregoing public documents consulted and referenced here are those deposited in the Legislative Library of Manitoba.

100 *Study of the Distribution of Medical Care and Public Health Services in Canada*, 12.

101 *Health in Manitoba*, 36.

102 "Health Insurance Survey Completed by McGill Expert," *CH*, 9 (June, 1932), 11; Irving, "The Doctors *versus* the Expert;" Struthers, 64–6.

103 *Report of the Royal Commission on Dominion-Provincial Relations*, Book II, *Recommendations* (Ottawa, 1940), 33–43.

104 Owram, *The Government Generation*, xi, 189.

105 Canada, House of Commons, Special Committee on Social Security, *Report on Social Security for Canada*, 16 March 1943, 55.

106 Ibid., citing the conclusions of the Rowell-Sirois Commission.

107 Ibid., 56.

108 Canada, House of Commons, Special Committee on Social Security, *Health Insurance*, 16 March 1943.

109 Canada, House of Commons, Special Committee on Social Security, *Minutes of Proceedings and Evidence*, no 6, 9 April 1943, 171–87.

110 Special Committee on Social Security, *Health Insurance*, 505–7.

111 "Three in Four Favour Health Insurance: Gallup Poll Across Canada," *CH*, 19 (May, 1942), 27.

112 Finkel, "Paradise Postponed: A Re-examination of the Green Book Proposals of 1945."

113 Sigerist, *Autobiographical Writings*, 189–90. Duffin, "The Guru and the Godfather," describes Sigerist's role in Douglas's decision to implement health care reform in Saskatchewan.

114 Saskatchewan Health Services Survey Commission, *Report*, esp. 4, 6, 7, 10.

115 McLeod and McLeod, *Tommy Douglas*, 148. Mombourquette, "'An Inalienable Right,'" 106–8; Thomas, *The Making of A Socialist*, 231; Ostry, "Prelude to Medicare: Institutional Change and Continuity in Saskatchewan, 1944–1962."

116 Owram, *Born At the Right Time*, ch 1.

117 For the history of this public policy initiative see Taylor, *Health Insurance and Canadian Public Policy*, ch 3; Hastings, "Federal-Provincial Insurance for Hospital and Physician's Care in Canada"; Naylor, *Private Practice*, 162–5.

CHAPTER FOUR

1 Bernier, *La médicine au Québec*, 1.

2 Gidney and Millar, *Professional Gentlemen*. Unless otherwise noted, this discussion is a gloss of Gidney and Millar's evidence and argument appearing on pages 6–24, 43–60, and 85–101.

3 Naylor, "Rural Protest and Medical Professionalism in Turn-of-the-Century Ontario," 9.

4 Bouchard, "Naissance d'une élite," 531–2.

5 Rosenberg, "The Therapeutic Revolution: Medicine, Meaning and Social Change in Nineteenth-Century America," 15.

6 Sullivan, "Sanguine Practices," 233.

7 Bonner, *Medicine in Chicago, 1850–1950*, 229.

8 See Gidney and Millar, "The Reorientation of Medical Education in Late-Nineteenth- Century Ontario," 52–78.

9 "The Claims of the Profession on the Public," *CL*, 15 (March, 1883), 219.

10 Connor, "'A Sort of *Felo-de-se*': Eclecticism, Related Medical Sects, and Their Decline in Victorian Ontario," provides an analysis of the eclectics' responsibility for their own extinction in late-Victorian Canada.

11 The history of this movement is documented in Hamowy, *Canadian Medicine: A Study in Restricted Entry*, esp. ch 4.

12 See Shortt, "Social Change and Political Crisis in Rural Ontario: The Patrons of Industry, 1889–1896"; Naylor, "Rural Protest and Medical Professionalism," 12–17.

13 "Physicians as Business Men," *CL*, 24 (August, 1892), 391.

14 Cited from *The Maritime Medical News* in Hamowy, *Canadian Medicine*, 173.

15 "The Claims of the Profession on the Public," *CL*, 15 (March, 1883), 219.

16 Andrews, "Medical Attendance in Vancouver, 1886–1920," 34.

17 See Maulitz, " 'Physician *versus* Bacteriologist,'" 92; C. Howell, "Medical Professionalization," 13–18; Bernier, *La médicine au Québec,* 139; Perkins, "Shaping Institution-based Specialism," 430; Sturdy, "The Political Economy of Scientific Medicine," 129.

18 Hayter, "The Clinic as Laboratory," 666–79; Maulitz, " 'Physician *versus* Bacteriologist,'" 95–104.

19 Mitchinson, "Agency, Diversity, and Constraints: Women and Their Physicians, Canada, 1850–1950," 131; Biggs, "The Case of the Missing Midwives," 29–30 notes that in 1899 only 3 per cent of all births in Ontario were attended by midwives, but suggests that there was a noticeable rural-urban dichotomy in the preference for midwives over doctors, and cautions against reading too much into data skewed by the tendency of beleaguered midwives to practise their calling covertly.

20 Bouchard, "Naissance d'une élite," 545–7.

21 Bernier, "Les practiciens de santé au Québec, 1871–1921," 48–9.

22 See, for example, the development of obstetrics in American hospitals as described in Borst, *Catching Babies,* 137–47.

23 These data are based on a quantitative analysis of the *Ontario Medical Register, 1877,* and a 20 per cent sample of the *Ontario Medical Register, 1907.*

24 Bernier, "Les practiciens de la santé au Québec, 1871–1921."

25 "Physicians as Business Men," *CL*, 24 (August, 1892), 391.

26 W.H. Moorehouse, "Presidential Address," *CL*, 37 (September, 1903), 11.

27 "An Urgent Need in the Medical Profession," *CL*, 37 (April, 1904), 751; "Improvement in the Character of the Medical Profession," *CL*, 23 (April, 1891), 249; "The Financial Position of the Medical Practitioner," *CL*, 41 (November, 1907), 240–1; and see Andrews, "Medical Attendance in Vancouver" for a description of one doctor's practice.

28 Willinsky, *A Doctor's Memoirs,* 47–57, 79–80.

29 "The Overcrowding of the Medical Profession," *CL*, 25 (January, 1893), 177.

30 Flexner, *Medical Education in the United States and Canada,* 332.

31 See Shortt, " 'Before the Age of Miracles,'" 126–7. These reforms represented the thrust of Flexner, *Medical Education in the United States and Canada,* submitted to the Carnegie Foundation for the Advancement of Teaching in 1910.

32 T.O. Summers, "Professional Courtesy," *CL*, 27 (November, 1894), 84.

33 "The Financial Position of the Medical Practitioner," 240–1.

34 "The Future of the Medical Profession," *CL*, 40 (November, 1906), 367–8.

35 Edward J. Moore, "The Why and Wherefore of Doctors' Bills," *Maclean's Magazine,* 25 (December, 1912), 56.

227 Notes to pages 108–12

36 J.S. Hart, "What the Average Medical Man Expects of the Hospital," HW, 1 (January, 1912), 36–41.
37 PAM, WGH, Medical Staff, Minutes, 7 May 1908.
38 R.H. Richards, "Manitoba Medical Matters," CL, 37 (July, 1904), 1030.
39 PAM, MSP, 1896, Report of the Department of Public Works, 1895.
40 VGH, Inquiry, 1912, *Investigative Proceedings*, 300–1.
41 "Toronto General Hospital," CL, 39 (September, 1905), 69–70.
42 Stevens, *American Medicine and the Public Interest*, 47; Rosenberg, *Care of Strangers*, 172–3.
43 "Hospital Troubles in Halifax," CMAJ, 1 (March, 1911), 256–7.
44 Hart, "What the Average Medical Man Expects from the Hospital," 36.
45 "Medical Staff Re-organization at the Toronto General Hospital," CP, 33 (March, 1908), 189–90.
46 "A Hospital Sunday," CL, 40 (August, 1907), 1111.
47 Hamilton Public Library, Hamilton City Hospital Scrapbook, Clipping, Hamilton *Daily Spectator*; 29 May 1894, 4 December 1894; HCA, HCH, Board of Governors, Minutes, 6 August 1896.
48 "The Charges and Privileges in the Toronto Hospitals," CL, 39 (May, 1906), 838–40; "Some Hospital Problems," CL, 41 (February, 1908), 465–6; "An Act Respecting the Toronto General Hospital," CL, 44 (April, 1911), 634.
49 "Hospital Abuses," DMJ, 10 (March, 1898), 128.
50 Starr, *Social Transformation of American Medicine*, 163–4.
51 See Stevens, *American Medicine and the Public Interest*, 51 for a summary of the experience of American hospitals.
52 "The Charity Abuse," DMJ, 9 (November, 1897), 854.
53 Ibid.; "Comment," DMJ, 29 (December, 1907), 278.
54 "The Ontario Hospital Association," CL, 36 (January, 1903), 357.
55 "Another Phase of Hospital Abuse," DMJ, 12 (January, 1899), 39; "Editorial," DMJ, 13 (November, 1899), 264; J.E. Jones, "Hospital Legislation," WCMJ, 3 (August, 1909), 296.
56 "The Pay System at Hospitals," CL, 27 (December, 1894), 127; W. Robson Nicholson, "Relations of Doctors to Dispensaries and Hospitals," WCMJ, 3 (November, 1909), 505.
57 "Editorial," DMJ, 13 (November, 1899), 263–4.
58 "The Pay System at Hospitals," 126.
59 "The Hospital Facilities for Clinical Teaching in the Centres of Medical Education," CL, 37 (December, 1903), 353.
60 "Municipal Hospitals," WCMJ, 12 (December, 1907), 555–6.
61 "An Important Decision," CL, 35 (No 3, 1901), 161–2; "Hospital Use and Abuse," CP, 26 (March, 1901), 169–70.
62 Perron, *Un siècle de vie hospitalière au Québec*, 57–87.

63 Hart, "What the Average Medical Man Expects from the Hospital," 39–40.
64 Shortt, " 'Before the Age of Miracles,' " 129, 138.
65 "Hospital Dietetics," CMAJ, 6 (May, 1916), 433.
66 PAM, MSP, 1919, Second Interim Report of the Public Welfare Commission of Manitoba, 1919, 24.
67 Ibid.
68 "In the Mail," CD, 1 (October, 1935), 4.
69 James R. Chadwick, "Medical Libraries, Their Development and Use," CL, 27 (April, 1896), 270.
70 "Hospitals and the Medical Profession," CL, 41 (September, 1907), 71–2; "Hospitals and the Diffusion of Knowledge," CL, 41 (December, 1907), 315–16; "Osler on 'The Organization of the Clinical Lab,' " WCMJ, 8 (October, 1914), 466–7; OSGM, Owen Sound Medical Society, Minutes, 1 November 1919.
71 Malcolm T. MacEachern, "How Hospitals Are Meeting Present Day Conditions," CH, 11 (January, 1934), 11.
72 "Hospital Bed Shortage," VMAB, 4 (March, 1928), 142.
73 Kathryn Meitzler, "Some of the Newer Developments in Hospital Equipment and Procedure," Proceedings of the Thirteenth Annual Convention of the British Columbia Hospitals' Association(Vancouver, 1931), 160.
74 James McKenty, "The Relations of the Medical Profession to Hospitals," CMAJ, 17 (February, 1927), 152.
75 PAM, MSP, 1919, Second Interim Report of the Public Welfare Commission of Manitoba, February, 1919, 2.
76 Risse, Mending Bodies, Saving Souls, 677.
77 Le Fanu, The Rise and Fall of Modern Medicine, 3.
78 Report of the Vancouver Hospital Survey Commission [typescript version], 117.
79 PAM, WGH, Annual Reports, 1920–1930.
80 J.O. Todd, "Canada and Hospital Administration," WCMJ, 11 (November, 1910), 485–8; PAM, WGH, Medical Staff, Minutes, 25 July 1911; PAM, MSP, 1919, Second Interim Report of the Public Welfare Commission of Manitoba, 1919, p.13.
81 R.H. Cameron, "Address of the President," CH, 5 (November, 1928), 12.
82 This is the substance of McKenty, "The Relations of the Medical Profession to Hospitals."
83 Connor, Doing Good, 211.
84 PAM, WGH, Medical Staff Minutes, 25 August 1914.
85 McKenty, 153–4.
86 PAM, MSP, 1919, Second interim Report of the Manitoba Public Welfare Commission, 16.
87 "Hospital Bed Shortage," VMAB, 4 (1928),143.

88 Ibid.

89 Report of the Vancouver Hospital Survey Commission [typescript version], 111–15.

90 Ibid., [print version], 42.

91 BCMA, Vancouver Medical Association, Minutes, 23 December 1929; Dr M. MacEachern to Dr J. Monro, 12 December 1929; MacDermot papers, "The Broad Aspects of the Hospital Question in Vancouver," typescript, 31 July 1930; "Hospital Committee," VMAB, 7 (May, 1931), 175–8.

92 Report of the Vancouver Hospital Survey Commission, [print version] 84–5.

93 Ibid., 71, 85.

94 "Hospital Committee," VMAB, 7 (May, 1931), 175–8.

95 G. Harvey Agnew, "The Relationship of the Medical Profession to the Hospital," CH, 7 (November, 1930), 15–16.

96 "A Confrere Sees Movement Further Affecting Position of General Practitioner and Urges Caution," CD, 3 (June, 1937), 23; C.F. Martin, "Medical Ethics and Medical Etiquette," CD, 2 (May, 1936), 9; Hilton C. Winternitz, "Young Doctors Urged to Avoid Specialization," CD, 2 (August, 1936), 84.

97 "Report of the Committee on Economics: A Plan for Hospital Insurance in Canada," CMAJ, 31 (September, 1934), Supplement, 51–2.

98 Irving, "Harry Morris Cassidy and the Health Insurance Dispute," 65.

99 Harris McPhedran, "The Difficulties of the Profession," CMAJ, 31 (July, 1934), 76.

100 "Changing Times," CD, 2 (June, 1936), 13.

101 "The Medical Officer and the 'Hospital Aid Act,'" MMAB, 13 (June, 1933), 505–7; H.I.P. O'Crates, "On Free Hospital Services: Unnecessary Waste of Public Funds," MMAB, 12 (July, 1932), 186–8; C.W. McCharles, "The Place of an Out-Patient Department in the Medical Services for a Community," MMAB, 13 (May, 1933), 461–2; Basil Cuddihy, "The Patients That Do Not Come to Me," CD, 2 (June 1936), 9–13.

102 "An Opportunity for Ontario Municipalities to Lighten the Doctor's Burden," CH, 10 (February, 1933), 9; Naylor, "Canada's First Doctors' Strike," 155. The Ontario scheme was subsequently revised in 1935 to replace half fees with flat fees, and to pro-rate monthly payments to physicians on the basis of a formula that calculated the total capitalization of the relief fund as a percentage of the total physicians' bills submitted. If funds available were equal, for example, to 40 per cent of the physicians' bills submitted, each participant received 40 per cent of his/her approved billings. Capitalization of the fund was set at $0.35 per capita. See Marsh, Health and Unemployment, 178–87.

103 PAM, WGH, Annual Reports, 1930–1932.

104 McCharles, "The Place of an Out-Patient Department in the Medical Services for a Community," 461.

105 The history of the Winnipeg doctors' job action has been exhaustively reconstructed in Naylor, "Canada's First Doctors' Strike." Unless otherwise noted, this summary relies on Naylor's analysis.

106 Carr and Beamish, *Manitoba Medicine*, 120.

107 R.F. Coliman, "Medical Economics," *VMAB*, 8 (March, 1932), 122–4.

108 "Report of the Committee on Economics," 26–60 (details of the actual plan are on 53–60 following lengthy background documentation).

109 Ibid., 37.

110 Ibid., 27, 40, 38.

111 Ibid., 58, 38. These concerns had been flagged two years earlier by Harvey Agnew, "The Possible Effect of Health Insurance Upon Hospitals," *CMAJ*, 26 (February, 1932), 182–6, in which he argued that research confirmed that health insurance led to more competition among doctors for hospital privileges, more intervention by hospital-centred specialists, more impersonal doctor-patient relationships, and a greater demand for technology-based diagnostic services.

112 Bothwell and English, "Pragmatic Physicians: Canadian Medicine and Health Care Insurance," 482–7; Bothwell, "The Health of the Common People," 211.

113 *VMAB*, 9 (September, 1933), 217, quoted in Andrews, "The Course of Medical Opinion on State Health Insurance in British Columbia," 135.

114 Irving, "Harry Morris Cassidy and the Health Insurance Dispute," 68–74.

115 H.F. Angus, "Health Insurance in British Columbia," *Canadian Forum*, 17 (No. 195, 1937), 13.

116 "B.C. Doctors and State Medicine," *CD*, 15 (November, 1948), 84–5.

117 King, *Industry and Humanity*, 223.

118 Ibid., 222.

119 MacDermot, *History of the Canadian Medical Association*, vol 2, 74–84.

120 Naylor, *Private Practice*, 162.

121 Swartz, "The Limits of Health Insurance," 259.

122 See, Le Fanu, *The Rise and Fall of Modern Medicine*, chs 1–3; Naylor, *Private Practice*, 99–100.

123 "Professional Status of the General Practitioner," *CD*, 13 (December, 1947), 84–5; "Why Specialization is Popular," *CD*, 13 (June, 1947), 78; James Stevenson, "What's Wrong with General Practice?" *CD*, 12 (August, 1946), 31–3.

124 W.V. Johnston, "The General Practitioner and His Neighbourhood Hospital," *CMAJ*, 63 (October, 1950), 379.

125 Shortt, "'Before the Age of Miracles,'" 125.

CHAPTER FIVE

1 McPherson, *Bedside Matters*, 51.
2 Kinnear, *In Subordination*, 181.
3 McPherson, *Bedside Matters*, 31.
4 Melosh, *The Physician's Hand*, 17–20.
5 Gibbon and Mathewson, *Three Centuries of Canadian Nursing*, 146.
6 Ibid., 122–30; McPherson, *Bedside Matters*, 27.
7 Gibbon and Mathewson, *Three Centuries of Canadian Nursing*, 131.
8 CVA, RCH, Vol. 31, File 65, Royal Columbian Rules For Patients.
9 Gibbon and Mathewson, *Three Centuries of Canadian Nursing*, 130.
10 F.J. Shepherd, as cited in Gibbon and Mathewson, *The Nursing School of Montreal General Hospital*, 146.
11 Bradbury, *Working Families*, 29–33.
12 Clarke, *History of the Toronto General Hospital* (Toronto: Ryerson Press, 1913), as cited by Gibbon and Mathewson, *Three Centuries of Canadian Nursing*, 151.
13 Reverby, *Ordered to Care*, 36.
14 Gibbon and Mathewson, *Three Centuries of Canadian Nursing*, 122.
15 Williams, "From Sarah Gamp to Florence Nightingale," 58.
16 Gibbon and Mathewson, *Three Centuries of Canadian Nursing*, 110, 151.
17 MacDermot, *History of the Montreal General Hospital*, 31.
18 See Roland, "The Early Years of Antiseptic Surgery in Canada," especially 237–41 for a discussion on the introduction of Listerism to Canada and the ensuing debates.
19 Baly, *Nursing and Social Change*, 131.
20 Reverby, *Ordered to Care*, 42.
21 Ibid., 80.
22 Ibid., 4; Tomes, "'Little World of Our Own,'" 473; R. Gagan, *A Sensitive Independence*, 40.
23 Riegler, *Jean I. Gunn*, 17.
24 PAO, SCGM, Decennial Report 1865–1875, 9.
25 McPherson, *Bedside Matters*, 27; Coburn, "'I See and Am Silent,'" 136–7; Jardine, "An Urban Middle-Class Calling," 178.
26 Gibbon and Mathewson, *Three Centuries of Canadian Nursing*, 144.
27 McPherson, "'Skilled Service and Women's Work,'" 9.
28 Ibid.
29 Mary A. Snively, "The Toronto General Hospital Training School for Nurses," CN, 1 (March, 1905), 7–8.
30 Coburn, "'I See and Am Silent,'" 141.
31 McPherson, *Bedside Matters*, 28–9; Gibbon and Mathewson, *Three Centuries of Canadian Nursing*, 146–7; MacDermot, *A History of the Montreal General Hospital*, 84.

32 McPherson, *Bedside Matters*, 29.
33 Baly, *Nursing and Social Change*, 124.
34 MacDermot, *A History of the Montreal General Hospital*, 84.
35 Gibbon and Mathewson, *Three Centuries of Canadian Nursing*, 149.
36 Statistics Canada, Historical Statistics of Canada, Health (Series B82-92), "Number of Physicians, Dentists, and Nurses ... Canada, 1871 to 1975."
37 See Strange, *Toronto's Girl Problem*, 27.
38 McPherson and Stuart, "Writing Nursing History in Canada," 12–14.
39 Frederica Wilson, "Notes on Nursing as Given to my Class," CN, 2 (September, 1906), 13.
40 *Women of Canada*, 59.
41 For a discussion of the difficulties of creating a united, self-regulating nursing profession in Quebec see, for example, Cohen and Bienvenue, "Émergence de l'identité professionelle chez les infirmières québecoises, 1890–1927;" and Petitat, *Les infirmières*, 67.
42 Roberts and Group, *Feminism in Nursing*, 3–7; Reverby, *Ordered to Care*, 41–2.
43 Kinnear, *In Subordination*, 98.
44 Dauphin, "Single Women," 440.
45 See Dean and Bolton, "The Admonition of Poverty and the Development of Nursing Practice in Nineteenth-Century England," 88, for a discussion of the association between the uniform and power in the hospital; Valverde, *The Age of Light, Soap, and Water*, 32.
46 McPherson, "'The Country is a Stern Nurse,'" 183.
47 André Mesureur, "The Mission of the Modern Nurse," CN, 3 (June 1907), 328.
48 Strong-Boag, "Making a Difference," 237.
49 For a recent examination of nursing history see D'Antonio, "Revisiting and Rethinking the Rewriting of Nursing History."
50 Reverby, *Ordered to Care*, 42.
51 Davies, "A Constant Casualty," 103.
52 Splane, *Social Welfare in Ontario*, 210.
53 Davies, "A Constant Casualty," 104.
54 McPherson, *Bedside Matters*, 44.
55 PAM, WGH, Oral History Project, Oral History, Winnipeg General Hospital 1920–1940, interview with Josephine Mann, Tapes C925-26, Side B.
56 TGH, School of Nursing, Graduate Applications, 1882–1889.
57 Boyd, *Josephine Butler, Octavia Hill, Florence Nightingale*, 194.
58 Weir, *Survey of Nursing Education in Canada*.
59 Jardine, "An Urban Middle-Class Calling," 178–9.
60 Kelly, *Quest for a Profession*, 8.
61 CVA, VGH, Series C, Vol 12, File 102, Isabella Smith, [unpublished typescript], 5.

62 See Baumgart and Kirkwood, "Social reform versus education reform," 511.

63 TGH, School of Nursing, Annual Report, 1890, 1.

64 Jardine, "An Urban Middle-Class Calling," 179.

65 TGH, School of Nursing, Annual Report, 1891, 6.

66 TGH, School of Nursing, Annual Report, 1892, 3.

67 TGH, School of Nursing, Annual Report, 1891, 2.

68 TGH, School of Nursing, Annual Report, 1896, 3.

69 Wilson, "Notes on Nursing as Given to my Class," CN, 2 (December, 1906), 51–2.

70 Adams, "Rooms of Their Own," 34.

71 PAM, WGH, Oral History Project, interview with Beryl Seeman. Tape 21, Side B; and see Petitat, Les infirmières, 126–8 for a discussion of both the subordinate relationships and the familial environment characteristic of nurses' encounter with the hospital.

72 PAM, WGH, Oral History Project, interview with Josephine Mann, Tape C 925 Side B.

73 C.A. Aikens, "Hospital Ethics and Discipline," CN, 3 (May, 1907), 247.

74 Snively, "The Canadian Society of Superintendents of Training Schools for Nurses First Annual Meeting: Excerpt of Address given by Miss Snively of Toronto General Hospital, President of the Society," CN, 3 (October, 1907), 541.

75 Aikens, "Hospital Ethics and Discipline," CN, 3 (May, 1907), 247.

76 Aikens, "Hospital Ethics and Discipline," CN, 3 (August, 1907), 420.

77 Ibid., 421.

78 PAM, MSP, Public Welfare Commission of Manitoba, Second Interim Report, February 1919, 5.

79 Tom Olson, "Apprenticeship and Exploitation"; Social Science History, 17 (Winter, 1993), 566.

80 Kelly, Quest for a Profession, 92.

81 Street, Watch-fires on the Mountains, 23.

82 Ibid., 25.

83 Ibid., 131; Riegler, Jean I. Gunn, 111; M.A. McKenzie, "The Employing of Graduate Nurses in Hospitals," CN, 2 (September, 1906), 19–20.

84 McKenzie, "Employing of Graduate Nurses,"19–20.

85 Coburn, "I See and am Silent," 152.

86 Whittaker, "The Search for Legitimacy," 320.

87 Kinnear, In Subordination, 107.

88 CVA, VGH, Series C, Vol. 12, File 102, Isabelle Smith [typescript], 9.

89 Grant Fleming, "The Survey of Nursing Education in Canada," CMAJ, 23 (April, 1932), 472.

90 PAO, CGH, Box 8, Training School, Student Files, Lecture Subjects, 1908.

91 Richardson, "Staffing the Hospitals," 138.

92   Ibid.
93   Gibbon and Mathewson, *Three Centuries of Canadian Nursing,* 156.
94   Richardson, "Staffing the Hospitals," 138.
95   PAM, WGH, Oral History Project, interview with Olive Irwin, Tape 32, Side A.
96   Kelly, *Quest for a Profession,* 97.
97   Strong-Boag and McPherson, "The Confinement of Women," 146.
98   Gidney and Millar, "Medical Students at the University of Toronto," 35–6 documents the overwhelming preponderance of sons of the professional and business classes among University of Toronto medical students 1910–1940.
99   H.W. Riggs, "The Doctor as a Factor in the Education of a Nurse," CN, 12 (October, 1916), 560.
100   Dr Dunlop, "Address to the Nursing Staff, Holy Cross Hospital, Chicago," CN, 21 (July, 1925), 364.
101   PAM, WGH, Oral History Project, interview with Josephine Mann, Tape 925, Side B.
102   Aikens, "Hospital Ethics and Discipline," CN, 3 (June, 1907), 313.
103   PAM, WGH, Oral History Project, interview with Mary Duncan, Tape C903, Side B.
104   PAM, WGH, Oral History Project, interview with Grace Parker, Tape 908, Side A.
105   PAM, WGH, Oral History Project, interview with Beryl Seeman, Tape 21, Side B.
106   Jean I. Gunn, "Trends of Nursing in Ontario: Summary," CN, 23 (September, 1927), 485.
107   Peter Twohig, " 'Local Girls' and 'Lab Boys': Gender, Skill, and Science in Interwar Nova Scotia," 15.
108   Melosh, "More Than 'The Physician's Hand,' " 491.
109   Dunlop, "Address to Nursing Staff," 363.
110   PAM, WGH, Oral History Project, interview with Myrtle Crawford, Tape 40 Side B
111   "Nurses, Stenography, and Matrimony," *Busy Man's Magazine,* (February, 1906), 78.
112   Aikens, "Hospital Ethics and Discipline," CN, 3 (June, 1907), 313.
113   PAO, CGH, Box 9, Training School Records, 1918. This file provides some reasons for nurses' dismissal from the training school in 1918, including being "too familiar with male patients."
114   PAM, WGH, Oral History Project, interview with Ingebjorg Cross, Tape C 922, Side B.
115   PAM, WGH, Oral History Project, interview with Isabel Cameron, Tape 14, Side A.
116   Aikens, "The Head Nurse and Her Patients," CN, 3 (March, 1907), 130.

117 Ibid.
118 Coburn, "I See and Am Silent," p .145.
119 Weir, *Survey of Nursing Eductaion in Canada*, 66.
120 McPherson, *Bedside Matters*, 51.
121 Ibid., 52.
122 Weir, *Survey of Nursing Education in Canada*, 429.
123 PAM, WGH, Oral History Project, interview with Myrtle Crawford, 5 August 1988, Tape 40, Side B.
124 Ibid.
125 McPherson, *Bedside Matters*, 79.
126 See PAO, CGH, Box 10, Class Record Book, Oct. 1928–Feb. 1931, Training School, for a list of the courses taken by the preliminary class of 1928–31.
127 See McPherson, *Bedside Matters*, 88–90 for an examination of the implementation of scientific management principles in Canadian hospitals.
128 Reverby, "The Search for the Hospital Yardstick," 219.
129 McPherson underscores this perception in "Skilled Service and Women's Work," 327, and in McPherson, "Science and Technique: Nurses' Work in Canadian Hospitals, 1920–1939," 81.
130 CVA, VGH, Vol. 11, File 94. Ethel Johns to M. MacEachern, 25 June 1921.
131 Riegler, *Jean I. Gunn*, 177.
132 Ibid., 107; Kelly, *Quest for a Profession*, 107. For example, the VGH board estimated that the shift to the eight-hour day in 1937 would require fifty additional general duty nurses at a total cost of $60,000 annually unless other economies could be identified.
133 McPherson, *Bedside Matters*, 86–7.
134 Weir, *Survey of Nursing Education in Canada*, 193.
135 Ibid.
136 McPherson, *Bedside Matters*, 88.
137 Risse, *Mending Bodies, Saving* Souls, 10.
138 S.R. Laycock, "Patients Are Persons," CN, 37 (December, 1941), 819.
139 PAM, WGH, Oral History Project, interview with Mabel Lytle, 30 June 1987, Tape C 910, Side A.
140 See Adams, "Rooms of their Own," for a description of the Royal Victoria Hospital's attempts to create a home-like atmosphere that would attract middle-class women into nursing.
141 PAM, WGH Oral History Project, interview with Olive Erwin, 3 August 1988. Tape 33 (C-9320), Side A.
142 M.T. MacEachern, *Survey of the Nursing Question: with special consideration of the problems arising therefrom and their application in the Vancouver General Hospital* (Vancouver: np, 1919), 8.
143 Ibid., 20–2.

144 TGH, School of Nursing, Annual Report, 1909, 1.
145 TGH, School of Nursing, Annual Report, 1931, 6.
146 Mary H. Tufts, "Hospital Discipline and Ethics," CN, 11 (September, 1915), 519.
147 MacEachern, *Survey of the Nursing Question*, 23.
148 CVA, VGH, Isabelle Smith Manuscript, 14.
149 Ethel Johns, "Let Us Try to Understand," CN, 32 (November, 1936), 504.
150 Weir, *Survey of Nursing Education in* Canada, 63.
151 Fleming, "The Survey of Nursing Education in Canada," 471; for commentary on the relationships between these two organizations see Julia Kinnear, "The Professionalization of Canadian Nursing, 1924–1932: Views in the CN and the CMAJ," 153–74.
152 Weir, *Survey of Nursing Education in Canada*, 7.
153 Baumgart and Kirkwood, "Social reform *versus* education reform," 510–13.
154 Fleming, "The Survey of Nursing Education in Canada," 472.
155 Ibid.
156 Weir, *Survey of Nursing Education in Canada*, 205.
157 Ibid., 204.
158 Ibid., 354.
159 Ibid., 203.
160 Ibid., 354.
161 Ibid., 217.
162 Ibid., 178.
163 Ibid., 191.
164 Ibid., 276.
165 Ibid., 298.
166 Ibid., 390.
167 Ibid., 197.
168 Ibid., 298.
169 Ibid., 381.
170 Ethel Johns, "A Sense of Value," CN, 26 (December, 1930), 403.
171 See, for example, Gertrude Johnson, "Educational Problems of the Small Hospital," CN, 28 (April, 1932), 194–5.
172 McPherson, *Bedside Matters*, 20–1.
173 Georgina E. Thompson, "Some Pointed Questions," CN, 32 (October, 1936), 454.
174 PAO, CGH, Box 28, File 8, School of Nursing Inspection Reports, 1935.
175 Ibid., 1937.
176 Ibid., 1942.
177 McPherson, *Bedside Matters*, 150, 159–60; Cohen and Bienvenue, "Émergence de l'identité professionnelle"; and see Boutilier, "Helpers

or Heroines? The National Council of Women, Nursing, and 'Women's Work' in Late Victorian Canada."

178   McPherson, *Bedside Matters*, 207.

179   Gibbon and Mathewson, *Three Centuries of Canadian Nursing*, 489.

180   Petitat, *Les infirmières*, 164.

181   Ibid., 379; McPherson, *Bedside Matters*, 159.

182   See H.B. Atlee, "The Future of Nursing," CN, 34 (September, 1939), 469.

183   McPherson, *Bedside Matters*, 211.

184   Kelly, *Quest for a Profession*, 83; McPherson, *Bedside Matters*, 213.

185   Rita Curley, "Is the General Staff Nurse Worthwhile," CN, 39 (October, 1943), 674–5.

186   Annie F. Laurie, "Hospitals and Schools of Nursing: A Plea for the General Duty Nurse," CN, 38 (June, 1942), 410.

187   E.C. McIlwraith, "What We Expect of General Staff Nurses," CN, 39 (August, 1943), 533–4.

CHAPTER SIX

1   Stevens, *In Sickness and in Wealth*, 110.

2   Sister John Gabriel, "The Hospital and the Changing Social Order," *The Hospital in Modern Society*, Arthur C. Bachmeyer and Gerhard Hartman, eds. (New York, 1943), 20.

3   "The Patient – A Personality, Not a Case," HW, 1 (January, 1912), 5.

4   PABC, VGH, Inquiry, 1912, *Investigative Proceedings*, 295.

5   Sister Harquil, "The Admission and Discharge of Patients," CH, 9 (September, 1932), 11.

6   For the purposes of the analysis that follows, we have made extensive use of records pertaining to patient experience in the Vancouver General Hospital. Other hospital records have been accessed where appropriate and as available; but as the result of two major public inquiries, separated by seventeen years, both of which canvassed patient opinion, these VGH sources are especially revealing.

7   *Report of the Vancouver Hospital Survey Commission*, 1931, 124 [typescript].

8   "The Hospital Field in Canada," CH, 8 (September, 1931), 52–5; Gagan, 'A Necessity Among Us,' 18; "New Owen Sound Hospital," CH, 6 (October, 1929), 28–9.

9   See Gagan, 'A Necessity Among Us,' 69; HCA, HCH, Board of Directors, Minutes, 20 February 1900, 29 December 1943.

10   See, for example, "Equipment of the New Toronto General Hospital," HW, 1 (April, 1912), 239–42; PAO, RG8, Department of the Provincial Secretary, Report on General Hospitals, 1916, 12–19; "The Place of the Dietitian in the Hospital," CH, 3 (January, 1926), 20; Meitzler, "Some of

the Newer Developments in Hospital Equipment and Procedure," 161.
A sample of contemporary hospital improvement literature might
include "Soya Beans, The Grain with a Hundred Uses," *CH*, 8 (January,
1931); "The Use of Concentrated Milks in the Hospital Diet," *CH*, 8
(February, 1931); "The Trend in Hospital Construction on the North
American Continent," *CH*, 9 (January, 1932); "Mechanical Equipment of
Hospitals Presents Many Complex Problems," *CH*, 12 (March, 1935);
"Important Advances Have Been Made in Hospital Lighting," *CH*, 8
(May, 1931); "Selecting Food Service Equipment for the Modern Hospi-
tal," *CH*, 8 (October–December, 1931).

11 Anne Anderson Perry, "The High Cost of Sickness," *The Chatelaine*, 2
(February, 1929), 13.

12 C.J. Decker, "The Business of Hospitals," *CH*, 14 (March, 1937), 37; Rev
T. Boyle, "Keep the Hospital in the Public Mind and Inspire Local
Pride," *CH*, 7 (February, 1930), 20–1.

13 Mrs Rex Eaton, "Hospitals from a Woman's Viewpoint," *Report of the
Twenty-Second Annual Convention of the British Columbia Hospitals'
Association* (Vancouver, 1939), 34.

14 Leonard Shaw, "Private Room Service in Keeping with Present Day
Needs," *CH*, 12 (March, 1935), 18.

15 Ibid.

16 "Public Relations," *CH*, 14 (October, 1937), 64.

17 Sister Harquil, "The Admission and Discharge of Patients," 11.

18 For equivalent American hospital distinctions see David Rosner,
"Business at the Bedside: Health Care in Brooklyn, 1895–1915."

19 *Survey of Public General Hospitals in Ontario*, Part 4, 1.

20 Weir, *Survey of Nursing Education in Canada*, 394–412.

21 Shaw, "Private Room Service in Keeping with Present Day Needs,"
18–19.

22 PABC, VGH, Inquiry, 1912, *Investigative Proceedings*, 100–19.

23 Ibid., 127–216; PABC, VGH, Inquiry, 1912, *Commissioner's Report*, 51.

24 "Public Relations," *CH*, 14 (October, 1937), 64.

25 Vancouver *Province*, 7 September 1912.

26 Risse, *Mending Bodies, Saving Souls*, 8–10.

27 PABC, "Rules and Regulations of the Vancouver General Hospital...1906," 1–56; Decker, "The Business of Hospitals," 37; Meitzler,
"Some of the Newer Developments in Hospital Equipment and Procedure," 161; CVA, VGH, Medical Board, Minutes, 8 April 1919.

28 *Report of the Vancouver Hospital Survey Commission*, 104 [print version];
Report of a Study of the Vancouver General Hospital, 11, 16.

29 "Hospital Noises," *CMAJ*, 20 (June, 1929), 669.

30 Robertson, Marcellus, and Dandy, *Mission's Living Memorials*, 49.

31 American Public Health Association, *Public Health in Manitoba*

(Winnipeg: King's Printer, 1941), 90–1; J.M. Kniseley, "Medical Social Work in the Toronto General Hospital," sw, 13 (February, 1931), 93–5; PAM, WGH, Annual Report, 1931, 17; CVA, VGH, Medical Board, Minutes, 12 March 1918, 14 January 1919; *Report of the Vancouver Hospital Survey Commission*, 85 [print version]; G.F. Stephens, "Problem of Patients," *MMAB*, no. 111(November, 1930), 4–5.

32 Manitoba Welfare Supervision Board, *Hospitals in Manitoba: Report of a Study* (Winnipeg, 1944), 45; PAM, WGH, Annual Reports, 1907, 16, and 1917, 13; PAM, Nurses and Their Work, Oral Histories of Nursing in Winnipeg, 1920–1940, Interview, Tape C923, I. Cross, 10 July 10 1988 re: Scarlet Fever Epidemic, Brandon General Hospital.

33 *Report of the Vancouver Hospital Survey Commission*, 156–7 [print version].

34 Ferguson, *A White Man's Country*, 4–6.

35 CVA, VGH, Board of Directors, Minutes, 14 November 1907; *Vancouver Daily Province*, 16 May 1912; CVA, VGH, Annual Report, 1908; PABC, VGH, Inquiry, 1912, *Commissioner's Report*, 23–4.

36 Walsh, "Report of a Study of the Vancouver General Hospital," 12.

37 PAM, Oral Histories of Nursing in Winnipeg, Interview, Myrtle Crawford, 5 August 1988, Tape 40.

38 Rosenberg, *Care of Strangers*, 291.

39 McPherson, *Bedside Matters*, 100.

40 C.A. Aitkens, "The Head Nurse and Her Patient," CN, 3 (March, 1907), 130–4; S.R. Laycock, "Patients Are Persons," CN, 37 (December, 1941), 816–19.

41 PAM, Oral Histories of Nursing in Winnipeg, Interview, Josephine Mann, 22 July 1988, Tapes C925-C926.

42 Ernest A. Hall, "Hospital Treatment and Some Cases in Practice," CL, 37 (May, 1904), 794.

43 Weir, *Survey of Nursing Education in Canada*, 394–6.

44 PABC, VGH, Inquiry, 1912, *Proceedings*, 7, 12, 14–22, 24, 64, 312–14, 610–11, 651; *Vancouver Sun*, 18 May 1912; *Report of the Vancouver Hospital Survey Commission*, 98 [print version].

45 PABC, VGH, Inquiry, 1912, *Investigative Proceedings*, 628.

46 TGH, Annual Report, 1891.

47 See Levenstein, *Revolution at the Table*, 23–5.

48 PABC, VGH, Inquiry, 1912, *Investigative Proceedings*, 43–52, 315, 601; *Commissioner's Report*, 57–8, 75. Vancouver *The Sun*, 11 June 1912; PAO, Cornwall General Hospital, Visiting Governors' Reports, 12 October 1909, 16 December 1909; Gagan, *'A Necessity Among Us,'* 42–6; "Hospital Dietetics," 432.

49 "Hospital Dietaries," CMAJ, 16 (February, 1926), 184.

50 "Food Service in the Small Hospital," CMAJ, 36 (January, 1937), 80.

51 PABC, VGH, Inquiry, 1912, *Investigative Proceedings*, 43–52, 606–8.

52 CVA, VGH, Newspaper Clippings, *Truth*, 12 March 1912.

53 "More Publicity is Needed," 11.

54 Decker, "The Business of Hospitals," 37–8.

55 Stewart, "The Care of the Sick," *CMAJ*, 16 (December, 1926), 1513.

56 *Survey of Public General Hospitals in Ontario*, Part 1, 13–23; Part 4, 10, 72; Part 5, Table 22.

57 G.F. Stephens, "Problems of Patients," *MMAB*, no. 111 (November, 1930), 4–5; PAM, WGH, Annual Report, 1931.

58 PAO, RG3, Mitchell Hepburn Papers, Box 199, File 162, "Survey of Long Stay Patients, 1936."

59 *Survey of Public General Hospitals in Ontario*, Part 5, Table 24.

60 PAO, "Survey of Long Stay Patients, 1936."

61 Lewis, "Reducing Maternal Mortality in British Columbia: An Educational Process," 344.

62 "Teaching Men to Legislate for Women," *The Chatelaine*, 1 (July, 1928), 16; Bertha E. Hall and Anne Elizabeth Wilson, "Must 1,532 Mothers Die?" *The Chatelaine*, 1 (July, 1928), 38.

63 Strong-Boag and McPherson, "The Confinement of Women," 154, 161; Leavitt, *Brought to Bed*, 187.

64 Oppenheimer, "Childbirth in Ontario," 66–7; *Survey of Public General Hospitals in Ontario*, Part 5, 22.

65 Robert Ferguson, "A Plea for Better Obstetrics," *CMAJ*, 10 (October, 1920), 902–4.

66 *Report of the Vancouver Hospital Survey Commission*, 88 [print version]; Strong-Boag and McPherson, "The Confinement of Women," 142.

67 "Is It Dangerous to Have a Baby in the Hospital?" *CH*, 14 (April, 1937), 21.

68 McLaren and McLaren, *The Bedroom and the State*, 47–51.

69 PAO, CGH, Register of Surgical Operations, 1908.

70 PAM, WGH, Annual Report, 1911.

71 *Survey of Public General Hospitals in Ontario*, Part I, 17–19; Part 5, 10, 17–22, Table 10.

72 Jasper Halpenny, "The Contribution of the Hospital to the Surgery of To-day," *CMAJ*, 9 (August, 1919), 681, 683.

73 PAM, WGH, Box 27, Gas Gangrene Infection 1921.

74 Halpenny, "The Contribution of the Hospital to the Surgery of Today," 681, 693.

75 .Johnston, "The General Practitioner and His Neighbourhood Hospital," 378.

76 *Report of the Vancouver Hospital Survey Commission*, 123–5 [typescript version].

77 PAO, RG3, "Survey of Long Stay Patients, 1936."

78 Weir, *Survey of Nursing Education in Canada*, 427–8.

79 Stewart, "The Care of the Sick," *CMAJ*, 16 (December, 1926), 1511.

80 Hayter, "The Clinic as Laboratory," 687; and see Hayter, "Medicalizing Malignancy: The Uneasy Origins of Ontario's Cancer Program, 1929–34."

81 Smith and Nickel, "From Home to Hospital," 53.

82 "The Writing of Medical Histories," *CMAJ*, 15 (October, 1925), 1060.

83 S.M. Fisher, "Some Thoughts on the Role of Anxiety in Ill Health," *University of Western Ontario Medical Journal*, 3 (December, 1932), 69.

84 Rosenberg, "Inward Vision," 45.

85 Anne Anderson Perry, "The High Cost of Sickness," *The Chatelaine*, 2 (September, 1929), 2–3, 14–15.

86 Perry, "The High Cost of Sickness," *The Chatelaine*, 2 (February, 1929), 12–15.

87 Perry, "What Can Women Do to Combat the High Cost of Sickness?" *The Chatelaine*, 3 (January, 1930), 19.

88 *Report on Social Security for Canada*, 55.

CHAPTER SEVEN

1 Canada, Dominion Bureau of Statistics, *Hospital Statistics, vol. VI: Hospital Expenditures, 1959* (Ottawa: Queen's Printer, 1962), Table 1; Canada, Dominion Bureau of Statistics, *Hospital Statistics, vol. VI: Hospital Expenditures, 1960* (Ottawa, Queen's Printer, 1963), Graph 1.

2 See Bennett and Krasny, "Health Care in Canada."

3 Risse, *Mending Bodies, Saving Souls*, 679.

4 "The Patient – A Personality, Not a Case," *HW*, I (January, 1912), 4–5.

Bibliography

INSTITUTIONAL, PROFESSIONAL, AND MEDICAL
RECORDS

British Columbia Medical Association Archives. Vancouver Medical Association. Minutes.
City of Vancouver Archives. Royal Columbian Hospital. Historical Records (ADD MSS 284).
– Vancouver City Hospital. Historical Records (ADD MSS 320).
– Vancouver General Hospital. Historical Records (ADD MSS 320).
Hamilton City Archives. Hamilton City Hospital. Hospital Committee Minutes.
– Hamilton City Hospital. Board of Directors' Minutes.
Hamilton Public Library. Hamilton City Hospital. Scrapbooks.
The Ontario Medical Register, 1877. Toronto: College of Physicians and Surgeons of Ontario, 1877.
The Ontario Medical Register, 1907. Toronto. College of Physicians and Surgeons of Ontario, 1907.
Owen Sound General and Marine Hospital. Historical Records.
– Owen Sound Medical Society. Minutes.
Public Archives of Manitoba. Winnipeg General Hospital. Historical Records (MG 10)
Public Archives of Ontario. Cornwall General Hospital. Historical Records (RG F1396)
St Catharines General and Marine Hospital. Historical Records.
Toronto General Hospital. Historical Records.
University of Manitoba Archives. Faculty of Medicine. Dean's Office Files.

HOSPITAL AND MEDICAL JOURNALS

Canada Lancet.
Canadian Doctor
Canadian Hospital
Canadian Medical Association Journal.
Canadian Nurse
Canadian Practitioner
Dominion Medical Journal
Hospital World
Manitoba Medical Association Bulletin
Manitoba Medical Association Review
Manitoba Medical Review
Social Welfare
Vancouver Medical Association Bulletin
Western Canada Medical Journal

GOVERNMENT RECORDS AND PUBLICATIONS

Canada. Department of National Health and Welfare. *Hospital Care in Canada: Recent Trends and Development.* Health Care Series, Memorandum no 12. Ottawa, 1960.

Canada. Department of National Health and Welfare. *Hospital Care in Canada: Trends and Development, 1948–1962.* Health Care Series, Memorandum no 19. Ottawa, 1964.

Canada. Dominion Bureau of Statistics and Department of National Health and Welfare. *Canadian Sickness Survey, 1950–51.* Ottawa, 1953.

Canada. Dominion Bureau of Statistics. *Hospital Statistics, VI, Hospital Expenditures, 1959.* Ottawa: Queen's Printer, 1962.

Canada. Dominion Bureau of Statistics. *Hospital Statistics, VI, Hospital Expenditures, 1960.* Ottawa: Queen's Printer, 1963.

Canada. Dominion Bureau of Statistics. *The Small General Hospital in 1957: A Statistical Summary.* Ottawa: Queen's Printer, 1960.

Canada. Dominion Bureau of Statistics. *The Large General Hospital in 1957: A Statistical Summary.* Ottawa: Queen's Printer, 1960.

Canada. House of Commons. Special Committee on Social Security. *Report on Social Security for Canada.* March 16, 1943.

Canada. House of Commons. Special Committee on Social Security. *Health Insurance.* March 16, 1943.

Canada. House of Commons. Special Committee on Social Security. *Minutes of Proceedings and Evidence,* no. 6. 9 April 1943.

Canada. *Report of The Royal Commission on Dominion-Provincial Relations.* Ottawa, 1940.

City of Vancouver Archives. City of Vancouver. Social Services. Series S. Director, Statistics.

Province of British Columbia. Legislative Assembly. Sessional Papers. Hospital Returns.

Province of Manitoba. Manitoba Health Advisory Survey Committee. *Report on Health Services, Facilities and Personnel, and Recommendations*, 1952.

Province of Manitoba. Welfare Supervision Board. *Hospitals in Manitoba: Report of a Study*, 1944.

Province of Manitoba. Royal Commission in Reference to the Costs of Hospitalization. *Report*, 1949.

Province of Ontario. Department of Health. *The Hospitals of Ontario: A Short History.* Toronto: King's Printer, 1934.

Province of Ontario. Department of Health. Division of Medical Statistics. *A Survey of Public General Hospitals in Ontario.* Toronto, 1939–40.

Province of Ontario. Legislative Assembly. Sessional Papers. Inspector of Hospitals and Charities. Annual Reports.

Province of Ontario. Minister of Health. *Report of the Ontario Health Survey Committee.* Toronto, 1951.

Province of Ontario. Royal Commission on Public Welfare. *Report to the Lieutenant-Governor in Council.* Toronto: King's Printer. 1930.

Province de Québec, *Annuaire statistique/Statistical year-book.* Québec: King's Printer, 1915–1945.

Public Archives of British Columbia. Province of British Columbia. Provincial Secretary. Hearings Committee on Health Insurance, 1935. Briefs. [GR-391]

Public Archives of British Columbia. Province of British Columbia. Royal Commissions and Commisions of Inquiry. Commission on Health Insurance (1919–1921). Report on Maternity Insurance, 1921.

Public Archives of British Columbia. Province of British Columbia. Royal Commissions and Commissions of Inquiry. Commission on Health Insurance (1919–1921). Report.

Public Archives of British Columbia. Province of British Columbia. Royal Commissions and Commissions of Inquiry. Public Inquiry. Vancouver General Hospital, 1912. *Investigative Proceedings.*

Public Archives of British Columbia. Province of British Columbia. Royal Commissions and Commissions of Inquiry. Public Inquiry. Vancouver General Hospital, 1912. *Commissioner' s Report.*

Public Archives of British Columbia. Province of British Columbia. Royal Commissions and Commissions of Inquiry. Public Inquiry. Vancouver General Hospital, 1912. *Investigative Proceedings.*

Public Archives of British Columbia, *Rules and Regulations of the Vancouver General Hospital*, 1906.

Public Archives of Manitoba. Province of Manitoba. Legislative Assembly. Sessional Papers. Public Welfare Commission. Reports.

Public Archives of Manitoba. Province of Manitoba. Legislative Assembly. Sessional Papers. Department of Health and Public Welfare. Reports.
Public Archives of Manitoba. Province of Manitoba. Legislative Assembly. Sessional Papers. Department of Public Works, Annual Reports.
Public Archives of Manitoba. Province of Manitoba. Legislative Assembly. Sessional Papers. Department of Agriculture. Reports.
Public Archives of Ontario. Province of Ontario. Department of the Provincial Secretary. Reports on General Hospitals.
Public Archives of Ontario. Province of Ontario. Department of the Provincial Secretary. Inspector of Hospitals and Charities. Annual Reports.
Public Health in Manitoba: Report of a Study by the American Public Health Association, 1941
Revised Statutes of Ontario, 1897.
Saskatchewan. Health Services Survey Commission. *Report of the Commissioner.* Regina: King's Printer, 1944.
Statutes of Manitoba, 1933.

NEWSPAPERS

Hamilton *The Spectator*
Owen Sound *The Sun*
Owen Sound *Sun Times*
Owen Sound *The Times*
Vancouver *Daily Province*
Vancouver *Daily World*

SECONDARY SOURCES

Achenbaum, Andrew W. "American Medical History, Social History, and Medical Policy." *Journal of Social History.* 18(June, 1985), 343–7.
Adams, Annmarie. "Rooms of Their Own: The Nurses' Residences at Montreal's Royal Victoria Hospital," *Material History Review,* 40(Fall, 1994), 29–41.
Agnew, G. Harvey. *Canadian Hospitals, 1920–1970: A Dramatic Half Century.* Toronto: University of Toronto Press, 1974.
Allen, Richard. *The Social Passion: Religion and Social Reform in Canada, 1914–1928.* Toronto: University of Toronto Press, 1973.
Anctil, Hervé et al. "La santé et l'assistance publique au Québec, 1886–1986." *Santé Société.* Edition Spéciale. Québec: 1986.
Andrews, Margaret W. "The Course of Medical Opinion on State Health Insurance in British Columbia, 1919–1939." *Histoire sociale/Social History,* XVI(May, 1983), 131–43.

– "Medical Attendance in Vancouver, 1886–1920." *B.C. Studies*, 40(Winter, 1978–9), 32–56.

Angus, H.F. "Health Insurance in British Columbia." *Canadian Forum.* XVII(no. 195, 1937), 12–14.

Angus, Margaret. *Kingston General Hospital: A Social and Institutional History.* Montreal: McGill-Queen's University Press, 1973.

Artibise, Alan F.J. *Winnipeg: A Social History of Urban Growth, 1874–1914.* Montreal: McGill-Queen's University Press, 1975.

Bacchi, Carol. "Race Regeneration and Social Purity: A Study of the Social Attitudes of Canada's English-Speaking Suffragists." *Histoire sociale/Social History*, XI(22, 1978), 460–74.

Baly, Monica E. *Nursing and Social Change.* 2nd Edition. London: William Heineman, 1980.

Barber, Marilyn. "The Women Ontario Welcomed: Immigrant Domestics for Ontario Homes, 1870-1930." *The Neglected Majority: Essays in Canadian Women's History*, vol. 2. Alison Prentice and Susan Mann Trofimenkoff, eds. Toronto: McClelland & Stewart, 1985. Pp. 102–21.

Bartlett, Eleanor. "Real Wages and the Standard of Living in Vancouver, 1901–1929." *B.C. Studies*, 51(Autumn, 1981), 3–61.

Baumgart, Alice J. and Rondalyn Kirkwood. "Social reform versus education reform: university nursing education in Canada, 1919–1960." *Journal of Advanced Nursing*, 15(1990), 510–16.

Bennett, James E. and Jacques Krasny. "Health Care in Canada." *Health and Canadian Society.* David Coburn, Carl D'Arcy, Peter New and George Torrance, eds., 40–66. Toronto, 1981.

Bernier, Jacques. *La médicine au Québec: Naissance et évolution d'une profession.* Québec: Les Presses de l'Université Laval, 1989.

– "Les practiciens de la santé au Québec, 1871–1921. Quelques données statistiques." *Recherches Sociographiques*, XX(I, 1979), 41–58.

Biggs, C. Lesley. "The Case of the Missing Midwives: A History of Midwifery in Ontario from 1795–1900." *Ontario History*, 75(March, 1983), 22–35.

Bonner, Thomas Neville. *Becoming a Physician: Medical Education in Britain, France, Germany, and the United States, 1750–1945.* New York: Oxford University Press, 1995.

– *Medicine in Chicago, 1850–1950.* 2nd edition. Chicago: University of Illinois Press, 1991.

Borst, Charlotte G. *Catching Babies: The Professionalization of Childbirth, 1870–1920.* Cambridge, Mass.: Harvard University Press, 1995.

Bothwell, Robert S. "The Health of the Common People." *Mackenzie King: Widening the Debate.* John O. Stubbs and John English, eds., 191–220. Toronto: Macmillan, 1977.

Bothwell, Robert S. and John English. "Pragmatic Physicians: Canadian Medicine and Health Care Insurance." *Medicine in Canadian Society: Historical Perspectives.* S.E.D. Shortt, ed., 479–93. Montreal: McGill-Queen's University Press, 1981.

Bouchard, Gérard. "Naissance d'une élite: les médecins dans la société saguenayenne (1850–1940)." *Revue d'Histoire de l'Amérique Française,* 49(Printemps, 1996), 521–50.

Boutilier, Beverly. "Helpers or Heroines? The National Council of Women, Nursing, and 'Woman's Work' in Late Victorian Canada," *Caring and Curing: Historical Perspectives on Women and Healing in Canada.* Dianne Dodd and Deborah Gorham, eds, 17–48. Ottawa: University of Ottawa Press, 1994.

Boyd, Nancy. *Josephine Butler, Octavia Hill, Florence Nightingale: Three Victorian Women Who Changed Their World.* London: Macmillan, 1982.

Bradbury, Bettina. *Working Families: Age, Gender, and Daily Survival in Industrializing Montreal.* Toronto: McClelland & Stewart, 1993.

Britnell, G.E. "Saskatchewan, *1930–35.*" *Canadian Journal of Economics and Political Science,* 1(May, 1936), 143–66.

Burke, Sara Z. *Seeking the Highest Good: Social Service and Gender at the University of Toronto, 1888–1937.* Toronto: University of Toronto Press, 1996.

Carr, Ian and Robert Beamish. *Manitoba Medicine: A Brief History.* Winnipeg: University of Manitoba Press, 1999.

Coburn, Judi. " 'I See and Am Silent': A Short History of Nursing in Ontario." *Women at Work: Ontario, 1850–1950.* Janice Acton et al., eds, 127–64. Toronto: Canadian Women's Educational Press, 1974.

Cohen, Yolande et Louise Bienvenue. "Émergence de l'identité professionnelle chez les infirmières québecoises, 1890–1927." *Canadian Bulletin of Medical History,* 11(1994), 119–51.

Comacchio, Cynthia R. *Nations Are Built of Babies: Saving Ontario's Mothers and Children, 1900–1940.* Montreal: McGill-Queen's University Press, 1995.

Connor, J.T.H. "The Adoption and Effects of X-Rays in Ontario." *Ontario History.* 79(March, 1987), 92–107.

– *Doing Good: The Life of the Toronto General Hospital.* Toronto: University of Toronto Press, 2000.

– "Hospital History in Canada and the United States." *Canadian Bulletin of Medical History,* 7(1990), 93–104.

– "Listerism Unmasked: Antisepsis and Asepsis in Victorian Anglo-Canada." *Journal of the History of Medicine,* 49(April, 1994), 207–39.

– "'A Sort of *Felo-De-Se'*: Eclecticism, Related Medical Sects, and Their Decline in Victorian Ontario." BHM, 65(1991), 503–27.

Cook, Ramsay. *The Regenerators: Social Criticism in Late-Victorian English Canada.* Toronto: University of Toronto Press, 1985.

Copp, Terry. *The Anatomy of Poverty: The Condition of the Working Class in Montreal 1897–1929.* Toronto: McClelland & Stewart, 1974.

Cortiula, Mark W. "Social Class and Health Care in a Community Institution: The Case of Hamilton City Hospital." *Canadian Bulletin of Medical History,* 6(Winter, 1989), 133–45.
– "The Social Transformation of the Clinic in Hamilton, 1880–1917." Unpublished PhD thesis, University of Guelph, 1992.
Craig, Barbara Lazenby. "The Canadian Hospital in History and Archives." *Archivaria,* 21(Winter, 1985–6), 52–67.
– "The Role of Records and of Record-Keeping in the Development of the Modern Hospital in London, England, and Ontario, Canada, c.1890–c.1940," *Bulletin of the History of Medicine,* 65(1991), 376–97.
Crosbie, W.G. *The Toronto General Hospital, 1819–1965: A Chronicle.* Toronto: Macmillan, 1975.
D'Antonio, Patricia. "Revisiting and Rethinking the Rewriting of Nursing History." *Bulletin of the History of Medicine,* 73(Summer, 1999), 268–90.
Dauphin, Cecile. "Single Women." *A History of Women in the West: IV, Emerging Feminism from Revolution to War.* Georges Duby and Michelle Perrot, eds, 427–42. Cambridge, Mass.: Harvard University Press, 1993.
Davies, Celia. "A Constant Casualty: Nursing Education in Britain and the USA to 1939." *Rewriting Nursing History.* Celia Davies, ed., 102–22. London: Croom Helm, 1980.
Dean, Mitchell and Gail Bolton. "The Admonition of Poverty and the Development of Nursing Practice in Nineteenth-Century England." *Rewriting Nursing History.* Celia Davies, ed., 76–101. London: Croom Helm, 1980.
Digby, Anne. *Making a Medical Living: Doctors and Patients in the English Market for Medicine, 1720–1911.* Cambridge: Cambridge University Press, 1994.
Dodd, Dianne. "Advice to Parents: The Blue Books, Helen MacMurchy, MD, and the Federal Department of Health, 1920–1934," *Canadian Bulletin of Medical History,* 8(1991), 203–30.
Duffin, Jacalyn. "The Guru and the Godfather: Henry Sigerist, Hugh MacLean, and the Politics of Health Care Reform in 1940s Canada." *Canadian Bulletin of Medical History* 9(1992), 191–218.
Duncan, Sara Jeanette. 'The Life of a Nurse," *Sara Jeanette Duncan: Selected Journalism,* Thomas Tauskey, ed., 29. Ottawa, 1978.
Fahmy-Eid, Nadia et Lucie Piché. "Le savoir négocié: Les strategies des associations de technologie médicale, de physiothérapie et de diététique pour l'accès à une meilleure formation professionnelle (1930–1970)." *Revue d'histoire de l'Amérique Française,* 43(printemps, 1990), 509–34.
Fahrni, Gordon S. *Prairie Surgeon.* Winnipeg: Queenston House, 1976.
Flexner, Abraham. *Medical Education in the United States and Canada: A Report to the Carnegie Foundation for the Advancement of Teaching (1910).* Reprint. Buffalo. Heritage Press, 1973.

Ferguson, Ted. *A White Man's Country: An Exercise in Canadian Prejudice.* Toronto: Doubleday, 1975.

Fingard, Judith. *The Dark Side of Life in Victorian Halifax.* Porters Lake, NS: Pottersfield Press, 1989.

Finkel, Alvin. "Paradise Postponed: A Re-examination of the Green Book Proposals of 1945." *Journal of the Canadian Historical Association,* 4(1993), 120–42.

Gagan, David and Rosemary Gagan. "Working-Class Standards of Living in Late-Victorian Urban Ontario: A Review of the Miscellaneous Evidence on the Quality of Material Life." *Journal of the Canadian Historical Association,* 1(1990), 171–93.

Gagan, David. 'A *Necessity Among Us': The Owen Sound General and Marine Hospital 1891–1985.* Toronto: University of Toronto Press, 1990.

– "For 'Patients of Moderate Means': The Transformation of Ontario's Public Hospitals, 1880–1950." *Canadian Historical Review,* 70(June, 1989), 151–79.

Gagan, Rosemary. "Mortality Patterns and Public Health in Hamilton, Canada, 1900–1914." *Urban History Review,* 57(February, 1989), 161–76.

– *A Sensitive Independence.* Montreal: McGill-Queen's University Press, 1992.

Gibbon, John Murray and Mary S. Mathewson. *Three Centuries of Canadian Nursing.* Toronto: Macmillan, 1947.

Gidney, R.D. and W.P.J. Millar. "Medical Students at the University of Toronto, 1910–1940: A Profile." *Canadian Bulletin of Medical History,* 13(1996), 29–52.

– *Professional Gentlemen: The Professions in Nineteenth-Century Ontario.* Toronto: University of Toronto Press, 1994.

– "The Reorientation of Medical Education in Late-Nineteenth-Century Ontario: The Proprietary Medical Schools and the Founding of the Faculty of Medicine at the University of Toronto." *Journal of the History of Medicine and Allied Sciences,* 49(1994), 52–78.

Godfrey, W.G. "'Into the Hands of the Ladies': The Birth of the Moncton Hospital." *Acadiensis,* XXVII(Autumn, 1997), 22–43.

Goulet, Denis. *Histoire de la Faculté de Médicine de l'Université de Montréal, 1843–1993.* Montréal: VLB Éditeur, 1993.

Goulet, Denis et André Paradis. *Trois siècles d'histoire médicale au Québec: Chronologie des institutions et des pratiques (1639–1939).* Montréal: VLB, 1992.

Granshaw, Lindsay. "'Upon This Principle I Have Based a Practice'. The Development and Reception of Antisepsis in Britain, 1860–90." *Medical Innovations in Historical Perspective.* John Pickstone, ed, 17–47. New York: St. Martin's Press, 1992.

Goebel, Thomas. "American Medicine and the 'Organizational Synthesis': Chicago Physicians and the Business of Medicine,1900–1920" *Bulletin of the History of Medicine,* 68(1994), 639–63.

Grob, Gerald. "The Social History of Medicine and Disease in America: Problems and Possibilities." *Journal of Social History*. 10(June, 1977), 391–409.

Guest, Dennis. *The Emergence of Social Security in Canada*. Vancouver: University of British Columbia Press, 1985.

Haber, Samuel. *Efficiency and Uplift: Scientific Management in the Progressive Era, 1890–1920*. Chicago: University of Chicago Press, 1964.

Hall, Bertha E. and Anne Elizabeth Wilson. "Must 1,532 Mothers Die?" *The Chatelaine*, I(July, 1928), 6–7, 38–9.

Haller, Jr, John S. *American Medicine in Transition, 1840–1910*. Chicago: University of Illinois Press, 1981.

Hamowy, Ronald. *Canadian Medicine: A Study in Restricted Entry*. Vancouver, 1984.

Hastings, J.E.F. "Federal-Provincial Insurance for Hospital and Physician's Care in Canada." *International Journal of Health Services*, 1(No. 4, 1971), 398–414.

Hayter, Charles R.R. "The Clinic as Laboratory: The Case of Radiation Therapy, 1896–1920." *Bulletin of the History of Medicine*, 72(4, 1998), 663–88.

– "Medicalizing Malignancy: The Uneasy Origins of Ontario's Cancer Program, 1929–34." *Canadian Bulletin of Medical History*, 14(1997), 195–213.

Health in Manitoba: A Presentation to the Canadian Council on Mental Hygiene. Manitoba Pool Elevators, 1939.

Horn, Michiel, ed. *The Dirty Thirties*. Toronto: Copp Clark, 1975.

Howell, Colin. *A Century of Care: A History of the Victoria General Hospital in Halifax 1887–1987*. Halifax: The Victoria General Hospital, 1988.

– "Medical Professionalization and the Social Transformation of the Maritimes, 1850–1950," *Journal of Canadian Studies*, 27(Spring, 1992), 5–20.

Howell, Joel D. *Technology in the Hospital: Transforming Patient Care in the Early Twentieth Century*. Baltimore: The Johns Hopkins University Press, 1995.

– "Machines and Medicine: Technology Transforms the American Hospital." *The American General Hospital: Communities and Social Contexts*. Diana Long and Janet Golden, eds, 109–134. Ithaca: Cornell University Press, 1989.

Innis, H.A. "Economic Conditions in Canada, 1931-32." *Economic Journal*. 42(March, 1932), 1–16.

Irving, Allan. "The Doctors *versus* the Expert: Harry Morris Cassidy and the British Columbia Health Insurance Dispute of the 1930s." *BC Studies*, 78(Summer 1988), 53–79.

Jardine, Pauline. "An Urban Middle-Class Calling: Women and the Emergence of Modern Nursing Education at the Toronto General Hospital, 1881–1914." *Urban History Review*, 17(February, 1989), 176–90.

Johnston, William V. *Before the Age of Miracles: Memoirs of a Country Doctor*. Toronto: Fitzhenry and Whiteside, 1972.

Katz, Michael, Michael Doucet and Mark. J. Stern. *The Social Organization of Early Industrial Capitalism*. Cambridge, Mass.: Harvard University Press, 1982.

Kealey, Greg, ed. *Canada Investigates Industrialism.* Toronto: University of Toronto Press, 1973.

Kelly, Nora. *Quest for a Profession: The History of the Vancouver General Hospital School of Nursing.* Vancouver: Evergreen Press, 1973.

King, William Lyon Mackenzie. *Industry and Humanity.* David Jay Bercuson, ed. Toronto: University of Toronto Press, 1973.

Kinnear, Julia. "The Professionalization of Canadian Nursing, 1924–32: Views in the CN and the *CMAJ.*" *Canadian Bulletin of Medical History,* 11(1994), 153–74.

Kinnear, Mary. *A Female Economy: Women's Work in a Prairie Province, 1870–1970.* Montreal: McGill-Queen's University Press, 1998.

– *In Subordination: Professional Women 1870–1970.* Montreal: McGill-Queen's University Press, 1995.

Kubat, Daniel and Donald Thornton. *A Statistical Profile of Canadian Society.* Toronto: McGraw-Hill-Ryerson, 1974.

Lawrence, Christopher. *Medicine in the Making of Modern Britain, 1700–1920.* London: Routledge, 1994.

Leavitt, Judith Walzer. *Brought to Bed: Childbearing in America, 1750 to 1950.* New York: Oxford University Press, 1986.

Le Fanu, James. *The Rise and Fall of Modern Medicine.* London: Little, Brown, 1999.

Levenstein, Harvey. *Revolution At the Table: The Transformation of the American Diet.* New York: Oxford University Press, 1988.

Lewis, Norah L. "Reducing Maternal Mortality in British Columbia: An Educational Process." *Not Just Pin Money: Selected Essays on the History of Women's Work in British Columbia.* Barbara K. Latham and Roberta J. Pazdro, eds, 337–57. Victoria: Camosun College, 1984.

Lindert, Peter. "The Rise of Social Spending, 1880–1930," *Explorations in Economic History,* 31(Jan., 1994), 1–37.

MacDermot, H.E. *History of the Canadian Medical Association.* Vol. 2. Toronto, 1956.

– *A History of the Montreal General Hospital.* Montreal, 1950.

Manitoba Federation of Agriculture. *Submission to the Hospital Survey Committee, 1943.*

Markowitz, Gerald E. and David Rosner, "Doctors in Crisis: Medical Education and Medical Reform During the Progressive Era, 1895-1915." *Health Care in America: Essays in Social History,* Susan Reverby and David Rosner, eds, 185–205. Philadelphia: Temple University Press, 1979.

Marsh, Leonard. *Health and Unemployment.* London: Oxford University Press, 1938.

Maulitz, Russell C. "'Physician *versus* Bacteriologist': The Ideology of Science in Clinical Medicine." *The Therapeutic Revolution: Essays in the Social*

History of Medicine, Morris J. Vogel and Charles E. Rosenberg, eds., 91–108. Philadelphia: University of Pennsylvania Press, 1979.

McGinnis, Janice P. Dickin, "The Impact of Epidemic Influenza: Canada, 1918–1919." *Historical Papers*, 120–41. Ottawa: Canadian Historical Association, 1977.

McKeown, Thomas. "A Sociological Approach to the History of Medicine." *Medical History and Medical Care: A Symposium of Perspectives*. Gordon McLachlan and Thomas McKeown, eds, 1–23. London: Oxford University Press, 1971.

McKillop, A.B. *A Disciplined Intelligence: Critical Inquiry and Canadian Thought in the Victorian Era*. Montreal: McGill-Queen's University Press, 1979.

McKinnon, N.E. "Mortality Reductions in Ontario, 1900–1942." *Canadian Journal of Public Health*, 36(July, 1945), 285–98.

McLaren, Angus and Arlene Tigar McLaren. *The Bedroom and the State: The Changing Practices and Politics of Contraception and Abortion in Canada, 1880–1980*. Toronto: McClelland & Stewart, 1986.

McLeod, Thomas H. and Ian M. McLeod. *Tommy Douglas: The Road to Jerusalem*. Edmonton: Hurtig, 1987.

McPhedran, N. Tait. *Canadian Medical Schools: Two Centuries of Medical History, 1822–1992*. Montreal: Harvest House, 1993.

McPherson, Kathryn. *Bedside Matters: The Transformation of Canadian Nursing, 1900–1990*. Toronto: Oxford University Press, 1996.

– "'The Country is a Stern Nurse': Rural Women, Urban Hospitals, and the Creation of a Western Canadian Nursing Work Force, 1920–1940." *Prairie Forum*, 20(Fall, 1995), 175–206.

– "Science and Technique: Nurses' Work in a Canadian Hospital, 1920–1939." *Caring and Curing: Historical Perspectives on Women and Healing in Canada*. Dianne Dodd and Deborah Gorham, eds, 71–101. Ottawa: University of Ottawa Press, 1994.

– "'Skilled Service and Women's Work': Canadian Nursing, 1920–1939." Unpublished PhD Thesis. Simon Fraser University, 1989.

McPherson, Kathryn, and Meryn Stuart. "Writing Nursing History in Canada: Issues and Approaches." *Canadian Bulletin of Medical History*, 11(1994), 3–22.

Meade, Richard H. *An Introduction to the History of General Surgery*. Philadelphia: Saunders, 1968.

Melosh, Barbara. *The Physician's Hand: Work, Culture and Conflict in American Nursing*. Philadelphia: Temple University Press, 1982.

Mitchinson, Wendy. "Agency, Diversity, and Constraints: Women and Their Physicians, Canada, 1850–1950." *The Politics of Women's Health: Exploring Agency and Autonomy*. Susan Sherwin, ed., 122–49. Philadelphia: Temple University Press, 1998.

- *The Nature of Their Bodies: Women and Their Doctors in Victorian Canada.* Toronto: University of Toronto Press, 1991.

Mombourquette, Duane. "'An Inalienable Right': The CCF and Rapid Health Care Reform, 1944–1948." *Saskatchewan History,* 43(Autumn, 1991), 101–16.

Moore, Edward J. "The Why and Wherefore of Doctors' Bills." *Maclean's Magazine,* 25(December, 1912), 53–7.

Morton, W.L. *Manitoba: A History.* Toronto: University of Toronto Press, 1957.

Naylor, David C. "Canada's First Doctors' Strike: Medical Relief in Winnipeg, 1932–4." *Canadian Historical Review,* 67(2, 1986), 151–80.

- *Private Practice, Public Payment: Canadian Medicine and the Politics of Health Insurance, 1911–1966.* Montreal: McGill-Queen's University Press, 1986.

- "Rural Protest and Medical Professionalism in Turn-of-the-Century Ontario." *Journal of Canadian Studies,* 21 (Spring, 1986), 5–20.

Olson, Tom. "Apprenticeship and Exploitation: An Analysis of the Work Pattern of Nurses in Training, 1897–1937." *Social Science History,* 17(Winter, 1993), 559–76.

Oppenheimer, Jo. "Childbirth in Ontario: The Transition from Home to Hospital in the Early Twentieth Century." *Delivering Motherhood: Maternal Ideologies and Practices in the 19th and 20th Centuries.* Katherine Arnup, Andrée Lévesque and Ruth Roach Pierson, eds, 51–74. New York: Routledge, 1990.

Ormsby, Margaret A. "T. Dufferin Patullo and the Little New Deal." *Politics of Discontent.* Ramsay Cook, ed., 28–48. Toronto: University of Toronto Press, 1967.

Ostry, Aleck. "Prelude to Medicare: Institutional Change and Continuity in Saskatchewan, 1944–1962," *Prairie Forum,* 20(Spring, 1995), 87–106.

Owram, Doug. *Born at the Right Time: A History of the Baby Boom Generation.* Toronto: University of Toronto Press, 1996.

- *The Government Generation: Canadian Intellectuals and the State, 1900–1945.* Toronto: University of Toronto Press, 1986.

Palmer, Brian D. *A Culture in Conflict: Skilled Workers and Industrial Capitalism in Hamilton, Ontario, 1880–1914.* Montreal: McGill-Queen's University Press, 1979.

Parr, Joy. "Rethinking Work and Kinship in a Canadian Hosiery Town, 1919–1950." *Canadian Family History: Selected Readings.* Bettina Bradbury, ed., 220–40. Toronto: Copp Clark Pitman, 1992.

Pellagrino, Edmund D. "The Sociocultural Impact of Twentieth-Century Therapeutics." *The Therapeutic Revolution: Essays in the Social History of American Medicine.* Morris J. Vogel and Charles E.Rosenberg, eds, 245–66. Philadelphia, 1979.

Perkins, Barbara Bridgeman. "Shaping Institution-Based Specialism: Early Twentieth-Century Economic Organization of Medicine." *Social History of Medicine,* 10(December, 1997), 419–36.

Perron, Normand. *Un siècle de vie hospitalière au Québec: Les Augustines et l'Hôtel-Dieu de Chicoutimi 1884–1984.* Sillery: Presses de l'Université de Québec, 1984.

Perry, Anne Anderson. "The High Cost of Sickness." *The Chatelaine* (February, 1929), 12–15.

– "The High Cost of Sickness." *The Chatelaine* (September, 1929), 2–3, 14–14.

– "What Can Women Do to Combat the High Cost of Sickness?" *The Chatelaine* (January, 1930), 19, 39, 41.

Petitat, André. *Les infirmières: de la vocation à la profession.* Montréal: Boréal, 1989.

Pickstone, John V. *Medicine and Industrial Society: A History of Hospital Development in Manchester and its Region, 1752–1946.* Manchester: Manchester University Press, 1985.

Piva, Michael. *The Condition of the Working Class in Toronto, 1900–1921.* Ottawa: University of Ottawa Press, 1979.

Proceedings of the Thirteenth Annual Convention of the British Columbia Hospitals' Association. Vancouver, 1931.

Reaume, Geoffrey. *Remembrance of Patients Past: Patient Life at the Toronto Hospital for the Insane, 1870–1940.* Toronto: Oxford University Press, 2000.

Reverby, Susan. *Ordered to Care: The Dilemma of American Nursing, 1850–1940.* Cambridge: Cambridge University Press, 1987.

– "The Search for the Hospital Yardstick: Nursing and the Rationalization of Hospital Work." *Health Care in America: Essays in Social History.* Susan Reverby and David Rosner, eds, 206–225. Philadelphia: Temple University Press, 1979.

Richardson, Sharon. "Staffing the Hospitals: Edmonton's Nurse Training Programs." *Edmonton: The Life of a City,* 135–41. Edmonton: NeWest Press, 1995.

Riegler, Natalie. *Jean I. Gunn. Nursing Leader.* Markham, ON: Fitzhenry and Whiteside, 1997.

Risse, Guenter B. *Mending Bodies, Saving Souls: A History of Hospitals.* New York: Oxford University Press, 1999.

Roberts, Joan and Thetis Group. *Feminism in Nursing: An Historical Perspective on Power, Status, and Political Activism in the Nursing Profession.* Westport, Conn. Praeger, 1995.

Robertson, Betty, Catherine Marcellus, and Betty Dandy. *Mission's Living Memorials.* Altoona, MB, 1992.

Robin, Martin. *Pillars of Profit: The Company Province, 1934–1972.* Toronto: McClelland & Stewart, 1973.

Roland, Charles G. "The Early Years of Antiseptic Surgery in Canada." *Medicine in Canadian Society: Historical Perspectives.* S.E.D. Shortt, ed., 237–54. Montreal: McGill-Queen's University Press, 1981.

Rosen, George. "The Efficiency Criterion in Medical Care, 1900–1925." *Bulletin of the History of Medicine,* 50(1976), 28–44.

– "The Hospital: Historical Sociology of a Community Institution." *The Hospital in Modern Society*. Eliot Freidson, ed. London: Collier Macmillan, 1963. 1–36.

Rosenberg, Charles E. "And Heal the Sick: Hospital and Patient in Nineteenth-Century America." *The Medicine Show*. P. Branca, ed., 121–40. New York, 1977.

– "George Rosen and the Social History of Medicine." *Healing and History: Essays for George Rosen*. Charles E. Rosenberg, ed., 2–12. New York: Science History Publications, 1979.

– "Inward Vision and Outward Glance: The Shaping of the American Hospital, 1880–1914." *Social History and Social Policy*. David J. Rothman and Stanton Wheeler, eds., 19–56. New York: Academic Press, 1981.

– "The Therapeutic Revolution: Medicine, Meaning and Social Change in Nineteenth-Century America." *The Therapeutic Revolution: Essays in the Social History of American Medicine*. Morris Vogel and Charles E. Rosenberg, eds., 2–20. Philadelphia, 1979.

– *The Care of Strangers: The Rise of America's Hospital System*. New York: Basic Books, 1987.

Rosner, David. "Business at the Bedside: Health Care in Brooklyn, 1890–1915." *Health Care in America: Essays in Social History*. Susan Reverby and David Rosner, eds., 117–131. Philadelphia: Temple University Press, 1979.

Rothstein, William G. *American Physicians in the Nineteenth Century: From Sects to Science*. Baltimore: Johns Hopkins University Press, 1972.

Rutty, Christopher J. "The Middle-Class Plague: Epidemic Polio and the Canadian State, 1936–1937," HTTP//www.healthheritageresearch.com/MCPlague.html.

Savage, Peggy. *To Serve With Honour: The Story of St. Joseph's Hospital, Hamilton, 1890–1990*. Toronto: Dundurn Press, 1990.

Shortt, S.E.D. "Social Change and Political Crisis in Rural Ontario: The Patrons of Industry, 1889–1896." *Oliver Mowat's Ontario*. Donald Swainson, ed., 211–35. Toronto: Macmillan, 1972.

– "'Before the Age of Miracles': The Rise, Fall, and Rebirth of General Practice in Canada, 1900–1940." *Health, Disease and Medicine: Essays in Canadian History*. Charles G. Roland, ed., 123–52. Toronto, 1983.

Sigerist, Henry. *Autobiographical Writings*. Nora Sigerist Beeson, trans. Montreal: McGill University Press, 1966.

Smith, Susan L. and Dawn D. Nickel. "From Home to Hospital: Parallels in Birthing and Dying in Twentieth-Century Canada." *Canadian Bulletin of Medical History*, 16(1999), 49–64.

Splane, Richard B. *Social Welfare in Ontario, 1791–1893: A Study of Public Welfare Administration*. Toronto: University of Toronto Press, 1965.

Starr, Paul. *The Social Transformation of American Medicine*. New York: Basic Books, 1982.

Stevens, Rosemary. *American Medicine and the Public Interest*. New Haven: Yale University Press, 1972.

- *In Sickness and In Wealth: American Hospitals in the Twentieth Century*. New York: Basic Books, 1989.

The Story of VGH. Vancouver: Vancouver General Hospital, 1977.

Strange, Carolyn. *Toronto's Girl Problem: The Perils and Pleasures of the City, 1880–1930* Toronto: University of Toronto Press, 1995.

Street, Margaret M. *Watch-Fires on the Mountain: The Life and Writings of Ethel Johns*. Toronto: University of Toronto Press, 1973.

Strong-Boag, Veronica. "Making a Difference: The History of Canada's Nurses." *Canadian Bulletin of Medical History*, 2(Autumn, 1991), 231–48.

Strong-Boag, Veronica and Kathryn McPherson. "The Confinement of Women: Childbirth and Hospitalization in Vancouver, 1919–1939." *British Columbia Reconsidered: Essays on Women*. Gillian Creese and Veronica Strong-Boag, eds., 143–71. Vancouver: Press Gang Publishers, 1992.

Struthers, James. *No Fault of Their Own: Unemployment and the Canadian Welfare State, 1914–1941*. Toronto: University of Toronto Press, 1983.

Study of the Distribution of Medical Care and Public Health Services in Canada. National Committee for Mental Hygiene, 1939.

Sturdy, Steve. "The Political Economy of Scientific Medicine: Science, Education, and the Transformation of Medical Practice in Sheffield, 1890-1922," *Medical History*, 26(April, 1992), 125–59.

Sullivan, John R. and Norman R. Ball. *Growing to Serve: A History of the Victoria Hospital, London, Ontario*. London: Victoria Hospital Corp., 1985.

Sullivan, Robert B. "Sanguine Practices: A Historical and Historiographical Reconsideration of Heroic Therapy in the Age of Rush." *Bulletin of the History of Medicine*, 68(1994), 211–34.

Swartz, Donald. "The Limits of Health Insurance." *The "Benevolent" State: The Growth of Social Welfare in Canada*. Allan Moscovitch and Jim Albert, eds., 255–70. Toronto: Garamond Press, 1987.

Tausky, Thomas, ed. *Selected Journalism: Sara Jeanette Duncan*. Ottawa: Tecumseh Press, 1978.

Taylor, Frederick W. *The Principles of Scientific Management*. New York: Harper and Brothers, 1911.

Taylor, Malcolm G. *Financial Aspects of Health Services*. Canadian Tax Papers, no. 12. Toronto, 1957.

Taylor, Malcolm G. *Health Insurance and Canadian Public Policy: The Seven Decisions that Created the Canadian Health Insurance System*. Montreal: McGill-Queen's University Press, 1978.

"Teaching Men to Legislate for Women." *The Chatelaine*, 1(July, 1928), 16.

Thomas, Lewis H. ed. *The Making of A Socialist: The Recollections of T.C. Douglas*. Edmonton: University of Alberta Press, 1982.

Tomes, Nancy. *The Gospel of Germs: Men, Women, and the Microbe in American Life*. Cambridge, Mass.: Harvard University Press, 1998.

– "'Little World of Our Own': The Pennsylvania Hospital Training School for Nurses, 1895–1907." *Women and Health in America*. Judith Walzer Leavitt, ed., 467–81. Madison: University of Wisconsin Press, 1984.

Twohig, Peter L. " 'Local Girls' and 'Lab Boys': Gender, Skill, and Science in Interwar Nova Scotia." Unpublished Manuscript, 2001.

– "Organizing the Bench: Medical Laboratory Workers in the Maritimes, 1900–1950.' Unpublished doctoral dissertation, Dalhousie University, 1999.

Urquhart, M.C. and K.A.H. Buckley, eds. *Historical Statistics of Canada*. Toronto: Cambridge University Press, 1965.

Valverde, Mariana. *The Age of Light, Soap, and Water: Moral Reform in English Canada, 1885–1925*. Toronto: McClelland & Stewart, 1991.

Vogel, Morris J. *The Invention of the Modern Hospital: Boston, 1870–1930*. Chicago: University of Chicago Press, 1980.

Warsh, Cheryl. " 'John Barleycorn Must Die': An Introduction to the Social History of Alcohol." *Drink in Canada: Historical Essays*. C. Warsh, ed., 3–26. Montreal: McGill-Queen's University Press, 1993.

Warner, John Harley. "Power, Conflict, and Identity in Mid-Nineteenth-Century American Medicine: Therapeutic Change at the Commercial Hospital in Cincinnati." *Journal of American History*, 73(March, 1987), 934–56.

Weir, G.M. *Survey of Nursing Education in Canada*. Toronto: University of Toronto Press, 1932.

Weisz, George. "Medical Directories and Medical Specialization in France, Britain, and the United States." *Bulletin of the History of Medicine*, 71(1, 1997), 23–68.

Whittaker, Jo Anne. "The Search for Legitimacy: Nurses' Registration in British Columbia, 1913–1935." *Not Just Pin Money: Selected Essays on the History of Women's Work in British Columbia*. Barbara K. Latham and Roberta J. Lazdro, eds, 315–26. Victoria: Camosun College, 1984.

Williams, Katherine. "From Sarah Gamp to Florence Nightingale: A Critical Study of Hospital Nursing Systems from 1840 to 1897." *Rewriting Nursing History*. Celia Davies, ed., 41–75. London: Croom Helm, 1980.

Willinsky, A.I. *A Doctor's Memoirs*. Toronto: Macmillan, 1960.

Women of Canada: Their Life and Work. National Council of Women of Canada. Ottawa, 1900 [reprint, 1975].

Woodward, John. *To Do the Sick No Harm: A Study of the British Voluntary Hospital System to 1875*. London: Routledge and Kegan Paul, 1974.

Woodward, John and David Richards. "Towards a Social History of Medicine." *Health Care and Popular Medicine in Nineteenth-Century England*. John Woodward and David Richards, eds, 15–55. London: Croom Helm, 1977.

Index

Mack, Dr Theophilus, 133
MacMurchy, Dr Helen: as
first female staff physician
of TGH, 144; on modern-
ization of hospitals, 43
McPherson, Kathryn, 137,
147, 149
management, of hospitals:
budget, 51–2, 116; chair-
man of medical staff, 51–2;
hospital boards, 42–7, 51,
52, 53–4; lady superintendent, 21, 51, 52, 53, 131,
136; managing secretary,
51, 52; medical superin-
tendent, 21, 51; physi-
cian/board relations, 116,
117; physicians, control of
medical priorities, 185; by
volunteers, 1900–20, 70
managing secretary, 51, 52
Manitoba: community hos-
pital crisis, during Great
Depression, 90–1; differ-
ence between urban and
rural medical services, 90;
effect of Great Depression
on hospitals, 79, 80–1;
hospital admissions,
increase during WWII, 86;
and hospital insurance,
88, 91; hospital usage,
1930, 4; increase in hospitals, 4; indigent patients,
as percentage of admis-
sions, 86–7. See also
names of specific hospi-
tals
Manitoba Commission on
Public Welfare: on nursing
schools, 141; objection to
physician mangement of
hospitals, 52; on role of
hospitals, 114–15
Manitoba Federation of
Agriculture, inquiry into
rural medical care, 90
Manitoba Medical Associa-
tion, support for govern-
ment payment of physi-
cians' fees for indigent
patients, 81
Manitoba Medical College:
Faculty of Medicine, 65;
students, as staff of outpatient clinics, 59
Mann, Josephine, 144

Margaret Scott Nursing
Mission, 143
Marsh, Leonard, 92–3
matrons, in late-Victorian era
hospitals, 21, 139
Medical Care Act (Canada,
1966), 180
medical schools, standardization and accreditation
of, 101, 106
medical science: bacteriology, and transition to scientific medicine, 31; and
emergence of medical
specialization, 14, 34–6;
and exclusion of irregular
practitioners, 103;
"heroic," 31, 100–1; laboratories, and transition to
scientific medicine, 31;
post-WWII technology
and research, 126; and
redefinition of hospital,
98, 114, 115; "research
ideal," 31, 32, 103. See also
antisepsis; asepsis; germ
theory; irregular practi-
tioners; laboratories,
hospital; technology,
medical
medical students: as cheap
source of labour in hospitals, 64–5; compulsory
internships, 65–6; curriculum, and hospital stan-
dardization initiative, 65;
staffing of outpatient
clinics, 66
medical superintendents, in
late-Victorian era hospi-
tals, 21, 51
medical technology. See technology, medical
Melosh, Barbara, 145
men: on hospital boards, 44;
as indigent patients, predominance of, 17–18; as
medically unfit for mili-
tary service, 77. See also
gendered relations
middle class patients. See
patients, paying
midwifery, lobbying against
by medical profession,
103–4, 172
Millar, W.P.J., 99
Moncton (NB) student nurses

as hospital labour force,
30–1
Montreal General Hospital:
and antisepsis proponent
Thomas Roddick, 28; first
x-ray technician, 1898, 32;
as late-Victorian metropolitan hospital, 14, 16;
medical specialization in,
35; nurses, ratio of graduate to student nurses, 155;
nurses' status, 19th
century, 131–2; nursing
school, 133, 134; operation
of first x-ray apparatus,
33; patient fees, as per-
centage of income, 61;
study of socio-economic
circumstances of indigent
patients, 1928, 76
Mott family, 44

National Council of Women
of Canada, 135
National Health Grants, 94
National Health Insurance Act
(Great Britain, 1911), 77
New Westminster: hospital
construction in, 15. See also
Royal Columbian Hospi-
tal
Nightingale, Florence: estab-
lishment of St Thomas'
Hospital training school,
132; and improvement of
nurses' training, 29; legacy
of nurses' exploitation by
hospitals, 136, 137; model
of nurse, difficulty of
achieving in 19th-century
Canadian hospitals, 138;
school standards, diffi-
culty of recreating in
Canada, 134
Nova Scotia, infant mortality
rate, 1926, 68
nurses: accommodation, 54;
as asset in attracting
paying patients, 186;
behaviour, as reported in
late-Victorian era, 22;
comraderie among, 150;
critical care, and increased
responsibilities, 145;
ethnic minorities, 156;
expectations of, by hospitals, 157; and gendered